Managing Pandemic Isolation With Literature as Therapy

Antonio Cortijo Ocaña
University of California, Santa Barbara, USA

Vicent Martines
ISIC-IVITRA, University of Alicante, Spain

Veronica Orazi
Università degli Studi di Torino, Italy

IGI Global
PUBLISHER of TIMELY KNOWLEDGE

A volume in the Advances in Psychology, Mental Health, and Behavioral Studies (APMHBS) Book Series

Published in the United States of America by
IGI Global
Information Science Reference (an imprint of IGI Global)
701 E. Chocolate Avenue
Hershey PA, USA 17033
Tel: 717-533-8845
Fax: 717-533-8661
E-mail: cust@igi-global.com
Web site: http://www.igi-global.com

Library of Congress Cataloging-in-Publication Data

Names: Cortijo Ocaña, Antonio, editor. | Martines, Vicent, DATE- editor | Orazi, Veronica, editor.
Title: Managing pandemic isolation with literature as therapy / Antonio Cortijo Ocaña, Vicent Martines, and Veronica Orazi, editors.
Description: Hershey PA : Information Science Reference, [2023] | Includes bibliographical references and index. | Summary: "This publication helps explain the positive medical and psychological effect of literature and writing during a disease/pandemic at a time when isolation prevents people from engaging with others socially with a secondary purpose of encouraging cross-disciplinary research involving the sciences and the humanities"-- Provided by publisher.
Identifiers: LCCN 2022015469 (print) | LCCN 2022015470 (ebook) | ISBN 9781668447352 (hardcover) | ISBN 9781668447369 (paperback) | ISBN 9781668447376 (ebook)
Subjects: LCSH: Psychology and literature. | Authorship--Psychological aspects. | COVID-19 Pandemic, 2020---Psychological aspects. | Bibliotherapy. | LCGFT: Essays.
Classification: LCC PN56.P93 M36 2023 (print) | LCC PN56.P93 (ebook) | DDC 801/.3--dc23/eng/20220526
LC record available at https://lccn.loc.gov/2022015469
LC ebook record available at https://lccn.loc.gov/2022015470

This book is published in the IGI Global book series Advances in Psychology, Mental Health, and Behavioral Studies (APMHBS) (ISSN: 2475-6660; eISSN: 2475-6679)

British Cataloguing in Publication Data
A Cataloguing in Publication record for this book is available from the British Library.

Advances in Psychology, Mental Health, and Behavioral Studies (APMHBS) Book Series

Harish C. Chandan
Argosy University, USA
Bryan Christiansen
Southern New Hampshire University, USA

ISSN:2475-6660
EISSN:2475-6679

Mission

The complexity of the human mind has puzzled researchers and physicians for centuries. While widely studied, the brain still remains largely misunderstood.

The **Advances in Psychology, Mental Health, and Behavioral Studies (APMHBS)** book series presents comprehensive research publications focusing on topics relating to the human psyche, cognition, psychiatric care, mental and developmental disorders, as well as human behavior and interaction. Featuring diverse and innovative research, publications within APMHBS are ideally designed for use by mental health professionals, academicians, researchers, and upper-level students.

Coverage

- Cognition
- Socialization
- Mental Health & Disorders
- Developmental Disorders
- Addiction
- Anxiety
- Neurological Disorders
- Eating Disorders
- Human Interaction
- Substance Abuse

IGI Global is currently accepting manuscripts for publication within this series. To submit a proposal for a volume in this series, please contact our Acquisition Editors at Acquisitions@igi-global.com or visit: http://www.igi-global.com/publish/.

The Advances in Psychology, Mental Health, and Behavioral Studies (APMHBS) Book Series (ISSN 2475-6660) is published by IGI Global, 701 E. Chocolate Avenue, Hershey, PA 17033-1240, USA, www.igi-global.com. This series is composed of titles available for purchase individually; each title is edited to be contextually exclusive from any other title within the series. For pricing and ordering information please visit http://www.igi-global.com/book-series/advances-psychology-mental-health-behavioral/110200. Postmaster: Send all address changes to above address.

Titles in this Series

For a list of additional titles in this series, please visit: http://www.igi-global.com/book-series/advances-psychology-mental-health-behavioral/110200

Latinx Mental Health From Surviving to Thriving
Edward A. Delgado-Romero (University of Georia, USA)
Medical Information Science Reference • © 2023 • 335pp • H/C (ISBN: 9781668449011) • US $305.00

Handbook of Research on Play Specialism Strategies to Prevent Pediatric Hospitalization Trauma
Giulia Perasso (University of Milano-Bicocca, Italy) and Yagmur Ozturk (University of Trento, Italy)
Medical Information Science Reference • © 2023 • 400pp • H/C (ISBN: 9781668450680) • US $425.00

The Role of Child Life Specialists in Community Settings
Genevieve Lowry (Bank Street College of Education, USA) Lindsey Murphy (Missouri State University, USA) and Cara Smith (Missouri State University, USA)
Information Science Reference • © 2023 • 435pp • H/C (ISBN: 9781668450970) • US $245.00

Counseling Strategies for Children and Families Impacted by Incarceration
Kenya Johns (Geneva College, USA)
Medical Information Science Reference • © 2022 • 365pp • H/C (ISBN: 9781799892090) • US $295.00

The Reproduction and Maintenance of Inequalities in Interpersonal Relationships
Tyler Ross Flockhart (Viterbo University, USA) Abigail Reiter (University of North Carolina at Pembroke, USA) and Matthew R. Hassett (University of North Carolina at Pembroke, USA)
Information Science Reference • © 2022 • 332pp • H/C (ISBN: 9781668441282) • US $215.00

Applying Mind Genomics to Social Sciences
Howard Moskowitz (Moskowitz Jacobs, Inc., USA) Arthur Kover (Fordham Business Schools, USA) and Petraq Papajorgji (European University of Tirana, Albania)
Information Science Reference • © 2022 • 281pp • H/C (ISBN: 9781799884095) • US $215.00

Developing, Delivering, and Sustaining School Counseling Practices Through a Culturally Affirming Lens
Sarah N. Brant-Rajahn (Messiah University, USA) Eva M. Gibson (Austin Peay State University, USA) and Mariama Cook Sandifer (Columbus State University, USA)
Information Science Reference • © 2022 • 383pp • H/C (ISBN: 9781799895145) • US $215.00

The Impact of the COVID-19 Pandemic on Child, Adolescent, and Adult Development
Nava R. Silton (Marymount Manhattan College, USA)
Information Science Reference • © 2022 • 262pp • H/C (ISBN: 9781668434840) • US $195.00

IGI Global
PUBLISHER of TIMELY KNOWLEDGE

701 East Chocolate Avenue, Hershey, PA 17033, USA
Tel: 717-533-8845 x100 • Fax: 717-533-8661
E-Mail: cust@igi-global.com • www.igi-global.com

Table of Contents

Preface xiv

Chapter 1
The Power of the Word That Leads to Healing: Forerunners of Bibliotherapy and Therapeutic Writing (Charles d'Orléans, Jordi de Sant Jordi, Joan Roís de Corella) 1
Vicent Martines, University of Alicante, Spain

Chapter 2
The Valencian Annals: Reflex of the Current Pandemic 14
Francisco José Conejero Pascual, Universitat d'Alacant, Spain

Chapter 3
A Song to Life in Pandemic Times: *Primavera extremeña* by Julio Llamazares (2020) 28
Barbara Greco, Università di Torino, Italy

Chapter 4
El tiempo que nos robaron (2021) de Rosa Huertas: Writing as a Lifeboat During COVID 19 Pandemic Confinement 43
Katiuscia Darici, University of Turin, Italy

Chapter 5
August Bover, "El contagi" (2021): Pandemic, Isolation, and the Therapeutic Power of Poetry 63
Veronica Orazi, Università degli Studi di Torino, Italy

Chapter 6
About Some Spanish Graphic Novels in Times of COVID-19 Pandemic: Cathartic Panels for the End of the World 86
Eduard Baile-López, Universitat d'Alacant, Spain

Chapter 7
Pandemics, Illness and Impairment as Reflected in Borges' Literature and as Key Factor to Shape His Authorial Style: Searching in Literature the Epic Fate Frailty Had Denied to Him 104
Belén Lozano Sañudo, Universidad de Valencia, Spain

Chapter 8
The Contribution of Children's Literature to the Development of the Child: Book Therapy and Narrative Therapy 118
Marinos Bouchtsis, Universidad de Alicante, Spain

Chapter 9
Algerian Literature as Socio-Educational Therapy During the 2020-2021 Pandemic 126
Mourad Kacimi, Universitat de València, Spain

Chapter 10
Coronavirus Pandemic and the Isolation of Deaf and Hard-of-Hearing Children in Greece 144
Evangelia Gkigkelou, University of the Basque Country, Spain

Chapter 11
E-Inclusion and the COVID-19 Pandemic: Inclusive Digital Classrooms and Collaboration Between General and Special Education Teachers 154
Maria Mouchritsa, University of the Basque Country, Spain
Ainara Romero-Andonegui, University of the Basque Country, Spain
Urtza Garay Ruiz, University of the Basque Country, Spain
Spyridon Kazanopoulos, University of the Basque Country, Spain

Chapter 12
Inclusion of Students With Special Educational Needs and the COVID-19 Pandemic: The Collaboration of School and Family in Distance Education Conditions 171
Spyridon Kazanopoulos, University of the Basque Country, Spain
Eneko Tejada, University of the Basque Country, Spain
Xabier Basogain, University of the Basque Country, Spain
Maria Mouchritsa, University of the Basque Country, Spain

Chapter 13
Distance Vocational Education and Training in the Pandemic: Adaptations and Challenges for Learners and Trainers in Europe – How the Pandemic Affected Distance Vocational Education and Training 189
Christos Lalos, University of Alicante, Spain

Chapter 14
Therapeutic and Learning Benefits of Reading During COVID-19 Among Spanish Secondary Students 198
Juan-Francisco Álvarez-Herrero, Universidad de Alicante, Spain

Chapter 15
Challenging Picturebooks and Domestic Geographies: A Multimodal Learning Path to Discuss the Consequences of the COVID-19 Lockdowns in the Classroom 213
Margarida Castellano Sanz, Universitat de València, Spain

Compilation of References 236

About the Contributors 274

Index 279

Detailed Table of Contents

Preface xiv

Chapter 1
The Power of the Word That Leads to Healing: Forerunners of Bibliotherapy and Therapeutic Writing (Charles d'Orléans, Jordi de Sant Jordi, Joan Roís de Corella) 1
Vicent Martines, University of Alicante, Spain

The authors study the contribution of some classics of medieval and renaissance romance literature to therapeutic writing and bibliotherapy as a means to encourage reading and writing during a pandemic lockdown (in times of pandemic, privation of freedom, or illness). They analyze the cases of the French duke Charles d'Orléans, the Valencian knight Jordi de Sant Jordi, and renaissance author Joan Roís de Corella. In addition, they reflect on the everlasting power and therapeutic value of the written word (reading and writing) since the time of the Egyptian pharaohs.

Chapter 2
The Valencian Annals: Reflex of the Current Pandemic 14
Francisco José Conejero Pascual, Universitat d'Alacant, Spain

Human nature has always experienced the need to count any facts close to or away in time from a subjective or objective perspective. The Valencian Annals is a work that collects events from the city of Valencia and its kingdom during the 14th and 15th centuries. The text is set in medieval autumn and is considered minor, as it is included in the genres of dietary or chronicons of memoralistic literature. All of them maintain a common denominator with the annotation of more or less relevant events in order to record the living, without any artistic intent. The purpose will be to establish a link between the vision of the 15th century population pandemics and today. COVID-19 has changed and transformed the world as humankind was living in this early 21st century. The metamorphosis caused by everything that this virus and disease has produced has prompted us to rethink certain individual and collective aspects of world society and, in particular, Western society.

Chapter 3
A Song to Life in Pandemic Times: *Primavera extremeña* by Julio Llamazares (2020)....................... 28
Barbara Greco, Università di Torino, Italy

The essay studies the work Julio Llamazares drafted during the months of confinement (March-June 2020) decreed by the Spanish state to counter the spread of the pandemic. Primavera extremeña: Apuntes del Natural is an illustrated book with watercolours by Laudenbahcher and recounts the experience of the author, confined in a "lagar" in the Extremaduran countryside, in a work that oscillates between a diary and a travelogue. The chapter studies the dual component of the text and the conception of the landscape, typical of Llamazares' work, which here acquires new meanings.

Chapter 4
El tiempo que nos robaron (2021) de Rosa Huertas: Writing as a Lifeboat During COVID-19 Pandemic Confinement... 43
Katiuscia Darici, University of Turin, Italy

The aim of this chapter is to analyse "El tiempo que nos robaron" (2021) by Rosa Huertas in the elements that can be most ascribed to pandemic writings. First of all, the author intends to underline the rise of the so called "pandemic narrative" to describe the traumatic experience during COVID-19 emergence. After presenting some theoretical considerations on journaling, the author will describe the salvific importance of writing and the primary importance of an interlocutor as an incentive for writing. The author intends to clarify to what extent the present and, in parallel, the past as it is recalled in the diary, is a stolen time. In addition, the importance of rituals must be taken into consideration. For this purpose, the author will describe the difficulty of filling the time as told by Huertas. The diary ends up being her main daily ritual. In this case, one can observe the importance of writing as a tool to objectify and distance oneself from the disease.

Chapter 5
August Bover, "El contagi" (2021): Pandemic, Isolation, and the Therapeutic Power of Poetry......... 63
Veronica Orazi, Università degli Studi di Torino, Italy

In November 2021, August Bover (Barcelona 1949) published the collection of poems El Contagi. His previous poetic works include En pèlag d'amor (1999); L'hivern sota el Cadí (2001); Mojave (2006); the bilingual anthology Vicino al mare (2006); Terres de llicorella. Imatges del Priorat (2008); the trilogy Cloc! (2011), Beabà (2014), and Tornaveu (2018); and the collection of poetry and prose Blau marí (2018). El Contagi contains 41 poems which, with the exception of the last one ("Senyal?"), were composed between March and June 2020, during the lockdown that was decreed in an attempt to contain contagions in the first phase of the pandemic. This contribution synthesises the results of the study of the text, according to the methodology based on the objectivisation, problematisation, and literarisation of the experience of the pandemic and its psychological consequences. This kind of investigation focuses on the use of literature as a therapeutic tool, in order to face, process, and progressively overcome the trauma caused by this impactful experience.

Chapter 6
About Some Spanish Graphic Novels in Times of COVID-19 Pandemic: Cathartic Panels for the End of the World 86
Eduard Baile-López, Universitat d'Alacant, Spain

The purpose of this chapter is to attend to comics produced during COVID-19 pandemic, especially those referring to the hardest moments of confinement and which may allow to observe the use of comics as a tool to analyze reality, both from a psychological point of view and from a sociopolitical one. Being such a recent phenomenon, corpus selection is introduced as temporary since new items continue to emerge, and furthermore, it is still early to assess its significance. As a pragmatic criterion, two vectors will be used: on the one hand, focus will be stressed on works belonging to the Spanish comics market in order to portray a particular cultural environment; on the other hand, four items will be selected to establish a coherent story which may adapt the stages of the hero's journey into a new paradigm (1. Fear, 2. Anger, 3. Humor, and 4. Healing).

Chapter 7
Pandemics, Illness and Impairment as Reflected in Borges' Literature and as Key Factor to Shape His Authorial Style: Searching in Literature the Epic Fate Frailty Had Denied to Him 104
Belén Lozano Sañudo, Universidad de Valencia, Spain

The first part of this chapter, consisting of Sections 1 and 2, aims at explaining the apparent scarce presence of Spanish Flu in modernist literature in general and in Borges' literary work in particular. The reason seems to be threefold: the degrading demise associated with illness in comparison to the glorifying destiny attributed to casualties from war, the different metaphorization processes undergone by distinct pandemics and epidemics, and the fact that this 1918 pandemic coincided in time with World War I and artists were trying to avoid evocating more suffering. The second part of the chapter, Sections 3 and 4, focuses on how the threat of Black Death and later Spanish Flu, which confined Borges at home, together with his frail health condition, made him prone to immersing in literature and dreams to escape from reality and experience adventures as real for him as those in the outside world.

Chapter 8
The Contribution of Children's Literature to the Development of the Child: Book Therapy and Narrative Therapy 118
Marinos Bouchtsis, Universidad de Alicante, Spain

The influence of children's literature on the general development of the child is important. The initiation of the child in the book contributes to the spiritual, cognitive, and linguistic development to the mental and emotional maturation, to the aesthetic cultivation, the wealth of ideas, and offers entertainment, improves expressive ability, and contributes to the formation of the reader's character. "Pandemic" may have been the word of the year 2020, but perhaps, it should have been "coped." Many families have had to adapt to home education, financial hardship, and losses as well as their daily stressors, and this has had an emotional impact on the children. It turns out that books can be powerful coping tools. Books can help children cope with conversations when difficult things happen. Books can also provide parents, guardians, or teachers around them with the best tools to help children during this pandemic time.

Chapter 9
Algerian Literature as Socio-Educational Therapy During the 2020-2021 Pandemic 126
Mourad Kacimi, Universitat de València, Spain

This chapter focuses on the therapeutic function of Algerian literary production during the pandemic between 2020 and 2021. It describes the socio-educational environment of the Algerian population before the lockdown and highlights the effect of the pandemic on the cultural life of Algerian intellectuals and citizens. Also it reveals the importance of new technological media such as television, the internet, social networks, and digital books for transmitting literary works as well and then reflects on the contribution of Algerian writers and artists in this exceptional period. Likewise, the use of digital media as an option to replace traditional media in the literary environment is valued.

Chapter 10
Coronavirus Pandemic and the Isolation of Deaf and Hard-of-Hearing Children in Greece 144
Evangelia Gkigkelou, University of the Basque Country, Spain

On March 11, 2020, the World Health Organization (WHO) declared the outbreak of COVID-19 as a worldwide pandemic affecting all people around the world. In order to control pandemic spread, governments, including Greece, took some public measures concerning health and social distancing. This has affected nearly every sector of the economy and education as well. Governments were forced to suspend students' attendance at schools and start distance education. As schools have been shuttered and the lives of students have been changed, it is crucial to consider the extreme isolation suddenly facing a special group of pupils: deaf and hard-of-hearing children who rely on sign language, lip reading, and facial expressions. That type of education and the obligatory use of facemasks acted as obstacles in their participation in school procedures and communication with their teachers and peers. However, those two years were transitional and have changed a lot of things regarding the data of these areas. There has been significant growth with innovations that should have been made long ago.

Chapter 11
E-Inclusion and the COVID-19 Pandemic: Inclusive Digital Classrooms and Collaboration Between General and Special Education Teachers 154
Maria Mouchritsa, University of the Basque Country, Spain
Ainara Romero-Andonegui, University of the Basque Country, Spain
Urtza Garay Ruiz, University of the Basque Country, Spain
Spyridon Kazanopoulos, University of the Basque Country, Spain

Extreme situations such as the COVID-19 pandemic have revealed important characteristics that can be used to improve inclusion in both face-to-face and distance modalities, such as strengthening connections between those involved and establishing activities in which technologies can be used to support inclusion effectively. This chapter aims to demonstrate that having a computer, tablet, or smartphone during a pandemic is not sufficient to ensure learning. To illustrate this point, several national online resources are inaccessible to students with disabilities, preventing them from participating in e-inclusion. Furthermore, because of a lack of collaboration and communication between classroom and special education teachers during COVID-19, teachers were unable to plan meaningful learning activities for their students. To achieve effective electronic inclusion, activities must be organized in such a way that they meet the needs of students with special needs, and modern, asynchronous tools must be available to assist in this process.

Chapter 12
Inclusion of Students With Special Educational Needs and the COVID-19 Pandemic: The Collaboration of School and Family in Distance Education Conditions 171
Spyridon Kazanopoulos, University of the Basque Country, Spain
Eneko Tejada, University of the Basque Country, Spain
Xabier Basogain, University of the Basque Country, Spain
Maria Mouchritsa, University of the Basque Country, Spain

With schools closed around the world during the pandemic, the use of technology and distance education has solved the problems and dysfunctions that have arisen. Students, their families, and school personnel have all been affected by the numerous challenges and barriers that have arisen because of distance education. This chapter seeks to evaluate school-family collaboration throughout the pandemic period. The study focuses on families with children who have special educational needs and disabilities (SEND) and their experiences with inclusive education. While the COVID-19 pandemic was underway, parents of children with SEND faced a variety of challenges, including a lack of resources, financial difficulties, communication difficulties, and a lack of attention from teachers. Parents believe that economic, social, and language limitations impede the effectiveness of online inclusion, whereas their digital abilities enable them to aid their children on both technical and psychological levels in overcoming distant learning difficulties.

Chapter 13
Distance Vocational Education and Training in the Pandemic: Adaptations and Challenges for Learners and Trainers in Europe – How the Pandemic Affected Distance Vocational Education and Training 189
Christos Lalos, University of Alicante, Spain

The COVID-19 pandemic has brought unprecedented challenges to all types and levels of learning, including vocational education and training. The chapter attempts to provide a preliminary analysis regarding the transition to ex distance education as a consequence of the closure of schools. Based on inputs from 14 informants, members of the Cedefop Ambassadors network for addressing early withdrawal from vocational education and training, covering five Member States and two non-EU countries, the work sheds light on aspects of this in order to highlight the challenges that trainees face in risk of early departure, but also their trainers, as well as the measures taken adopted for their support. Cedefop published a study in English, which the authors translated and summarized in the present work. The study shows that there is no digital integration without social integration. Vulnerable learners are less likely to participate in distance education, while their detachment from the learning process can lead to their early withdrawal from vocational education and training.

Chapter 14
Therapeutic and Learning Benefits of Reading During COVID-19 Among Spanish Secondary Students 198
Juan-Francisco Álvarez-Herrero, Universidad de Alicante, Spain

During the confinement due to COVID-19, the educational centers tried to cope as much as possible with the continuity of the teaching-learning processes. In this research, it was tried to verify if the implementation of a proposal that promoted reading among secondary school students of a science subject, characteristic to improve their learning as well as benefit their mental health. The comparison of the results obtained in a test before and after carrying out the proposal confirmed that there was an improvement in learning and a perception of therapeutic effects of reading in this difficult situation. It is necessary to continue carrying out proposals of this type, even without being subjected to situations of anxiety and stress, in order to improve both learning and the mental health of students.

Chapter 15
Challenging Picturebooks and Domestic Geographies: A Multimodal Learning Path to Discuss the Consequences of the COVID-19 Lockdowns in the Classroom 213
Margarida Castellano Sanz, Universitat de València, Spain

The COVID-19 pandemic has brought new ways of facing the world and its multiple realities. Picturebooks, as a crossover genre, help in the process of understanding new contexts while offering literature as therapy. The new challenges of the 21st century require the implementation of methodologies that focus both on words and on other modes of representation to construct knowledge, and to this end, literacy education through challenging picturebooks involves paying attention to the diverse pedagogical demands of a global, aesthetic, and multimodal world. This chapter supports the notion of visual literacy as a multidimensional concept and proposes the approach to different picturebooks dealing with neighbours and neighbourhoods through the pedagogy of the multiliteracies, in order to enhance the transformation of the self and the global and local understanding of the current world. A learning path for teachers is designed according to the four knowledge processes: experiencing, conceptualizing, analyzing, and applying.

Compilation of References 236

About the Contributors 274

Index 279

Preface

This book focuses on the effects the current COVID-19 pandemic has had on the population at large and the use of reading and writing as educational and therapeutic tools to help ease the effects of isolation and trauma. The many academic areas covered in this publication include, but are not limited to: Anxiety, Brain Neurology, Children's Literature, Clinical Psychology, Distance Education, Isolation, Literature, Stress, Therapy, Reading & Writing. In addition, the articles hereby contained could be of use for a variety of professionals such as psychologists, medical personnel, policy makers, government officials, researchers, scholars, academicians, practitioners, instructors, and students.

Literature has always played an important role in dealing with catastrophic events, including pandemics, as the case of Boccaccio´s *Decamerone* makes clear. A number of contributors to this volume analyze different literary works, genres, and periods in order to determine the curative and balsamic effect of literature in times of crisis. Vicent Martines ("The Power of the Word that Can Lead to Healing") focuses on the contributions of some medieval and Renaissance writers towards what he terms therapeutic writing and bibliotherapy and studies some compositions by the French Duke Charles d'Orléans, the Valencian knight Jordi de Sant Jordi and Renaissance author Joan Roís de Corella. He analyses the concept of literature as therapy to overcome personal (sentimental) setbacks (Corella). Charles d´Orléans and Jordi de Sant Jordi wrote works during their imprisonment requesting their freedom, either asking for ransom money or using artistic words as balsam for processing his personal situation. Francisco Conejero Pascual ("The Valencian Annals, Reflex of the current Pandemic") studies a work that chronicles events that took place in the city of Valencia during the 15th and 16th c. Just as our contemporary society faces a "new reality" after the onset of the COVID-19 epidemic, the author explores how late medieval society moved towards a new outlook on life in the midst of the fears provoked by intellectual crisis, plague and social upheavals and restructuring. Barbara Greco ("A song to life in pandemic times: *Primavera extremeña* by Julio Llamazares (2020)") focuses on Julio Llamazares´s *Primavera extremeña* as the author is confined during the pandemic to a country farm. Through a diaristic and odeoporistic text that reflects on the landscape and the essence of life, "he experiences, for the first time, the arrival and blossoming of spring, of which he absorbs smells, colors and sounds. The sensory adventure that Llamazares experiences to the full, invites him to reflect on the meaning of existence, to remember time gone by and the homeland lost under the waters of a dam, but also to simply enjoy the landscape, its tranquility and to penetrate its mystery." Following in the footsteps of the foundational works by Cicero, St. Augustin or Boethius, and as the author recalls, literature has a consolatory effect, both for the writer and the reader. Katiuscia Darici ("*El tiempo que nos robaron* (2021) utilizes Rosa Huertas´s book as an excuse to theoretically study "pandemic narrative" to describe the traumatic experience during Covid-19 emergence. In her diary, Huertas highlights that rituals in general during confinement are salvific mainly because "aplacan los malos pensamientos." The diary ends up being Rosa main daily ritual. Thus, we can observe the importance of writing as a tool to objectify and distance oneself from the disease. The long period of introspection also leads the writer to the conviction of personal change as well as a reconciliation with the past. Veronica Orazi ("August Bover, *El contagi* (2021)": Pandemic, isolation and the therapeutic power of poetry") focuses on a collection of 41 poems mostly composed between March and June 2020 during the lockdown that was decreed in an attempt to contain contagions in the first phase of the pandemic. The poems reveal the prevalence of the theme of isolation, taken up with a number of variations in most of the them, the need for a behavioral and psychological response (resilience) in order to manage and contain the fallout from a dramatic situation, and the function of artistic creation and, in particular, of literary production, as a powerful tool for conceptualizing and problematizing the lived experience and the trauma that results from it. Eduard Baile-López ("About some Spanish Graphic Novels in Times of COVID-19 Pandemic: Cathartic Panels for the End of the World") studies comics produced during the COVID-19 pandemic and how they are utilized to comment on reality from psychological and sociopolitical standpoints. In addition, the author observes how fiction as an analytical tool about reality can also become a tool to transform it. The comics are studied according to several axes: fear (the bewilderment before *status quo* is changed); anger, a feeling associated with stupefaction and the inability to find solutions; humor as a defensive weapon or an antidote to cope with misfortune; and healing (a light at the end). Belén Lozano Sañudo ("Pandemics, Illness and Impairment as Reflected in Borges´s Literature and as a Key Factor to Shape his Authorial Style: Searching in Literature the Epic Fate Frailty had Denied to Him") analyzes the seemingly scarce presence of the topic of Spanish Flu in literature, contrary to other pandemics and illnesses like the plague or tuberculosis. In stark contrast, war is seen as something glorifying and is more prevalent in literature. In addition, pandemics and epidemics have undergone processes of metaphorization and mystification that have associated, for instance, plagues to divine punishment and phthisis to profound spirituality and sensitivity. In addition, after the II World War writers did not want to dwell on suffering. Finally, the author studies the role Spanish Flu (and a frail health) and home confinement had in Borges´s immersion in literature as a escape from reality.

Education also plays an important role in trying to overcome the effects on the pandemic. Two more articles focus on literature but this time paying attention to the sociological and educational contexts in which it can be articulated. Marinos Bouchtsis ("The contribution of Children's Literature to the development of the child - Book therapy and narrative therapy") conceives of the "book" as essential for the development of the child because it contributes to the spiritual, cognitive and linguistic development, mental and emotional maturation, and aesthetic cultivation. Book therapy and therapeutic writing play a leading role in psychoanalysis and help individuals overcome their phobias or traumas. In sum, reading books can help children cope with worries, feel better and deal with difficult times, always using a list of books chosen and recommended by leading health professionals in cooperation with children and families. Mourad Kacimi ("Algerian Literature as Socio-Educational Therapy during the 2020-2021 Pandemic") focuses in general on the therapeutic function of Algerian literary production during the pandemic between 2020 and 2021. Algerian authors engaged at this time in the writing of works of literary studies and criticism, poetry, novel, as well as numerous articles that flooded journals and social media. The author also analyzes the role of these media (television, the internet, social networks and digital books) in transmitting literary works that have made people aware of the situation and contributed to alleviating their pain, making them forget their loneliness and the restrictions imposed on them.

Finally, a group of articles continues to focus on the psychological and therapeutic effect of reading and learning at large, although this time they adopt a more educational focus (in particular on populations at risk) than those of the previous section. Evangelia Gkigkelou ("Coronavirus Pandemic and the Isolation of Deaf and Hard-of-Hearing Children in Greece") focuses on the difficulties faced by deaf and hard-of-hearing children in Greece during the closure of in-person and face-to-face attendance to schools, since this population relies heavily on their facial expressions for communication. Masks and social distance have also proved to be very challenging for them, increasing their feelings of isolation. The article discusses several improvements over the last two years in distance learning, digital literacy and the use of technology in order for people to come closer to each other and leave no students excluded from the educational process. Maria Mouchrista, Ainara Romero-Andonegui, Urtza Garay Ruiz, and Spyridon Kazanopoulos ("E-Inclusion and COVID-19 Pandemic: Inclusive Digital Classrooms and Collaboration Between General and Special Education Teachers") also focus on distance learning, this time arguing that more efforts should be made to help special education students improve their learning. For these authors, computers, tablets, or smartphones during a pandemic are not sufficient to ensure learning. To achieve effective electronic inclusion, activities must be organized in such a way that they meet the needs of students with special needs, and modern, asynchronous tools must be available to assist in this process. They also argue that some national platforms' online materials and resources are inaccessible to students with disabilities or learning disabilities. For the most part, education providers have not received additional training to better serve students with disabilities, and as a result, the vast majority of teachers are unqualified to provide inclusive education materials to distance learning students. Spyridon Kazanopoulos, Eneko Tejada, Xabier Basogain, and Maria Mouchrista ("Inclusion of Students with Special Educational Needs and COVID-19 Pandemic: The Collaboration of School and Family in Distance Education Conditions") set out to evaluate school-family collaboration throughout the pandemic period. Their conclusion is that distance learning methods have shattered the conventional knowledge of in-person learning, while parents´ educational level and time commitment to their children's education have been critical to the educational process's efficacy under these crucial circumstances. The findings revealed that interactions between students and their families were especially critical during the pandemic. Distance learning approaches have shattered the form of knowledge about in-person learning. Christos Lalos ("Distance Vocational Education and Training During the Pandemic. Adaptations and Challenges for Learners and Trainers in Europe: How the Pandemic affected Distance Vocational Education and Training") focuses on another group of at-risk educational population whose practices were developed on the basis of physical presence of the trainee. Vulnerable learners are less likely to participate in distance education, while their detachment from the learning process can lead to their early withdrawal from Vocational Education and Training. The author analyzes the challenges this particular population has posed to the educational system, while affirming that this crisis can provide an opportunity to focus on creating a workforce of teachers and cocational trainers of Highly qualified Education and Training. Juan-Francisco Álvarez-Herrero ("Therapeutic and Learning Benefits of Reading During the COVID-19 Among Spanish Secondary Students") studies once again the therapeutic value of reading, this time with a focus on a particular student group in the educational system. He concludes that the promotion of reading is not exclusive to the areas of languages. Also in the areas of science, reading should be encouraged among the students, even from an early age. With the promotion of reading in the areas of science, not only is it possible to improve the reading competence of the students, but an improvement in motivation and interest in learning these subjects can also be achieved. Finally, Margarida Castellano Sanz ("Challenging Picturebooks and Domestic Geographies: A Multimodal Learning Path to Discuss the Consequences of the Covid-19 Lockdowns in the Classroom") is a perfect representative of the combination of literature and education that has been the leitmotif of this book. As a crossover genre, picturebooks perform both an educational and therapeutic function. A new modal, aesthetic, and multidimensional world can use visual literacy to offer an understanding of the world of the educational subjects and their search for their self.

In sum, a variety of approaches and a focus on numerous geographical areas and time periods and cultures point to the same conclusion, the validity and effectiveness of reading, literature, and writing for educational purposes and in times of distress and trauma. Literature (as well as reading and writing), then, is not only valid for its aesthetic value but finds a deep imbrication in human life as a way of making sense of the world and of engaging the reader in a process of self-knowledge, trauma healing, and coping with reality at large. As this book has explored, epidemics like COVID-19 are not new to the human race. And in all of them, the power of the word has always been crucial to help us cope with and learn from our travails and difficulties.

Antonio Cortijo Ocaña
University of California, Santa Barbara, USA

Vicent Martines
ISIC-IVITRA, University of Alicante, Spain

Veronica Orazi
Universita degli Studi di Torino, Italy

Chapter 1
The Power of the Word That Leads to Healing:
Forerunners of Bibliotherapy and Therapeutic Writing (Charles d'Orléans, Jordi de Sant Jordi, Joan Roís de Corella)

Vicent Martines
https://orcid.org/0000-0002-2186-4815
University of Alicante, Spain

ABSTRACT

The authors study the contribution of some classics of medieval and renaissance romance literature to therapeutic writing and bibliotherapy as a means to encourage reading and writing during a pandemic lockdown (in times of pandemic, privation of freedom, or illness). They analyze the cases of the French duke Charles d'Orléans, the Valencian knight Jordi de Sant Jordi, and renaissance author Joan Roís de Corella. In addition, they reflect on the everlasting power and therapeutic value of the written word (reading and writing) since the time of the Egyptian pharaohs.

INTRODUCTION

The Power of Words: First Reflections "avant la léttre" on Bibliotherapy and Therapeutic Writing

The scribes of the Egyptian pharaohs were conscious of the power they had to dominate the word, the techniques and channels of communication at that time. We are told about this in the *Praise of the Scribe*. This is an anonymous text written ca. 1,300 AD during the New Kingdom (1570-1090 AD), the Nineteenth Dynasty (that of the "Biblical" pharaoh Ramesses II the Great –1335-1200–) (Lichtheim (tr.) 1978, pp. 176-177)[1]:

DOI: 10.4018/978-1-6684-4735-2.ch001

As to those learned scribes,

Of the time that came after the gods,

They who foretold the future,

Their names have become everlasting,

While they departed, having finished their lives,

and all their kin are forgotten.

[…]

Their portals and mansions have crumbled.

The ka-servants are [gone];

Their tombstones are covered with soil

Their graves are forgotten.

Their name is pronounced over their books,

Which they made while they had being;

Good is the memory of their makers,

It is for ever and all time!

Words are powerful. Not only to write state agreements and contribute to the solution (or to the problem). Words can also be therapeutic not just on a public but also on a personal level. Regarding the latter, it is well known the inscription on the frontispiece of Ramesses´s library that described its contents as "medicine for the soul" (*ψῦχῆς ἰατρεῖου*). Diodorus Siculus (I c. AD) transmitted this information in his *Βιβλιοθήκη Ἱστορική* because words could be "therapeutic" for so many things (Lutz, 1978). Written words are powerful precisely because they are not just words, but they involve the complex universe of cultural references, knowledge and feelings that surrounds them. It is about managing (with the narrative itself of a past event or of something imagined by a person) the processing of that complex universe. *Storytelling* can organize, order, or sequence events from the catharsis to the overcoming of the cause of the infirmity, or can even manage happiness (Martínez-Roig, Merma-Molina & Urrea-Solano, 2020; Martínez-Roig, Urrea-Solano & Hernández-Amorós, 2021).

Classical, medieval, and Renaissance literature offers us numerous examples of its cathartic value. The creation of the *topos* of ´literature as therapy´ is considered an innovative element, a proof of being at the threshold of the literary Renaissance, for instance in the case of Roís de Corella, as we will see below. Currently, it is not a trivial topic, but an emerging line of research in both literary writing –especially in lyric– as well as in reflections about it (even with a therapeutic goal). The salutary effects of literature, reading and writing are not minor nor random, in terms of the improvement of cognitive skills and capabilities, and even in the case of serious psychological issues. Reading and writing (with or without artistic purposes) play a not-so-minor role in the so-called expressive therapies. These use creative arts as forms of therapy, either in the form of expressive therapies or in the form of creative arts therapy (art, dance, theater, music, writing, poetry, psychodrama). Creative writing has proven to be useful as clinical support in cancer treatments (Wu, Liu, Zheng, Xu, Chen *et al.*, 2021; Antoni & Dhabahar, 2019; Zachariae & O'Toole 2015) as well as in depression and emotional illness (Singer & Singer, 2008; Nazarian & Smyth, 2013; Travagin, Margola, Dennis & Revenson, 2016; Fioretti, Mazzocco, Riva, Oliveri, Masiero & Pravettoni, 2016). Bibliotheratpy is also similar in terms of its therapeutic goals and virtues (Rottenberg, 2022; Gualano, Bert, Martorana, Voglino, Andriolo, Thomas, Gramaglia, Zeppegno & Siliquini, 2017; Betzalel & Schechtman, 2017; Cannon 2018).

The Power of Poetry in *Prime Time*

The excellent BBT TV program entitled Intelligence Squared includes debates on universal and contemporary topics which are quite frequently polemical. It is noteworthy the fact that the BBC promotes a tradition of debate in the media, during *prime time* and featuring first-rate world figures in politics, economy, sports, and culture. It can be interpreted as a sign of the maturity of the society that produces and broadcasts these programs. Among the episodes of *Intelligence Squared*, we would like to highlight one devoted to the therapeutic power of words (of the "artistic word", of literature in general and more particularly of poetry). In fact, this power was also mentioned by the 15th-c. Valencian classic who wrote in Catalan, Joan Roís de Corella –*vid. infra* paragraph. 5–.

The episode we are referring to is entitled The Power of Poetry. As other episodes of the same series, it was recorded in the famous Central Hall of Westminster, full to capacity on March 2nd, 2018 (Intelligence[2]) and it was broadcast in prime time. The summary of the episode is rather eloquent (our *bold text*) –the therapeutic power of the word, of poetry–, as well as the cultural relevance of the participants and poets that intervened (which does not undermine in the least the objective and target audience of the program):

[…]. Argument and debate, we believe, can move, persuade, and create real change. Now, in these anxious and divided times, we held a special event that celebrated the positive, transformative force of another kind of spoken word – poetry.

William Sieghart told the extraordinary story of his bestselling book, *The Poetry Pharmacy: Tried-and-True Prescriptions for the Heart, Mind and Soul.* This is no conventional collection, but one created from Sieghart's own, personal experience of prescribing real poems to real people in need. Every poem is matched to a specific condition: fear of the unknown, unrequited love, stagnation, purposelessness, convalescence, oppression.

Joining him in conversation were novelist and poetry devotee Jeanette Winterson. **Together they explored poetry's uncanny ability to calm, console and, above all, connect us to the minds and feelings of others. Finding the right poem at the right moment is not just a problem shared, Sieghart says, but a problem transformed. It is 'to discover a powerful sense of complicity, and that precious**

realisation: I'm not the only one who feels like this.' It is to forge a connection with 'this stranger who understands – and what results is a sort of peace.'

Bringing the poems to dramatic life were a cast of star actors including Helena Bonham Carter, Sue Perkins, Jason Isaacs and Tom Burke.

Poetry as Refuge: Charles d'Orléans

Charles d'Orléans (Paris, 1394- Amboise, 1465) was Duke of Orléans and Valois, brother of King Charles VI of France and father to Louis XII, King of France. To this, he added his connection with the Duke of Milan through his mother, Valentina Visconti, who was related to this duchy. In 1415, he was in command of the French royal army that fought against Henry VI of England during the crucial battle of Azincourt. This battle was an absolute disaster for the French troops and resulted in over 6,000 casualties and 1,000 soldiers taken captive by the English. One of these prisoners was Charles d'Orléans himself, who remained in custody until 1440. Nonetheless, his was not a captivity of pain and torture. A grandee of France like him constituted enough booty in his own right. The English established his ransom at the astronomical figure of 22,000 *écus*. The English Crown was then interested in keeping him in perfect condition. Charles d'Orléans entertained his long sojourn by composing poetry. A large part of his works was written in captivity (ballads, rondeux, rondels, etc.); he even learned English and wrote poetry in the language of his captors (Figure 1).

Figure 1. Charles d'Orléans prisoner at the Tower of London. He is not represented suffering, rather he is assisted by a royal retinue and is writing at his desk (British Library, MS Royal, 16 fo 73).

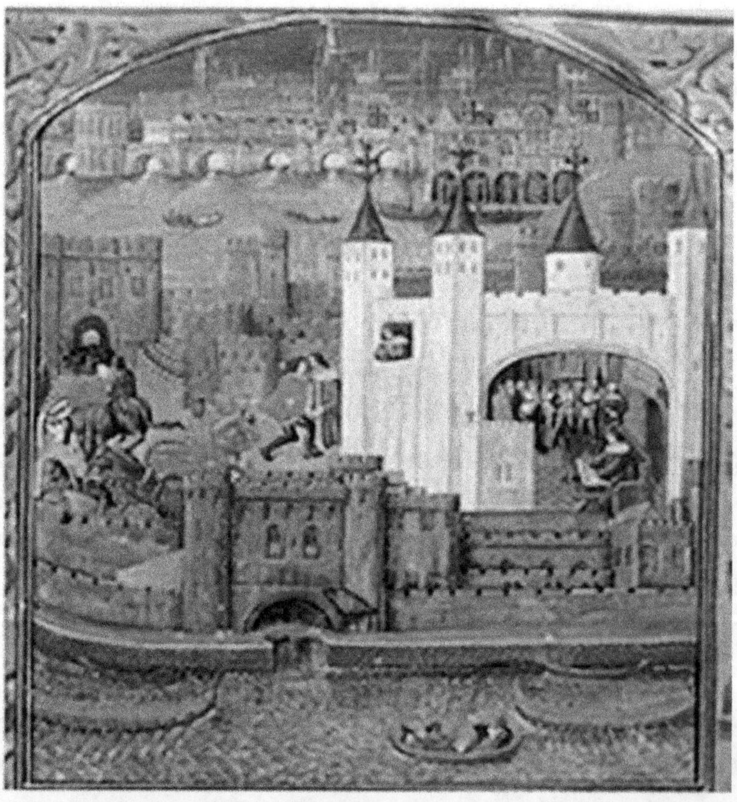

He did not use poetry to request his liberation, as was done by his contemporary Jordi de Sant Jordi (*vid. infra*). To do so he used writing, but more prosaic texts, deprived of mimesis (Figure 2).

Figure 2. Letter by Charles d'Orléans, dated July 16th, 1438, while still in prison, in which he lists the ecclesiastical offices of his fiefdom and the corresponding sums they must provide in order to come up with the amount of his ransom (Archives nationales de France, AE/II/450).

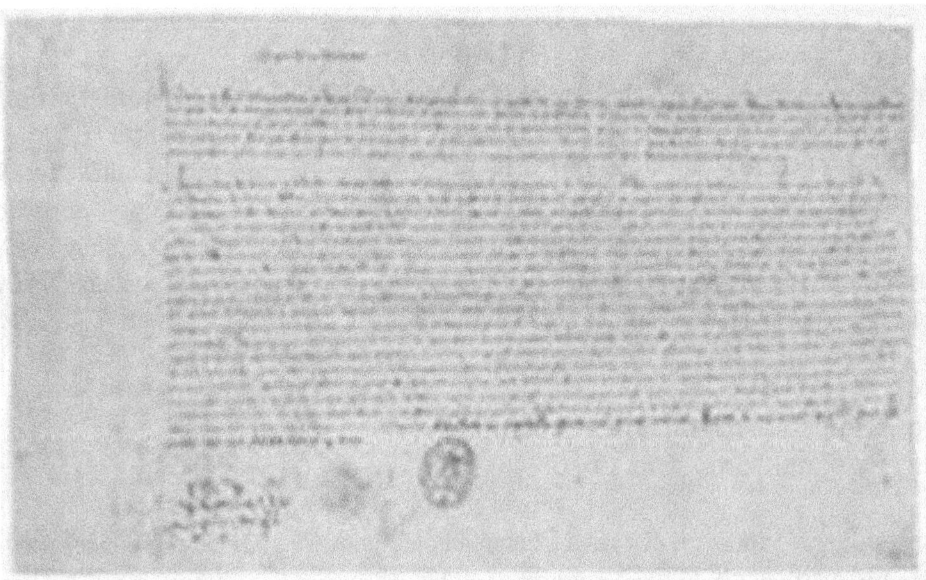

For Charles d'Orléans, while his imprisonment was not painful –nothing like the case of Cervantes in Algiers nor that of Jordi de Sant Jordi—, it was not a delightful experience either. For him, while prison was not paradise, it became an "accepted" refuge. It was a sort of proof of maturity that occupied much of his life (he was 20-years-old at the time of his captivity) until he was liberated in 1440, at the age of 45. He expressed this in his poem "Merencolie" (Andrade Boué, 2000), describing his prison as a non-permanent refuge while awaiting "full freedom":

Fruit suis d'yver qui a meins de tendresse

Que fruit s'esté; si suis en garnison,

Pour amolir ma trop verde duresse,

Mis pour meurir ou feurre de prison (Ballade LXXX)

[Fruit am from yver which has less tenderness

What fruit has sprung; if I am in garrison,

To soften my too green hardness,

Put to die or go to jail]

For Charles d'Orléans, prison is understood as a forest, a departure from society, a place of "Merencolie" and "Longue Actente". Three of his poems express this idea in a clear manner: Ballad XXVII (Mon cueur a envoyé querir / Tous ses biens vueillants et amis, / Il veult son grant conseil tenir / Avenc euix, pour avoir advis / Comment pourra ses annemis, / Soussy, Dueil et leur aliance, / Surmonter et tot desconfire, / Qui desirent de la destruiré / En la prisión de Desplaisance" (vv. 1-9)); "Complainte" II ("Ayez de lui souvenance / Et le venz deslongier / De la prison de Dangier / Ou il meurt en desplaisance" (vv. 18-21)); and "Carole" II ("Car Dangier qui desire / De la nocire du tout a mort / L'a mis pour plus tost le destruiré / En la prison de Desconfort" (vv. 17-20)). These poems point to different concepts of prison: from an imprisonment of "Desplaisance" (displeasure) to "Gangier" (afliction) and "Desconfort" (discomfort). In the three poems, the poet addresses his heart in love, "imprisoned" by his "enemies". The numbering of the three poems indicates that they are early compositions, written shortly upon his arrival in England, and hence their total agreement with the courtly love tradition (García Bascuñana, 2010: 324-325).

Liberating Poetry: Jordi de Sant Jordi: Desert of Friends, Possessions, and Lord

Jordi de Sant Jordi (*ca.* 1400-*ca.* 1424) is a Valencian classic of Catalan letters. For his services to the Crown of Aragon, particularly to the Kingdom of Valencia during the reign of King Alfons the Magnanimous, to whom he served since a young age, the king rewarded him with the title of knight (Mosén), as well as with lands and lordships: alcaide (chatelain) of the Castillo del Valle de Uixó, Castellón, and Lord of Polop, la Nucía and Xirles (Alacant/Alicante) (Figure 3).

Figure 3. Ideal representation of Jordi de Sant Jordi used in the dedication of the Aula Magna of the Seu Universitària de la Nucia to him (Universitat d'Alacant/Universidad de Alicante [UA]), adorned with a white Milan harness similar to those wore by contemporary figures from the mid-15th c. represented on the Triumphal Arch of King Alfons of Magnanimous in Castel Nuovo, Naples. Historical Advisor: Dr. Dr. Abel Soler. Illustrator: Josep-Miquel Martínez. Photo by Rosabel Martínez-Roig (UA).

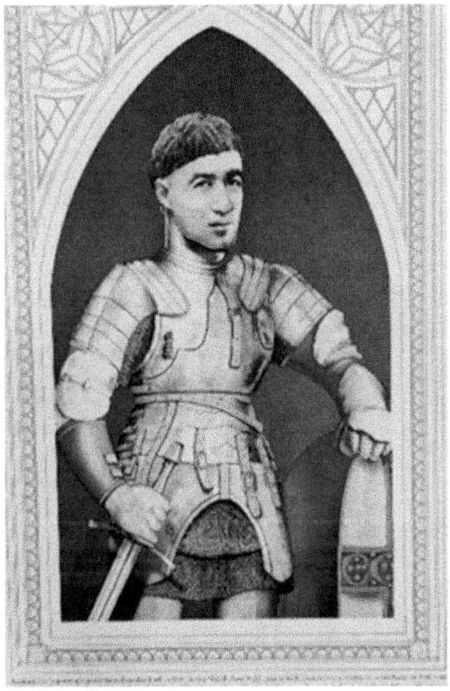

Jordi de Sant Jordi was the son of freed slaves from the Maghreb who became fully integrated into 15th-c. Valencian society. In fact, his parents acquired wealth and Jordi de Sant Jordi´s sister professed as a nun in one of the most elitist convents of Valencia, the Saidia; Jordi de Sant Jordi, because of his talent as poet and musician since an early age, and then because of his superb physical prowess, gained the confidence and protection of the king. A successful case of social integration: freed slaves from the Maghreb that did well –after converting to Christianity– and placed their children in positions that secured them a better life, in fact much better than the majority of their contemporary old Christians.

Jordi de Sant Jordi was a valiant soldier, dubbed into knighthood by his merits in war, a faithful and ardent man of action at the service of the Magnanimous. He was imprisoned in Naples after protecting his monarch´s retreat during the attack of the Milan troops of Francesco Sforza that came to help the Angevine French rights. The geostrategic situation did not favor a forceful resistance and the Magnanimous opted wisely in the last moment for a strategic retreat. Jordi de Sant Jordi was part of the troops that protected the monarch during the orderly retreat. He was taken prisoner. His imprisonment was not luxurious like that of his contemporary Charles d'Orléans in London. Jordi de Sant Jordi explains to us the condition he is in and his feelings about it, and at the same time he asks the king for help in rescuing him, for he has also paid his tribute to his monarch. He does so through poetry, in his impressive poem "Presoner". He indicates the terrible conditions of his imprisonment with such effectiveness that his monarch paid his ransom and Jordi de Sant Jordi immediately put his sword back at the service of the monarch. The powerful expression and the precision with which he describes the physical reality and his feelings, in clear language and without any resort to artifice, following the norms of contemporary poetic composition, make of "Prisoner" one of most outstanding poems on captivity. At the same time, the poem has a very concrete goal in mind, as can be seen in the *ritornello*, that addresses directly the king ("Rei virtuós, mon senyor natural" / 'Virtuous king, who are my lord by nature'):

Table 1.

PRESONER (Sant Jordi, 2011; RIALC)	THE PRISONER (Sant Jordi, 2023 [in press])
Desert d'amics, de béns e de senyor, en estrany lloc i en estranya contrada, lluny de tot bé, fart d'enuig e tristor, ma voluntat e pensa caitivada, me trob del tot en mal poder sotsmès, no vei algú que de mé s'haja cura, e soi guardats, enclòs, ferrats e pres, de què en fau grat a ma trista ventura.	Bereft of friends, possessions and my natural lord, In a foreign land and and in a strange dwelling, Far from any good and full of pain and suffering, My will and thoughts imprisoned, I am totally subjected to the power of evil, With no one to care for me, (well guarded and shackled in my cell) And nothing to offer some pleasure to this my ill fortune.
Eu hai vist temps que no em plasia res; ara em content de ço que em fai tristura, e los grillons lleugers ara preu més que en lo passat la bella brodadura. Fortuna vei que ha mostrat son voler sus mé, volent que en tal punt vengut sia; però no em cur, pus hai fait mon dever amb tots los bons que em trob en companyia.	There was a time when nothing seemed to please me, And I am happy now about what makes me sad, And my not-heavy fetters I have in esteem now more Than some fine brocades in the past. Fortune decided to impose herself On me, wanting to see me so utterly defeated. I do not care, though, I have fulfilled my duty With those so valiant in whose company I am.
Tots aquests mals no em són res de sofrir en esguard d'u qui al cor me destenta e em fai tot jorn d'esperança partir: com no vei res que ens avanç d'una espenta en acunçar nostre deslliurament, e mes que vei ço que ens demana Sforza, que no sofir algu raonament, de que llangueix ma virtut e ma força.	To suffer all these pains is nothing Compared to one that perturbs my heart And takes me daily far from having any hope, As I think we are barely moving forward Towards the attainment of our freedom, and I strive to keep on persevering not to allow in me any thought whatsoever that might weaken my courage nor my strength.
Per que no sai ni vei res al present que em puixa dar en valor d'una escorça, mas Déu tot sol, de qui prenc fundament e de qui fiu, i-z amb qui mon cor s'esforça; e d'altra part del bon rei liberal, qui em socorrec per gentilesa granda, lo qui ens ha mes del tot en aquest mal, qu'ell me'n traura, car soi jus sa comanda.	For I can't see nor think about anything presently That might encourage me somehow, Safe only God, who is my unique foundation, In whom I trust, and with whom I take heart, Who succours me out of his extreme generosity As well as my lord, a king of great largesse, Whose cause has taken us to this unfortunate situation From which he'll free me, for I am in his hands.
Reis virtuós, mon senyor natural, tots al present no us fem altra demanda, mas que us record que vostra sang reial mai defalli al qui fos de sa banda.	Virtuous king, who are my lord by nature, presently I beseech you about just this one thing, for you to keep in mind that your blood, that is kingly, do not be weary of those who fought well on your side.

Jordi de Sant Jordi resorted to poetry. He did not write a letter to his subordinates ordering them to collect the ransom money as did Charles d'Orléans. Neither was he as wealthy as his monarch. He used what he thought would be the most efficient and striking way when dealing with his natural lord, Alfons the Magnanimous, who was very sensitive to cultural and verbal productions, as the humanist king that he was. As a cathartic composition and one that was written with the goal of attaining his freedom, this work has become an identity reference. It has been able to transcend and become a trans-media product because of singer Raimon´s musical version of it. As a result, it has become a reference for Valencian identity in Catalan language as well as for Catalan language in general, as is also the rest of Raimon´s musical versions of Valencian classics such as Jordi de Sant Jordi, Ausiàs March, or Joan Roís de Corella (Raimon, 1993, 2010*a*, 2010*b*).

The Pen, a Frequent Respite from Misfortunes: Joan Roís de Corella

Valencian classic *Mossén* Joan Roís de Corella (Gandía or Valencia, 1435 - Valencia, 1497), a stylist and a herald of the Renaissance in Hispanic letters and not only in the Catalan-speaking world, offers a clear example of therapeutic literature, and even of personal overcoming, in several of his works, for instance in his profane proses (Martínez-Roig, Gavilán-Martín & Merma-Molina, 2020). On the other hand, in his famous *Tragèdia de Caldesa*, when the author (although this is probably autobiographical fiction) realizes at the end that the lady with whom he wanted to enjoy himself in her room has deceived him, he writes, following the translation into English by Antonio Cortijo (Cortijo & Martines, 2013: 225-230) (bold types are our):

¿Com, doncs, serà causa de tanta dolor escriure's puga? ¿Quin paper soferrà ésser tint de lletgea de tant crim?

[...]

Ab diversitat de tan impossibles pensaments, me partí de la cambra o sepulcre a on tanta pena sofert havia. **Acceptant la ploma, que sovint greus mals descansa,** *la present ab ma pròpia sang pinte, perquè la color de la tinta ab la dolor que raona se conforme.*

[How then could it be possible to write about such pain? Which paper could withstand to put in writing such criminous action?

[...]

Absorbed in the disparity of such impossible thoughts, I took leave of the room (nay the sepulcher) where I had suffered such great pain. ***I picked up the pen, which often alleviates great grief****, and depicted the present story with my own blood, so that the color of the ink would fit the pain it recounts.]*

The therapeutic value of literature is also present in authors of such relevance as Petrarch (Martines, 2015).

CONCLUSION

We have analyzed the contribution of several classics of medieval and Renaissance Romance literature to therapeutic writing and bibliotherapy as an encouragement to reading and writing during lockdowns (because of a pandemic, imprisonment, or illness). We have reviewed the cases of the French Duke

Charles d'Orléans, the Valencian knight Jordi de Sant Jordi and the Valencian Renaissance author Joan Roís de Corella. We have also reflected on the everlasting and therapeutic power of the written word (reading and writing), already documented in the Egypt of the Pharaohs.

The first author we have studied, Charles d'Orléans, was imprisoned in England, and the second, the Valencian Jordi de Sant Jordi, in Naples. Both were taken captive in battle: Charles d'Orléans in the decisive battle of Azincourt, which was a disaster for the English troops in the Hundred Years War; Jordi de Sant Jordi by the Milanese troops of Francesco Sforza when the latter attacked Naples in defense of the French house of Anjou´s rights against the Crown of Aragon´s army of Alfons the Magnanimous.

As we have seen, there were similar causes for both captivities, which also happened almost at the same time, although both were resolved in a different manner. Jordi de Sant Jordi´s case was solved in a short time, while Charles de Orléans´s took 25 years and only ended after the payment of an astronomical sum. Jordi de Sant Jordi indicated in his poem "Presoner" the harsh conditions of his imprisonment and requested at the same time from his monarch to free him as just compensation for his service and sacrifice in action while protecting the king´s retreat from battle. Charles d'Orléans composed much of his work in captivity, even in English, the language of his captors. He did not use fictional literature to request his freedom, rather artistic words were used as balsam for processing his personal situation during his long captivity, which took place in comfortable circumstances.

We have also analyzed the concept of literature as therapy to overcome personal (sentimental) setbacks. We used as an example the case of the work of Renaissance Valencian author Joan Roís de Corella, for whom "the pen is a frequent respite from misfortunes".

As can be observed, reflecting on the healing and the overcoming power of the word (artistic words) and literature (either reading or writing) has always been done from the beginnings of literature. Bibliotherapy, and especially therapeutic writing, can be effective in overcoming personal setbacks as well as long-lasting and more serious tribulations.

ACKNOWLEDGMENT

This study was done at the Institut Superior d'Investigació Cooperativa IVITRA [ISIC-IVITRA] (Programa per a la Constitució i Acreditació d'Instituts Superiors d'Investigació Cooperativa.

REFERENCES

Andrade Boué, P. (2000). Quelques aspects de la Merencolie de Charles d'Orléans [Some aspects of Charles d'Orléans' Merencolia]. *Thélème. Revista Complutense de Estudios Franceses, 15*, 167. https://revistas.ucm.es/index.php/THEL/article/view/THEL0000110167A

Antoni, M. H., & Dhabhar, F. S. (2019). The impact of psychosocial stress and stress management on immune responses in patients with cancer. *Cancer, 125*(9), 1417–1431. doi:10.1002/cncr.31943 PMID:30768779

Betzalel, N., & Shechtman, Z. (2017). The impact of bibliotherapy superheroes on youth who experience parental absence. *School Psychology International, 38*(5), 473–490. doi:10.1177/0143034317719943

Cannon, P. (2018). Rethinking bibliotherapy: A neurorhetoric narratology model for addiction treatment. *Health Information and Libraries Journal, 35*(4), 331–335. doi:10.1111/hir.12239 PMID:30499173

Cortijo, A., & Martines, V. (Eds.). (2013). Multilingual Joan Roís de Corella. The Relevance of a Fifteenth-Century Classic of the Crown of Aragon Joan Roís de Corella Multilingüe. La importància d'un clàssic de la Corona d'Aragó del segle XV. Publications of eHumanista-University of California at Santa Barbara.

de Sant Jordi, J. (2011). Poesia [Poetry]. Edició crítica d'Aniello Fratta, versió en català modern de Carles Duarte. Barcelona: Barcino.

de Sant Jordi, J. (2023). Poems (A. Cortijo, A. Cortijo-Rodgers, & V. Martines, Eds.). Academic Press.

Fioretti, C., Mazzocco, K., Riva, S., Oliveri, S., Masiero, M., & Pravettoni, G. (2016). Research studies on patients' illness experience using the Narrative Medicine approach: A systematic review. *BMJ Open, 6*(7), 112–120. doi:10.1136/bmjopen-2016-011220 PMID:27417197

García Bascuñana, J. F. (2010). *Por otra lectura de Charles d'Orléans: el valor de la imagen* [For another reading of Charles d'Orléans: the value of the image] [Doctoral thesis]. Universitat de Barcelona. https://www.tesisenred.net/handle/10803/1735#page=1

Gualano, M. R., Bert, F., Martorana, M., Voglino, G., Andriolo, V., Thomas, R., Gramaglia, C., Zeppegno, P., & Siliquini, R. (2017). The long-term effects of bibliotherapy in depression treatment: Systematic review of randomized clinical trials. *Clinical Psychology Review, 58*, 49–58. doi:10.1016/j.cpr.2017.09.006 PMID:28993103

Intelligence^2. (2018). *Intelligence Squared: The Power Of Poetry*. https://intelligencesquared.com/events/the-power-of-poetry/

Lichtheim, M. (Ed.). (1978). The Immortality of Writers [M. Lichtheim, Trans.). In Ancient Egyptian Literature, II. The University of California Press.

Lutz, C. (1978). The Oldest Library Motto: Ψῡχῆς Ἰατρεῖον. *The Library Quarterly, 48*(1). Advance online publication. doi:10.1086/629993

Martines, V. (2015). La escritura literaria como terapia y didáctica sentimental [Literary writing as therapy and sentimental didactics]. *Quaderni di didattica della scrittura, 12*(1), 25-37. DOI: doi:10.7369/80660

Martínez-Roig, R., Gavilán-Martín, D., & Merma-Molina, G. (2020). Transmedia storytelling que reporta y supera casos de marginados. Clásicos como muestra de didáctica y psicología social para la superación personal [Transmedia storytelling that reports and overcomes cases of marginalized. Classics as a sample of didactics and social psychology for self-improvement]. In A. Cortijo & J. M. Antolí (Eds.), Approaches to New Trends in Research on Catalan Studies (pp. 235-268). Peter Lang, Romance Literatures & Cultures.

Martínez-Roig, R., Merma-Molina, G., & Urrea-Solano, M. (2020). The power of storytelling. Some aspects of James I's Llibre dels Fets as a transmedia storytelling with educational purposes and social and political psychology. In V.J. Escartí, V. J., & R. Roca (Eds.), En los márgenes de la Historia: marginales y minorías (pp. 261-268). Zaragoza: Pórtico.

Martínez-Roig, R., Urrea-Solano, M., & Hernández-Amorós, M. (2021). Transmedia Storytelling i coneixement en obert. Clàssics i psicología social en favor de les virtuts del bon govern [Transmedia Storytelling and open knowledge. Classics and social psychology in favor of the virtues of good governance]. In A. Cortijo, & E. Sánchez López (Eds.), De la innovació al cànon. Noves tendències de recerca en Filologia Catalana: llengua, literatura, educación i cultura (pp. 395-427). Editorial Afers.

Nazarian, D., & Smyth, J. M. (2013). An experimental test of instructional manipulations in expressive writing interventions: Examining processes of change. *Journal of Social and Clinical Psychology*, *32*(1), 71–96. doi:10.1521/jscp.2013.32.1.71

Raimon. (1993). *Veles e vents* [Sails and winds]. https://www.youtube.com/watch?v=JEpKnkhTj-0

Raimon. (2010a). *Desert d'amics* [Friend Deserts]. https://www.youtube.com/watch?v=lJNRMOXCf50

Raimon. (2010b). *Balada de la garça i l'esmerla* [Ballad of the garza and the emerald]. https://www.youtube.com/results?search_query=raimon+ro%C3%ADs+de+corella

RIALC-Repertorio Informatizzato della Letteratura Catalana Antica. (n.d.). [RIALC-Computerized Repertoire of Ancient Catalan Literature]. Università degli Studi di Napoli Federico II. http://www.rialc.unina.it/inc-santjordi.html

Rottenberg, B. (2022). Bibliotherapy as an integrative psychotherapeutic channel. *Journal of Poetry Therapy*, *35*(1), 27–41. doi:10.1080/08893675.2021.2004371

Singer, J., & Singer, G. H. S. (2008). Writing as Physical and Emotional Healing: Findings from Clinical Research. In *Handbook of Research on Writing: History, Society, School, Individual, Text* (pp. 485–498). Lawrence Erlbaum Assoc.

Skočić Mihić, S., Maich, K., Belcher, C., Perrow, S., Barišić, A., & Ramić, N. N. (2017). The Role of Bibliotherapy and Therapeutic Storytelling in Creating Inclusive Classroom Communities. In C. M. Curran & A. J. Petersen (Eds.), *Handbook of Research on Classroom Diversity and Inclusive Education Practice*. IGI Global. doi:10.4018/978-1-5225-2520-2.ch016

Travagin, G., Margola, D., Dennis, J. L., & Revenson, T. A. (2016). Letting Oneself Go Isn't Enough: Cognitively Oriented Expressive Writing Reduces Preadolescent Peer Problems. *Journal of Research on Adolescence*, *26*(4), 1048–1060. doi:10.1111/jora.12279 PMID:28453210

Wu, Y., Liu, L., Zheng, W., Zheng, C., Xu, M., Chen, X., Li, W., Xie, L., Zhang, P., Zhu, X., Zhan, C., & Zhou, C. (2021). Effect of prolonged expressive writing on health outcomes in breast cancer patients receiving chemotherapy: A multicenter randomized controlled trial. *Supportive Care in Cancer*, *29*(2), 1091–1101. doi:10.100700520-020-05590-y PMID:32601853

Zachariae, R., & O'Toole, M. S. (2015). The effect of expressive writing intervention on psychological and physical health outcomes in cancer patients: A systematic review and meta-analysis. *Psycho-Oncology*, *24*(11), 1349–1359. doi:10.1002/pon.3802 PMID:25871981

ENDNOTE

1 I wish to thank Prof. Cortijo (CCS, UCSB) for providing me with information about this reference.

Chapter 2
The Valencian Annals: Reflex of the Current Pandemic

Francisco José Conejero Pascual
Universitat d'Alacant, Spain

ABSTRACT

Human nature has always experienced the need to count any facts close to or away in time from a subjective or objective perspective. The Valencian Annals is a work that collects events from the city of Valencia and its kingdom during the 14th and 15th centuries. The text is set in medieval autumn and is considered minor, as it is included in the genres of dietary or chronicons of memoralistic literature. All of them maintain a common denominator with the annotation of more or less relevant events in order to record the living, without any artistic intent. The purpose will be to establish a link between the vision of the 15th century population pandemics and today. COVID-19 has changed and transformed the world as humankind was living in this early 21st century. The metamorphosis caused by everything that this virus and disease has produced has prompted us to rethink certain individual and collective aspects of world society and, in particular, Western society.

INTRODUCTION

The current situation that we are living around the world with the COVID-19 pandemic is not a unique and unique event as society today can think but has been repeated before. So, we could define an epidemic as a temporary disease with an immediate and extraordinary rise in deaths (Moll, 2002) which mankind has experienced throughout history. If we take a look at the history of the European territories, we can notice that our ancestors also suffered a similar situation to the one we have currently. Even history has classified this situation into three major cycles: the Black Death between the 14th and 18th century and cholera in the 19th century with other diseases such as tuberculosis, typhus, etc., and as early as the 20th century, with the influenza so called Spanish influenza in 1918.

The consideration of an epidemic is linked not only to an extraordinary rise in mortality, but also to the change of behavior in the face of suspicion of the occurrence or presence of the disease in a particular place. The psychosis caused by the suspicion of the presence of the disease in a community is much

DOI: 10.4018/978-1-6684-4735-2.ch002

more dangerous than the effects of the disease itself. We have experienced this situation not only in the past with the previous diseases, but nowadays with the COVID-19 with attitudes of rejection towards people affected or even towards health workers transmitters as possible direct of the disease.

The onset of the disease or plague known as the Black Death, by the mid-14th century, caused a very high mortality rate up to reach between 55%-60% of the European population at the time (Benedictow, 2011). The demographic decline was very significant, as the increase in the population of the 12th and 13th centuries with the development of urban nuclei, social and commercial relations, thanks to the fact that trade routes through the Mediterranean suffered a strong stagnation.

So, the impact that it brought to society as a whole was evident in all areas, both socioeconomic, political and cultural. Along with the high mortality of population caused by the disease, it affected the number of laborers working in the countryside and wages were proportionally increased wages. Thus, tenants experienced decreased a decline in income, whereas cereal producers increased.

Depopulation led to the abandonment of many areas of cultivation and populations lost qualified inhabitants in certain trades. From a social point of view, fear, insecurity, and instability took over people, becoming a social event (Rubio, 1979).

Similarly, if we look at the current pandemic, we find significant and singular parallelisms between the humankind of those times and the present. During the second decade we have been personally faced with the consequences of a virus, which is still a great unknown at this stage, despite the technology available to us. As we reflect on this current pandemic, we first at the etymological origin of the word, whose Greek origin means "that affects the whole people". So, the current situation that we are experiencing affects the whole humanity, without escape, regardless the economic or social level of the country, the personal situation or any other variables that demonstrate the diversity and multiculturalism of this planet's population.

In this sense, COVID-19, the Black plague, is an unknown disease with a mortality rate of millions of people, which is causing metamorphosis in all countries' societies. Unfortunately, neither the cause nor treatment are known to heal it, except for the use of masks, handshaking with hydroalcoholic hand cleaning gel, and the innovative vaccines from different countries and clinical laboratories[1].

Just as people in the Middle Ages thought that plague was a divine punishment for sins committed (Parrilla, 2019), present day society is fluctuating from social networks, and apocalyptic and conspiratorial theories about the appearance of this disease. All of them are so implausible and improper of in a reef considered advanced society, that they are very close to those exposed by people in medieval times.

Francesc Gavaldà en diferents llocs de la seua obra, però també ho podem trobar en altres autors. La pesta, certament, era un dels quatre genets de l'apocalipsi, una plaga per a les societats judeocristianes que temptaven d'aplacar la voluntat de càstig d'un Déu ferotge amb processons i rituals religiosos. (Escartí, 2020, pp. 16-17)

Francesc Gavaldà in different places of his work, but we can also find it in other authors. The plague, certainly, was one of the four horsemen of the apocalypse, a plague for Judeo-Christian societies that tried to appease the punishing will of a fierce God with religious processions and rituals.

Among them, current unlikely arguments about the onset of the disease include that the virus that claims that came from Chinese laboratory and that it has been transferred from there to the rest of the world, because the Earth the is overpopulated and some people must be eliminated. Another theory states that vaccines are completely unnecessary, as they introduce microchips under the skin, or third world countries that propose to fight the virus by praying or inhaling herbal vapors.

These pernicious are typically ignorant and impact on the societies that condition the lives of the theories Conspiracy may correspond with individual attitudes or beliefs, but with traits of a personality of social psychology (Abalakina-Paap et al., 1999). Media usually play a prominent role in spreading of these theories, which expend an idea of information overload, resulting in information fatigue syndrome (IFS) with the spread of harmful and intoxicating thoughts.

The result is therefore a narrative that spreads everywhere. However, both, democratic or authoritarian and communities often take refuge in false theories or rumors for party-political purpose for their own interests (Mutsvairo and Bebawi, 2019). The resulting product is the discredit that causes challenges when there is a manifest uncertainty in a political or pandemic crisis such as that we have now suffered (Golob, Makarovi, and Rek, 2021).

On different scales, a parallel is observed between the pandemic medieval society of the Crown of Aragon, specifically in Valencia, and the current pandemic Valencian Country. Intoxication with conspiracy theories stems from people's nature that have always experienced the need to relate any facts close to or away in time from a subjective perspective. For this reason, many groups in society suffered a great marginalization, such as the women's collective and their innate malignant character (Conejero, 2017).

Both 14th-21st centuries, people intend to tell a fact or an event, and that this is an object of knowledge among other people in order to approve or disapprove of the common. The most remarkable contrast is based on the current immediacy of the messages and their content. Whereas in the Valencia society of the 14th century, the news and the events passed through the subjective pen of a dieter who from a subjective perspective, moves the impressions from the events surrounding him.

At present, if we wish to say so, we enjoy a great deal, as far as the media are concerned and as they were understood in the last century. With the technological revolution via the Internet, we have access to everything and from anywhere in the world. Technological globalization has caused a new phenomenon in our lives and societies. The appearance of social platforms such as *Twitter*, *Facebook*, *WhatsApp*, *Instagram* or *TikTok*, *YouTube* etc. has been a turnaround in the way information is transmitted. The new Internet channel has brought about a change in interpersonal relations as in social relations. So, due to these platforms, events, news, facts of people's lives and society have been documented from a subjective point of view without objective historical rigor.

Materials created are valuable documents from different disciplines that, as in previous times, showed us a photograph of society of that time. The designation of these written products is very difficult, and in this sense, we completely agree with the label given by Professor V. Scartine of 'remembrance literature (Escartí, 2010). *On* the pests in Valencia there were reports in the form of dietary books or memoirs, in which news was left of legislative episodes, painful or deadly caused by epidemics.

En definitiva, els valencians –com la resta dels europeus en un moment o en un altre– tenien una llarga experiència en malalties contagioses epidèmiques i, per tant, les seues autoritats disposaven de mecanismes de defensa –no sempre efectius–, que, en la seua legislació i aplicació ens han deixat una sèrie de documents, com ara les crides o els textos de les deliberacions i, fins i tot, memòries específiques destinades a la descripció de la malaltia i les actuacions sanitàries efectuades. (Escartí, 2021, p.53)

[In short, Valencians – like the rest of Europeans at one time or another – had a long experience in contagious epidemic diseases and, therefore, their authorities had defence mechanisms – not always

effective – which, in their legislation and application, have left us with a series of documents, such as calls or texts of deliberations and, Even specific reports aimed at describing the disease and the health actions carried out.]

The parallel between texts written in the 21st century and those between the 14th and 18th centuries consists of the author's will to make it clear to everyone's memory what he lived or told him. Thus, the bond of union is obvious and clear, as these texts expose noticeable facts from a subjective point of view.

So, we will try to find the similarities between these current texts and the Valencian Annals, of anonymous authorship, and which focuses on of the society of the city and Kingdom of Valencia between the 14th and 15th centuries. The work is part of the texts of the Valencian memorialist genre literature, which reflects events of various typology. My task will be to rediscover the motives, the intentions, the purpose of choosing and showing those facts that happened at a time of a specific past, giving a feeling of remembrance about what had happened.

The text is set in medieval and is considered as a minor text it is included among the genres of the dietary or chronicons of memorialist literature. All of them maintain a common denominator with the annotation of more or less relevant events in order to record facts lived or told with no artistic intent, but with variability in the extent and frequency of occurrence.

The *Valencian Annals* are part of the so-called Valencian historiography, (Escartí, 1998) written around the 15th century, in which a plurality of events is presented with great heterogeneity and thematic singularity and practically unknown. The Valencian society's character is distinguished by a mix of very miscellaneous moments, ranging from universal character with references to the flood or the Babylonian Tower, to emblematic monarchs such as James I, Alfonso V the Magnanimous, Peter and to more particular ones such as home episodes, named by Professor Vincent Escartí as local or *regnicultural* (Escartí, 2010).

The set of news, facts or events demonstrated by the author of the work, is based on first person experience, or because he has noticed them from various channels:

En nom de nostre senyor Déu Jeshucrist y de la Santíssima Verge Maria, aquest llibre és memòria de les coses passades d'aquest Regne de València, des de l'any MCCCXXXXVIII. fins a la jornada de les coses senyalades.[2]

[In the name of our lord God Jesus Christ and the Blessed Virgin Mary, this book is a memory of the past things of this Kingdom of Valencia, since the year MCCCXXXXVIII. until the day of things marked.]

If the study of the text continues, it can be seen that the original manuscript of the text has not been found, since it has reached us to this day through two copies. The first one since manuscript 694, the oldest one from the Archive of the Royal College-Seminary of Corpus Christi of Valencia by Agustí Sales in 1745. The other one is from the manuscript 83 of the Royal Convent of Predictors of Valencia by Bartomeu Ribelles in 1805. Both refer to an original that had not been found[3] and with a different appearance, though with a similar news content. This situation of copies and anonymous authorship only reveals how little importance has been attached to the work, which brings us closer to find out the Catalan social cosmos of that time. From a personal point of view, however, I find this document extremely important, as it is a kind of test for the creation of larger and more important ventures. Although, from Valencian historiography, this document is of great significance, since it constitutes the preliminary stage, that is, the test for the creation of larger and more important companies.

Among this type of contemporary protodietaristic (Escartí and Ribera, 2019) writings in the *Valencian Annals* are the *Dietary of Alfonso the Magnanimous* priest attributed to Melcior Miralles and the so-called *Chronicle of Pere Maça*, the universal Chronicle of 1427, that form the corpus of Valencian historiography among the most outstanding. All these texts are essential for understanding, through cross-disciplinary ways, history, philology, writing, women and ultimately, the social skeleton of the people of that society at that time.

In all this range of research possibilities, my purpose will be to establish a link between the population's vision of pandemics throughout the 15th century and ar present, the one that we have had to go through to live. The COVID-19 has changed and transformed the world as we perceive humanity in this new century. The metamorphosis caused by everything that this virus has produced, and which causes us to rethink certain individual and collective aspects of world society. Similarly, the people living in 15th century Valencia suffered from diseases, pandemics, and a great death toll which led to a shift in their optics and understanding of the relationship between alike people.

La pesta bubònica causava estralls demogràfics, però, també hi tenia efectes psicològics considerables, per la mateixa virulència de la mortalitat, que era ben elevada, i per les reaccions de les poblacions afectades. (Escartí 2020, p.15)

[The bubonic plague wreaked demographic havoc, however, it also had considerable psychological effects, due to the same virulence of mortality, which was very high, and the reactions of the affected populations.]

A very similar context between societies of so different countries is the apocalyptic view of fear towards the unknown. In addition, if we add to the recipe ingredient the opinion of visionaries with apocalyptic theories with the echo of new technologies, they mask thoughts beyond reason. So, after so many centuries and with the very advanced means we have at present, we don't look so far away from the thoughts of our ancestors.

DISEASES

19[4] disease is caused by a coronavirus called SARS-CoV-2, which is part of the family of viruses that affect both humans and animals, but which we did not know about, because it was only circulating among animals. Similarly, the plague came from the "Yersinia pestis or Pasteurella pestis" bacteria that it was discovered by Alexandre Yersin around 1894, primarily affected rodent mammals such as rats, mice, squirrels, etc. and that passed to people through a spike of a stitch. We therefore have a shared origin of both diseases through zoonosis, which will eventually be passed on from animals to humans.

Another surprising fact is its origin, as both appear to come from Asia. In the case of COVID-19, the epicenter is placed in Wuhan, China, first notified on 31st December 2019. It was spread from this city and throughout the world. Whereas, in the case of the plague, around 1346 in the siege of the city of Caffa, present-day Phoodosia in Ukraine, the Mongols used the body of men contaminated by the disease to infect Christians. It has since spread throughout the Mediterranean and from there to the rest of Europe.

Thus, transmission immediacy in both epidemics was very characteristic, as in the case of the plague, commercial cities were the main focus of irradiation towards the population centers. Similarly, COVID-19 has been transmitted thanks to the mobility of today's society not only of goods but also of people. The globalization of the present era has acted as a springboard so that nowhere on the planet has escaped the tentacles of the disease. Given the large geographical extent of the disease and the large number of people affected, on 30 January 2020, the WHO[5] Director-General (World Health Organization) convened the Emergency Committee of this international body, making the decision that the outbreak constituted a ESPII[6] and declaring the outbreak a pandemic.

The current medical treaties are multiple and varied, but the WHO has a key role to play in drawing up standards, treatments and indications regarding diseases of the world population. In this respect, a whole set of research articles on new developments and explorations are available on the medical community's website.[7]

In the 14th century, around the plague, treaties were also developed that studied the origin and effects of the disease, among them highlighting in the Crown of Aragon the work of Jaume Agramont. This physician and professor at the University of Lleida wrote the Regiment of Preservation of the Pestilence (1348). This treatise written in Catalan revealed a unique fact, since Latin was the language of prestige that occupied the field of science almost exclusively. It is stated in Chapter II:

De les maneres en les quals pot haver mudament e alteració ho destemprament en l'àer, en l'Article I: Què vol dir pestilència, en què s'escriu:

[I] *Segueix-se lo tractat lo qual comprèn VI articles, en lo primer dels quals se declare què vol dir pestilència e ha II capítols*

Lo segon capítol és de la enterpretació de pestilència.

[Of the ways in which there may be a change and alteration, it is stated in the àe r, in Article I: What does pestilence mean, in which it is written:

[I] *Follow the treatise which comprises VI articles, in the first of which it is declared what pestilence means and has II chapters*

The second chapter is about the interperetation of pestilence.]

E pus avem posada e declarada la diffinició de pestilència, rahó és que posem la enterpretació del seu nom. Hon dich que pestilència, segons verdadera enterpretació, vol dir aytant com temps de tempesta que ve de clardat, ço és a saber, de les esteles. Per la primera sil·laba sua, que és «pes», entench «tempesta». E per la segona síl·laba sua, que és «te», entench «temps». E per la terça sil·laba sua, que és «lència», entench «clardat» car «lencos» en grech vol aytant dir com «clardat» ho «lum» en latí.[8]

[And now that we have put and declared the definition of pestilence, the reason is that we put the interpretation of its name. They say that pestilence, according to the true interpretation, means as much as stormy weather that comes from clarity, that is, from the wakes. By its first syllable, which is "weight", you mean "storm". And by its second syllable, which is «te», you mean «time». And by its third syllable,

which is "lència", you understand "clarity" because "lencos" in Greek means what "clarity" means "light" in Latin.]

In the Treaty of J. Agramont, he distinguished two types of pestilence, a natural product produced by a qualitative or substantial change in air, an alteration or putrefaction of air. While the other was the moral pestilence resulting from a change of mind that caused confrontation, destruction, and death.

[VI] Lo. VIèn. article principal és de la pestilència moralment entesa, lo qual ha solament. I. capítol en lo qual se pose la diffinició d'aytal pestilència

[VI][Lo. Vien main article is of pestilence morally understood, which has only I. chapter in which the definition of such pestilence is given]

Dich primerament que, moralment parlan, «pestilència és mudament contra natura de coratge e de pensament», car axí com la pestilència natural fa mudament contra natura e infecció en la sanch del cor e en la vertut del cor, axí la pestilència moral semblantment fa mudament contra natura en lo coratge e en lo pensament de les gents[9]

[He says first that, morally speaking, "pestilence is change against the nature of courage and thought", for just as natural pestilence works against nature and infection in the sanch of the heart and in the virtue of the heart, so moral pestilence similarly does change against nature in the courage and thinking of the people.]

The Treaty of Agramont was based on the union of two perspectives, one of which was a medical and the other philosophical/moral aspect characteristic of the mentality of the time. However, there were other treatises concerning pestilence: *Regimen de epidemia editum a Magistro Sancio de Riva Aurea* [*A decree on the epidemic issued by Master Sancius de Riva Aurea*] (1365), *Preservatio contra pestiletcia* [*Preservation against pestilence*] by Juan de Torquemada (1370), *Regimen contra epidimiam siue pestem* [*Government against epidemic or pestilence*] by Johannes Jacobi de Johannes Jacobi (1370), Lluís Alcanyís with *Regiment preservatiu e curatiu de la pestilència* [*Preservative and curative regiment of pestilence*] (1490), *Utilíssim prompte y fàcil remei e memorial per a preservar-se y curar de la pesta* [*Very useful quick and easy remedy and memorial to preserve and heal from the plague*] (1587) by Antoni Girauld, *Discurs sobre la pesta* [*Discourse on the plague*] by Lluís Fabra (1589) or *Compendi de la peste* [*Fish compendiums*] (1590) by Francesc Terrades or la *Memòria* [*Memory*] by Francesc Gavaldà (1651) in all of them recommended as the main remedy, the flight as quickly as possible of a place, where it was suspected that there was plague, even immortalized with a Spanish proverb such as:

Huir de la pestilencia con TRES eles es prudencia: luego, lexos y luengo tiempo (Castillo, 1976).

[Fleeing from the pestilence with THREE L's is prudence: later, lessons and long time.]

The isolation was the most important measure they took because the technology had not developed any other miracle cures. Currently, the measure is in fact recognized not only in the 14th century but is used. Maintaining a distance between people has been one of the first effects of COVID-19, avoiding direct contact between people.

Despite the attempt to keep the distance so as not to be infected many times was and is a difficult task, because we have contact with people who are involuntarily contaminated and do not know.

The effects of the two diseases are evident, on the one hand the coronavirus SARS-CoV-2 in infected people causes the effects of a species of fever-ined flu, muscular soreness, cough, loss of smell or taste, vomiting, thin decompositions with extreme cases of respiratory inadequacy, etc. If the sick person has other conditions, the virus appears to affect him to a greater degree and entails the complications that have caused the collapse of hospitals.

On the other hand, in the case of the plague, symptomatically manifested itself in the axles, grooves or necks with the outflow of beads, coughs and a very high fever. Although there were other variations such as septicemic plague or pneumonic plague with spotting eruption throughout the body, or with continuous expectation. Also, in the case of COVID-19, there has not been a single variant of the virus since its inception, but the Alpha, Beta, Gamma, Delta, and present-day Omicron have appeared, all resulting from mutations of the virus in order to survive and escape the vaccines that are being put on people.

Effects and Consequences

The plague caused serious effects in medieval society as in modern society. In the first place, the demographic decline is thought to be between 60 and 70%, as demographic control did not have the right mechanisms. Among the people who lost their lives were not only those who took it, but also those who cared for the sick as priests, apothecaries, caregivers, etc.

The decline in population caused the more biased classes to be able to fall on some improvement, because they took on a central role and needed for the higher classes who had to pay for the corresponding tithes. This alteration in the known order resulted in peasant revolts such as those in France in 1358 and London 1381, the guild rebellion in Florence 1378.

The critical approach to the authority of the known, was also shown that not only the Ramon Galeno, Hippocrates or Aristoteles maintained the status of knowledge, but other perspectives regarding medicine began to be taken into account. For this reason, he increased the practice of surgery and anatomical dissections that were rarely performed before the plague.

Hospitals will undergo a transformation towards the conception of treatment sites, where hygienic conditions improved, saving distances at this time. The plague favored a new purpose of these spaces, not as isolation of sick people, but as a response to the sick. The new reality influenced that Latin even lost exclusive hegemony as the only language of prestige, so the vulgar languages began to take part in spheres of knowledge.

As far as religious and spiritual matters were concerned, there were also very significant consequences, the most notable being mistrust. The lack of knowledge of the origin of the plague made a set of highly varied hypothesis. One of them was the supernatural origin, attributed to a Jewish sniper with the support of the Church in making them guilty led to his persecution, torture and convictions (Cuadrada, 2012).

Thus, the guilt of the Jews grew, a product of the thoughts of Christians inculcating them as murderers of Jesus Christ, which caused superstitions and mania. For example, the one who killed children by witchcraft rituals, or also who polluted the water wells for which Christians were contaminated. Anti-Semitism insulating and oppression increased despite the bull issued by Pope Clement VI who acquitted Jews and condemned the attacks on their communities.

In the current pandemic, COVID-19 is having a very clear and specific effect on people who have suffered from the disease, which is totally different from patients. Symptom persistence has focused on the population of 40 years and mainly on women. Symptomatology is varied in scale, lack of appetite, fatigue, dizziness, eye problems with conjunctivitis, breathing with persistent dried cough, lack of air, oppression in the chest. This causes a multitude of musculoskeletal, otorhinolaryngological, gastrointestinal, and neurologic pains.

But among all the secondary effects, the most important thing is mental health. Anxiety and depression have experienced a significant increase in population[10] Constraining, the situation of fear, insecurity, emotional stress, and media pressure are factors that suggest mental illnesses[11] (Pirkis et al., 2012) that in some cases have led to suicide. Among the population segments most affected by mental problems, both youths and people who lost their jobs and their social, economic status. Among young people, the lack of socialization by the period of confinement and restrictions has caused serious psychological problems, as well as addicted behavior with increased consumption of medicines, alcohol, drugs etc.

DEMONSTRATIONS

The *Valencian Annals*, as we have already commented on above, is one of the first documents that reflect events, significant news from the city of Valencia. Among these are the episodes of the great deaths caused by plague and other diseases. This was reflected in writing in this format:

En juny de l'any MCCCXXXXVIII, fon la primera y major mortaldat.

Fon l'altra mortaldat, en l'any MCCCLXII.

Fon l'altra mortaldat, que dien dels infants en l'any MCCCLXXV.

Fon l'altra mortaldat, en l'any MCCCLXXXIIII[12]

[In June of the year MCCCXXXVIII, the first and highest mortality occurred.

Fon the other mortality, in the year MCCCLXII.

Fon the other mortality, which they say of children in the year MCCCLXXV.

Found the other mortality, in the year MCCCLXXXIII]

Despite his brevity, the various episodes that the city suffered in different periods of its history are exhibited. One of the possible causes that would favor the spread of la pandemia was the lack of grain, which was a major entanglement for the population at the time. Fully adverse climatic conditions must also be added between 1333 and 1375, which culminated in a great deal of expensiveness. A sample of the fact is this news gathered in the Annals.

En l'any MCLCCCCIII, fon gran carestia de blats e grans mortaldats[13]

[In the year MCLCCCCIII, there was a great shortage of wheat and deadly grains]

The immediate consequences in the economy were based on rising prices

En l'any MCCCXXXIIII, fon gran carestia de forment, que pujà a pus de 110 sous lo cafís de València. E en dit any, ach grans mortaldats, e gran guerra de catalans ab genovesos, e tots perderen naus e gents. [14]

[In the year MCCCXXXIII, there was a great shortage of cash, which rose to over 110 sous for coffee in Valencia. And in that year, there were great deaths, and a great war between the Catalans and the Genoese, and they all lost ships and people.]

Despite the virulence of the epidemic, people had to live with it and in parallel with COVID-19, the first harsh episodes went on to normalize.

En dit any, fon gran mortaldat en València e en lo regne; e lo jorn de Sant Pere, moriren en la ciutat 260. 1395. [15]

[In that year, there was great mortality in Valencia and in the kingdom; and on Saint Peter's day, they died in the city 260. 1395]

Acceptance of a difficult situation that despite its danger, did not impede the course of life. The fact that the disease was to be combated from a more religious attitude was accepted, thereby increasing the cult of the Virgin Mary. The malicious news was already a constant in the era and as in the present one spread to favor a stamina or thought. The church with such a prominent role in the society of the XIV found it necessary to argue the arrival of the disease by bad habits or by customs that departed from the canon established by it. However, together with this news, more empirical solutions were also mixed, such as cleaning up the areas affected by the outbreaks, essentially as regards the streets. Covered areas of the cities were also created, where visitors passed quarantine that prevented infection in the rest of the population.

Another measure was to form groups of people who watched for parishes that had not affected the disease. In a natural and progressive manner, immunization towards the disease occurred. However, not the extinction of this one that appeared in different pandemic waves, with greater or lesser intensity

Fon l'altra mortaldat, en l'any MCCCCXXXVIIII, en les quals moriren VII MD persones, dins València en V mesos. Fon l'altra mortaldat, en l'any MCCCCL, en les quals moriren dins València ab la contribució XI mil persones; començà mijant mag y durà fins a per tot octubre. Fon l'altra mortaldat, en l'any MCCCCLVIIII, en l'estiu. [16]

[There was the other mortality, in the year MCCCCXXXVIII, in which VII MD people died in Valencia in V months. There was the other mortality, in the year MCCCCL, in which eleven thousand people died in Valencia with the contribution; It started in mid-May and will last until the whole of October. The other death was in the year MCCCCLVIII, in the summer.]

The arrival and return of the disease caused uncertainty during the period of suffering, while the rest of the time continued to live as if there was no distressing concern. The remedies that doctors had at the time were based on the application of simple drugs or compounds in the form of antidotes that attempted to remove the poison from the plague[17]. Blood or phlebotomies were common practice when symptoms of the disease appeared.

With the COVID-19 pandemic, wing-like measures have been implemented at the time such as border control, restrictive measures taken to enter foreign countries or cities, confinements and of course pharmacological remedies to mitigate the side effects produced by the virus. Drugs used with primary care, hospitals and intensive care units have been focused on mitigating side effects, but unfortunately not with care, because no solution has yet been found.

The advent of vaccines has been a certain victory in the battle of immunization towards the virus, as they have served as a prevention instrument. As in all areas of our society, the economic prism has provoked the struggle of interests between multinationals and countries to see who leads this open war.

CONCLUSION

Through this research a parallel has been established between two pandemic moments in the city of Valencia. The fact is that people have acted in a similar way between the 14th and 21st century. Throughout the article, it has been raised as in a previous and current society, a pandemic disease has altered the thinking of the individual making up it, with consequences in all areas.

The disease of COVID-19 has transformed the world as we were living in, albeit in a different way in some countries than in others. From the perspective of the Western developed world, then, restrictions on individual freedom have been imposed with restrictions on mobility, the economic status that has led to numerous cuts with dossiers and redundancies that have left these societies very much in touch.

In addition, the psychological footprint left in the population by disease and confinement with a considerable increase in anxiety and depression.

While the underdeveloped countries have suffered the same stringency of the pandemic as regards disease, they have increased restrictions and freedoms on the part of the most powerful social classes and thus manipulated the population.

The social anguish surrounding us has resulted in the appearance of old totalitarian, sectarian and discriminatory ghosts radiating antidemocratic postulates. The pandemic has acted as a shield, and ultraconservative postulates have been demonstrated, taking advantage of the context in which we find ourselves.

Thus, as in the 14th–XV centuries, society experienced a metamorphosis towards a new optics in the midst of a fear installed by the crisis of thought, plague and social restructuring; the starting society of this new century is directed towards a distinct new society, different from the previous 20th century in the midst of a pandemic, economic, political and social crisis, in which women will have a fundamental role.

Humanity is wary of the uncertain future that will make it live, and for this reason it has a sense of distress, of fear of instability in front of the unknown where it is heading. Let us hope that it is a time when we do not regret better past times and we can move to a new status without the imbalances that have been suffered and still suffer from it by many people on this planet.

REFERENCES

Abalakina-Paap, M., Stephan, W., Craig, T., & Gregory, W. (1999). Beliefs in Conspiracies. *Political Psychology*, *20*(3), 637–647. doi:10.1111/0162-895X.00160

Benedictow, O. J. (2011). La peste negra (1346-1353) [The Black Death (1346-1353)]. In La historia completa, (p. 589). Akal SA.

Castillo, A. D. L. (1976). Selección de refranes médicos de la obra de Pedro Valles [Selection of medical sayings from the work of Pedro Valles]. *Medicamenta*, *482*, 455–462.

Conejero, P.F.J. (2017). Lletraferides als convents, una escriptura femenina al segle XVI [Letters to convents, a female writing in the sixteenth century]. *Mirabilia/MedTrans. Mirabilia/Mediterranean and Transatlantic Approaches to the Culture of the Crown of Aragon*, (2), 38-70.

Conejero, P.F.J. (2019). Els delits prohibits als cenobis femenins [Forbidden delights in female cenobis]. *Mirabilia/MedTrans: Mirabilia/Mediterranean and Transatlantic Approaches to the Culture of the Crown of Aragon*, (1), 52-76.

Cuadrada, C. (2012). El llibre de la pesta [The Book of the Plague] (R. Dalmau, Ed.). Academic Press.

Escartí, V.J. (1998). Memòria privada [Private memory]. In *Literatura memoralística valenciana dels segles XV al XVIII.* Tres i Quatre.

Escartí, V.J. (2010). Notícia sobre la literatura memorialística al País Valencià, del segle XIV al XIX [News about memorial literature in Valencia, from the fourteenth to the nineteenth century]. *Manuscrits: Revista d'història moderna*, (28), 181-205.

Escartí, V. J. (2020). *La pesta a València (1647-1648)* [The plague in Valencia (1647-1648)]. Diputació de València, Institució Alfons el Magànim.

Escartí, V.J. (2021). La memòria de les pestes a l'antic Regne de València: de la nota marginal a la centralitat (s. XV-XVII) [The memory of the plagues in the ancient Kingdom of Valencia: from marginal note to centrality (s. XV-XVII)]. *Mirabilia/MedTrans: Mirabilia/Mediterranean and Transatlantic Approaches to the Culture of the Crown of Aragon, 53.*

Escartí, V. J., & Ribera, R. J. (2019). *El llibre de memòries de la ciutat de València (1308-1644)* [The book of memoirs of the city of Valencia (1308-1644)]. Edició Ajuntament de València.

Golob, T., Makarovi, M., & Rek, M. (2021). Meta-reflexivity for resilience against disinformation. *Comunicar*, (66), 107-118.

Gunnell, D., Appleby, L., Arensman, E., Hawton, K., John, A., Kapur, N., Khan, M., O'Connor, R. C., Pirkis, J., Appleby, L., Arensman, E., Caine, E. D., Chan, L. F., Chang, S.-S., Chen, Y.-Y., Christensen, H., Dandona, R., Eddleston, M., Erlangsen, A., ... Yip, P. S. F.COVID-19 Suicide Prevention Research Collaboration. (2020). Suicide risk and prevention during the COVID-19 pandemic. *The Lancet. Psychiatry*, *7*(6), 468–471. doi:10.1016/S2215-0366(20)30171-1 PMID:32330430

Hawton, K., Marzano, L., Fraser, L., Hawley, M., Harris-Skillman, E., & Lainez, Y. X. (2021). Reporting on suicidal behaviour and COVID-19-need for caution. *The Lancet. Psychiatry*, *8*(1), 15–17. doi:10.1016/S2215-0366(20)30484-3 PMID:33160581

Klomek, A. B. (2020). Suicide prevention during the COVID-19 outbreak. *The Lancet. Psychiatry*, *7*(5), 390. doi:10.1016/S2215-0366(20)30142-5 PMID:32353271

Moll, B. I. (2002). Epidemiologia des de l'Edat Mitjana fins a l'actualitat [Epidemiology from the Middle Ages to the present day] *Gimbernat: Revista d'Història de la Medicina i de les Ciències de la Salut*, *37*, 21–54.

Mutsvairo, B., & Bebawi, S. (2019). Journalism educators, regulatory realities, and pedagogical predicaments of the "fake news" Era: A comparative perspective on the middle east and Africa. *Journalism & Mass Communication Educator*, *74*(2), 143–157. doi:10.1177/1077695819833552

Parrilla, V. F. (2019). La pesta negra del 1348 a la corona d'Aragó. Una revolució social, econòmica i salubrista [The Black Death of 1348 in the Crown of Aragon. A social, economic and health revolution]. *Gimbernat. Revista d'Història de la Medicina i de les Ciències de la Salut.*, (71), 13–22.

Pirkis, J., John, A., Shin, S., DelPozo-Banos, M., Arya, V., Analuisa-Aguilar, P., Appleby, L., Arensman, E., Bantjes, J., Baran, A., Bertolote, J. M., Borges, G., Brečić, P., Caine, E., Castelpietra, G., Chang, S. S., Colchester, D., Crompton, D., Curkovic, M., Deisenhammer, E. A., … Spittal, M. J. (2021). Suicide trends in the early months of the COVID-19 pandemic: an interrupted time-series analysis of preliminary data from 21 countries. *The Lancet. Psychiatry*, S2215-0366(21)00091-2.

Rubio, V.A. (1979). Peste negra, crisis y comportamientos sociales en la España del siglo XIV [Black Death, crisis and social behaviors in fourteenth-century Spain]. In *La ciudad de Valencia (1348 – 1401)* (pp. 22-48). Universidad of Granada.

ENDNOTES

1. Retrieved from https://www.who.int/emergencies/diseases/novel-coronavirus-2019/covid-19-vaccines on February 22, 2022. When it comes to the different vaccines, the following composition, three, differences and similarities, the WHO intends to be the target organization that donates the necessary guidelines for humanity on this malaise.
2. ARCSCCV ms. 694 copiat per Agustí Sales el 1745.
3. I have now located the original 15th century manuscript. In the doctoral thesis I am working on, I will transcribe it and carry out a study and edition, since we only have the edition of the work made by Cabanes Català, M. L (Ed.) (1983) *Anales valencianos*. Saragossa: Anubar.
4. Retrieved from https://canalsalut.gencat.cat/ca/salut-a-z/c/coronavirus-2019-ncov/ciutadania/que-es-coronavirus/
5. Organization specialized in managing prevention, promotion and intervention policies worldwide in health, defined in its Constitution as a state of complete physical, mental and social well-being, and not only as the absence of conditions or diseases. It was initially organized by the Economic and Social Council of the United Nations, which promoted the drafting of the first statutes of the

WHO. The first meeting of this organization took place in Geneva (Switzerland) in 1948. The 195 member states of the WHO govern the entity through the World Health Assembly, which is made up of representatives from each of these countries. His website is https://www.who.int/

6 Assessment of the declaration of the outbreak of the new coronavirus 2019 (n-CoV) a Public Health Emergency of International Importance (ESPII). [02/01/2022]

7 Retrieved from https://www.who.int/es/health-topics/coronavirus#tab=tab_3

8 Retrieved from http://www.lluisvives.com/obra-visor/regiment-de-preservacio-de-pestilencia-lleida-1348-0/html/fefbefdc-82b1-11df-acc7-002185ce6064_23.html#I_20.

9 Retrieved from http://www.lluisvives.com/obra-visor/regiment-de-preservacio-de-pestilencia-lleida-1348-0/html/fefbefdc-82b1-11df-acc7-002185ce6064_23.html#I_20.

10 First international study on the consequences of the COVID-19 pandemic and the psychological relationship between depression and suicide. There has been no increase in this because of rapid government action, but also because of the growth of a sense of community.

11 In people with no previous psychiatric history, a diagnosis of COVID-19 was associated with increased incidence of a first psychiatric diagnosis in the following 14 to 90 days compared with six other health events. Strengthening mental health responses to COVID-19 in the Americas: A health policy analysis and recommendations. https://www.sciencedirect.com/science/article/pii/S2667193X21001149?via%3Dihub#bib0029

12 ARCSCCV ms. 694- Arxiu Convent copied per Agustí Sales el 1745, f.4.

13 ARCPV, ms.83 – Arxiu Convent de Predicadors de València. f.1b.

14 ARCPV, ms.83 – Arxiu Convent de Predicadors de València. f.3b

15 ARCPV, ms.83 – Arxiu Convent de Predicadors de València f.4.b

16 ARCSCCV ms. 694- Arxiu Convent del Patriarca de València copied per Agustí Sales el 1745, f.4.

17 Retrieved from https://historia.nationalgeographic.com.es/a/peste-lucha-medicos-contra-epidemia_16782

18 Among the simple medicines were bolarmenic, terra sigillata, and agaric; and among the compounds stood out the triac, the mitridate, the emerald, and the pills of aloe, saffron, and myrrh. There were also compounds that served to prevent infection. For example, another 16th century Spanish doctor, Andrés Laguna, prescribed a potion with the most colorful ingredients: sandalwood, coral, red roses, artichoke, gemstone powder (rubies, emeralds, sapphires ...), ivory and horn deer, grain and cotton seed, spices, ox tongue ... "Taken a tablet of this on an empty stomach every morning," said the doctor, " that no poison or infected air is enough to offend them."

Chapter 3
A Song to Life in Pandemic Times: *Primavera extremeña* by Julio Llamazares (2020)

Barbara Greco
Università di Torino, Italy

ABSTRACT

The essay studies the work Julio Llamazares drafted during the months of confinement (March-June 2020) decreed by the Spanish state to counter the spread of the pandemic. Primavera extremeña: Apuntes del Natural is an illustrated book with watercolours by Laudenbahcher and recounts the experience of the author, confined in a "lagar" in the Extremaduran countryside, in a work that oscillates between a diary and a travelogue. The chapter studies the dual component of the text and the conception of the landscape, typical of Llamazares' work, which here acquires new meanings.

INTRODUCTION

In March 2020, two days before the national confinement due to the health emergency, Llamazares and his family decide to leave Madrid and move for a few days to an old *lagar*, a farmhouse near Trujillo, in Extremadura, while waiting for a return to normality. The stay lasts three months, the duration of the first lockdown and the social restrictions, coinciding with the arrival and explosion of the Extremaduran spring, with its colours and scents, in which the author immerses himself and that contrasts with the anguished and tragic atmosphere of pandemic Madrid, confirming that "Mientras el mundo se desmoronaba, la naturaleza volvía a revivir igual que cada año al llegar la primavera" [As the world crumbled, nature came back to life as it does every year at the arrival of spring] (Llamazares, 2020a, p. 28).

The result of this experience was *Primavera extremeña. Apuntes del natural*, published by Alfaguara in 2020. It is a personal chronicle of the pandemic, a poetic and intimate diary where the author sings of the beauty of nature that rises up despite the tragedy that threatens human life. A text that is also a song to life, to the miracle of nature and in which Llamazares' sensitivity once again emerges, in tune with rural and

DOI: 10.4018/978-1-6684-4735-2.ch003

archaic Spain, that of forgotten territories, abandoned by man and crushed by the weight of modern world; anchored in ancient traditions and a way of life in contact with the land, which so few still cultivate. The diary seems to take the form of a travel book, limited by the restrictions of the health emergency and the suspicious gaze of the locals, around deserted fields and mountain villages, where spring, heedless of the danger facing humanity, tints the landscape in pastel colors. It is simultaneously an inner journey in which the author reconciles with himself through the contemplation of a beautiful and evocative spring (which takes him back to the happy time of his childhood) and through the exercise of writing, which takes on a cathartic and therapeutic function, of consolation in the face of the drift of the defenseless and powerless human race. The scenic beauty of the Extremaduran spring is portrayed in Llamazares' lyrical words and made even more vivid by the watercolors accompanying the text, painted by Konrad Laudenbahcher, an artist and friend of the author, who spends his confinement in the same place, on the other side of the mountain. The grafting of the two codes, the hybridization of word and image, endows this pandemic diary with a dual artistic value: it praises life and its essence, banishes the grey shadow of the virus and restores to man the springtime, the rebirth, that the covid has taken away from him.

In its sense of a travel notebook, *Primavera extremeña* is part of a rich production devoted to "travel literature" (a definition used by the author, who claims to be interested in a type of testimonial and sentimental writing, where the memory of places is filtered through the eyes of the writer), inaugurated in 1990 with *El río del olvido*, a travel diary through the Curueño river made in 1981 on foot, following the route of the river that crosses the Leonese mountains and where Llamazares spent his childhood. This genre, which Llamazares has cultivated with continuity and dedication since the beginning of his literary career, also includes *Trás-os-Montes. Un viaje portugués* (1998), *Cuaderno del Duero* (1999), the two complementary volumes dedicated to Spanish cathedrals, *Las rosas de piedra* (2008) and *Las rosas del sur* (2019), whose pages the author "leaf through as if they were architectural roses", *Atlas de la España imaginaria* (2015), a book with illustrations and photographs where the author retraces mythical places in Spanish literature, and *El viaje de Don Quijote* (2016), also illustrated and inspired by Azorín's *La ruta de Don Quijote*. Llamazares' travel literature demonstrates the author's renewed attention to lesser-known Spain, the ancestral, rural and mountainous Spain that man has gradually abandoned and returned to the power of nature, but where it is possible to find oneself and give meaning to life, even in the darkest moments of the 21st century.

Considering the above, the aim of this essay is to study the genesis and meaning of *Primavera extremeña*, its combination of diaristic and travelogue genres and the conception of landscape, developed in a unique text, where the journey experience is set in the dramatic context of a world pandemic, and which sanctions the salvific value of both literature and nature.

LLAMAZARES' PERSONAL VERSION

In the interviews he gave on the occasion of the book's presentation, Llamazares dwells on the genesis of the work, which was the result of the unforeseen circumstances he found himself experiencing during the long lockdown that confined the Spaniards (and with them half the world) to their homes, and which for him, who was lucky enough to leave the capital, coincided with a three-month stay in a country cottage, where he experienced the most extraordinary springtime of his life, as he states, with ill-concealed guilt, in the prologue. More precisely, Llamazares explains that for him there do exist three types of books, corresponding to as many creative impulses: the books that "te pide el cuerpo" [asks for your body] in which he inserts his travel literature production, conceived as an almost physical urgency to give expression to a passion; the books that "te pide el alma" [asks for your soul]and that he feels *condemned* to write, such as novels, in which there is an almost predestined inclination to write and, finally, the books that "determina el azar" [Determine chance], or those dictated by case. We know, in fact, that the author had to interrupt the drafting of a novel he was working on and which he felt unable to continue because of the state of disorientation and concern caused by the pandemic, and that he felt compelled by the desire to tell the story of reality, *his* reality. It is after receiving a gift of a watercolor painted by his neighbor and lockdown companion Konrad when Llamazares has a revelation and realizes that the mountainous landscape surrounding them in Extremadura, which the painting depicts, is to be the subject of his new literary project, consisting of twenty-five 'written watercolors' in dialogue with the pictorial landscapes accompanying the book, which originates from the collaboration between the two friends and their desire to pay homage to spring. For this reason, the publication is not intended to be a book *about* the pandemic and is quite distinct from the rest of the profuse creative production (literary and not) developed during the months of confinement. Rather, the pandemic scenario that we learned about during the forced quarantine, with its new spaces and rituals that eliminated the public-private border, is here an almost evanescent background, in transparency, which the author sketches using oppositional pairs: on the one hand, the countryside, a source of peace, harmony and wellness, and on the other, the Madrid from which he fled and which has become a sinister place of horror, perturbations and illness.

The *locus amoenus* that is the Extremaduran country and that gives Llamazares a sensory experience of unrepeatable beauty, nucleus of the book, contrasts with the urban reality he has left behind, where spring does not bring with it rebirth and life but on the contrary the deadly virus, an invisible threat to mankind. This dichotomy between rural space, tangible and concrete, and urban space, evoked by TV images and calls to relatives and friends left behind in the city, emerges right from the prologue, significantly titled "Una primavera extraña" [A strange spring]:

Quizá parezca obsceno hablar en términos elogiosos de una primavera que para mucha gente fue trágica y para todos, sin excepción, muy dura, pero es que la que a mí me regaló Extremadura, y más concretamente la sierra de los Lagares, junto a Trujillo, en tierras de Cáceres, sin imaginar que la viviría entera cuando llegué, fue sin lugar a dudas la más extraordinaria que he vivido. (Llamazares, 2020a, pp. 9-10)

[It may seem obscene to speak in laudatory terms of a spring that for many people was tragic and for all, without exception, very hard, but the spring that Extremadura gifted me, and more specifically the Sierra de los Lagares, next to Trujillo, in the lands of Cáceres, without imagining that I would experience it all when I arrived, was undoubtedly the most extraordinary spring I have ever experienced]

The contrast between the two realities, the pleasant one experienced in the luxuriant nature of the camp and the frightening one of the coronavirus, kept outside but no less distressing and visible in the sense of guilt that runs through the pages, is marked by a clear timeline that separates the day, spent in the "libertad y ligereza del campo en plena explosión" [freedom and lightness of the exploding countryside], from the evening, when, says the narrator, "ante la televisión, volvíamos a caer en la angustia y el miedo" [in front of the television, we fell back into anguish and fear] (Llamazares, 2020a, pp. 28-29).

A play of antinomies characterizing all the reflections invoked by the exceptional historical circumstance framing the text (in this sense, the repeated reference to the *Decameron* is eloquent) that pushes the author to critical reasoning on the reactions of the Spanish people and of the "España negra" [Black

Spain] of hatred and violence, that re-emerges overbearingly in social crises (Llamazares, 2020a, pp. 89-90) and against which the placid and slow atmosphere of the isolated countryside is contrasted. This dual feeling, fluctuating and wandering, reaches its climax in the final part of the work (especially in chapters 21 and 22), where the author describes the feeling of return and at the same time offers a renewed vision of the two conflicting dimensions:

En la sierra de los Lagares éramos felices a pesar de las circunstancias [...] estábamos disfrutando de una primavera que jamás olvidaríamos [...] pero ya se iba acercando el momento de regresar a la realidad, una realidad perdida y transformada de arriba abajo [...] Lo que nos preocupaba era qué nos encontraríamos a la vuelta y, sobre todo, cómo nos adaptaríamos a ello después de tanto tiempo viviendo en una burbuja, la de la sierra extremeña y el viejo lagar convertido en refugio en el que llevábamos ya dos meses y medio viendo la realidad desde lejos a través de la televisión. (Llamazares, 2020a, pp. 105-106)

[In the Sierra de los Lagares we were happy despite the circumstances [...] we were enjoying a spring that we would never forget [...] but the time was approaching when we had to return to reality, a reality that had been lost and transformed through and through [...]. We were worried about what we would find on our return and, above all, how we would adapt to it after so long living in a bubble, that of the mountains of Extremadura and the old vineyard converted into a refuge where we had been watching reality from afar through the television for two and a half months]

En cualquier caso, lo que parecía claro era que ya teníamos que empezar a pensar en irnos, lo que nos producía un sentimiento contradictorio. Por un lado, estábamos deseando volver a nuestra verdadera vida, pero, por otro, nos generaba inquietud. En Madrid las cosas no parecían claras aún y, además, estábamos tan a gusto en nuestro lagar disfrutando de la tranquilidad del campo y de la primavera que nos producía melancolía tener que romper con ellas. (Llamazares, 2020a, p. 109)

[In any case, what seemed clear was that we already had to start thinking about leaving, which gave us a contradictory feeling. On the one hand, we were looking forward to returning to our real life, but on the other, it caused us anxiety. In Madrid the situation didn't seem clear and, what's more, we were so comfortable in our vineyard, enjoying the tranquility of the countryside and the spring, that it made us feel melancholy to have to leave them behind]

From the above passages, we can well understand the author's feeling of being protected and sheltered in a kind of happy "bubble" outside time - the *burbuja* Llamazares refers to has nothing to do with its "covidian" meaning, where it is understood as a restricted space of sharing - and that makes it a non-reality (or *irrealidad*, as he repeatedly defines it), a joyous and luminous nebula, a kind of dream made possible by disgrace. In other words, Llamazares' contribution to the creative effluvium of the pandemic months returns to the public a song to nature, meant as an inexhaustible source of life, and to the small things that we tend to neglect, immersed as we are in the frenzy of modern society, through a skillful use of language and words. The poetic prose, which is a distinctive feature of all Llamazares' work, accompanies the story of a unique experience, collected in a text that is both an intimate diary and a travel notebook.

A POETIC WATERCOLOR BETWEEN THE PRIVATE DIARY AND THE TRAVEL NOTEBOOK

As we have seen, Llamazares' highly personal account of his confinement flows into the creation of an illustrated volume, accompanied by Laudenbahcher's watercolors, which are part of a text-image dialogue already present on the cover and capable of radiating new meanings, without considering the aesthetic pleasure experienced by the reader and deriving from the juxtaposition of the two languages, textual and figurative, which intertwine in a hybrid work similar in some segments to visual poetry. The book's iconic component, complementary to the verbal one, offers "artistic postcards" of the described landscape, depicting its vegetation, fauna and in some cases its architecture, while arousing multiple feelings (melancholy, solitude, joy, serenity, inner peace, etc.), in accordance with the text and conveyed through the use of a wide color scale.

Figure 1.

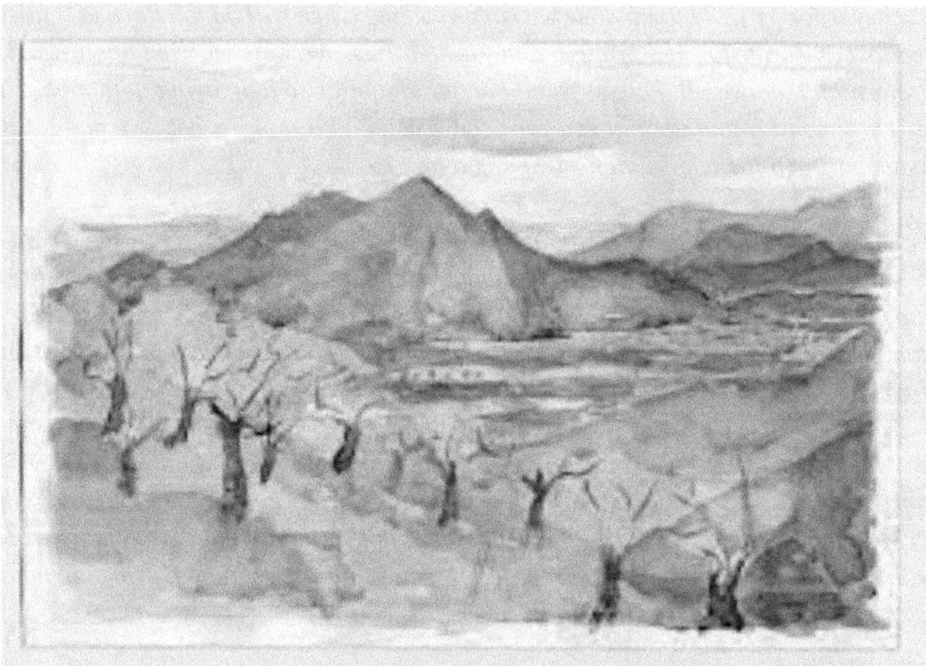

Figure 2.

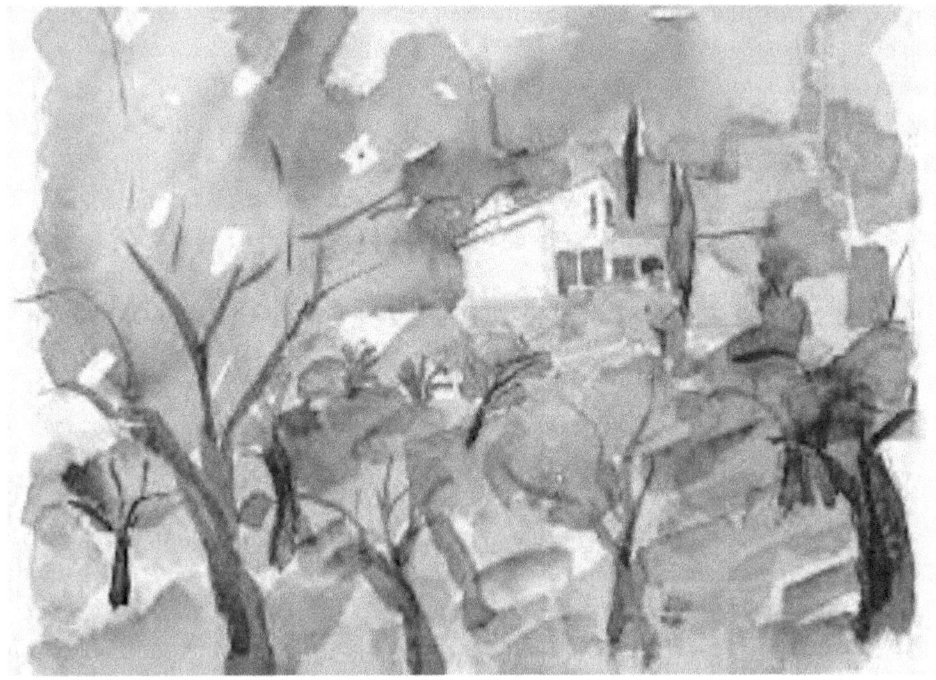

The centrality of nature, exalted by the paintings and protagonist of many descriptive pages in which Llamazares indulges in front of the astonishing beauty of the landscape, can be deduced from the subtitle of the work, which reads "Apuntes del natural" [Notes from nature] and raises the question, by no means idle, of the genre in which it can be inscribed. As we have said, the author's intention is to create "written watercolors" - the paintings are the inspiration - to record the three months he spent in the Extremaduran *lagar*, following the course of time. The desire to preserve the memory of these moments of life, sometimes epiphanic, sometimes simply ordinary but worthy of being saved from oblivion and collected in chronologically organized notes, is the first essential element that leads us back to the diary genre, characterized by a fragmentary, open and simultaneous structure, which makes it resemble a mosaic or a collage (Luque Amo, 2016, p. 294) and where the exercise of writing is carried out in the present time. Freixas suggests that the diary should be characterized by everyday life and intimacy, not merely in the sense of the author-narrator's inner excavation, but also in relation to the subjective perspective of the self and its scrutinizing gaze that rests on reality and filters it, returning "el magma cotidiano y las epifanías que lo iluminan, la observaciones sociológicas, la reflexión moral, la idea, la sensación, el sentimiento" [the daily magma and the epiphanies that illuminate it, sociological observations, moral reflection, the idea, the sensation, the feeling], and sometimes embracing "una reflexión, en primera persona y enraizada en la cotidianidad, sobre la condición humana y el sentido de la vida" [a reflection, in the first person and rooted in everyday life, on the human condition and the meaning of life] (Freixas, 2016, p. 12).

This last possibility, to which the diary may open up, can be found in certain pages of *Primavera extremeña*, containing an existential meditation triggered by contemplation of the elements of nature, which fuels the author's lyrical afflatus, as in the following passage:

Aquella noche, salí a mirar el cielo. Había luna creciente y su luz iluminaba todo el paisaje como la noche americana de las películas. A lo lejos se escuchaban unas ovejas y los ladridos de un perro, pero, fuera de eso, el silencio era total. Sobre las dos palmeras la noche se recortaba llena de estrellas, tan solitarias como el mundo ahora. Imaginé que muchas personas desde sus ventanas en las ciudades estarían mirando el mismo cielo con angustia y con la sensación también de estar fuera del mundo como yo y sentí una solidaridad con ellas que iba más allá del pensamiento y de las noticias que había visto en la televisión. Había cumplido sesenta y cinco años, una edad en la que muchos abandonan sus trabajos para siempre y que señala el comienzo de la última etapa de la vida, y lo hacía muy lejos del lugar en el que vine al mundo y al que no podría volver aunque quisiera, porque ya no existe, y en unas circunstancias que jamás imaginé que viviría, con la humanidad sumida en una gran inquietud y el mundo entero en suspenso, expectante ante un futuro que de repente se había convertido, como el cielo, en un montón de preguntas. En medio de ese silencio, yo miraba la noche sin saber qué pasaría al día siguiente, pues el libro del que Rilke dijo era el mejor, que era el cielo estrellado, se había parado también como la vida desde hacía semanas. (Llamazares, 2020a, pp. 46-47)

[That night, I went out to look at the sky. There was a crescent moon and its light illuminated the whole landscape like the American night in the movies. In the distance I could hear some sheep and the barking of a dog, but, apart from that, the silence was total. Above the two palm trees, the night was lined with stars, as lonely as the world now. I imagined that many people from their windows in the cities would be looking at the same sky with anguish and with the feeling of being out of the world as I was, and I felt a solidarity with them which went beyond the thought and the news I had seen on television. I had turned sixty-five, an age when many leave their jobs for good and which marks the beginning of the last stage of life, and I was doing so far from the place where I came into the world and to which I could not return even if I wanted to, because it no longer exists, and in circumstances I had never imagined I would experience, with humanity plunged into great unrest and the whole world in suspense, expectant of a future that had suddenly become, like the sky, a heap of questions. In the midst of that silence, I looked at the night, not knowing what would happen the next day, for the book that Rilke said was the best, which was the starry sky, had also stopped like life for weeks]

This passage is a good example of an intimate diary, in which the exceptionality of the historical moment is intersected with a private episode (the author's sixty-fifth birthday) and the majesty of the starry sky, enlivened by the silence of the countryside, awakens a profound feeling of solidarity and belonging to the human race. Llamazares seems to be coming to terms with his life, recalling his homeland to which he will never be able to return - the author was born in Vegamián, a Leonese village submerged by the waters of the Porma dam in 1969 and which he would define as a "sombra bajo el agua" [shade under water] (Llamazares, 2015b)[1] and the uncertainty of the future, made even more doubtful by the threat of the virus. In this state of confusion and anguish, the sight of the sky gives him a sense of peace and reconciliation with the world and seems to overwhelm him with its immensity and beauty. In this regard, the reference to Rilke seems illuminating for a better understanding of the meaning of the above quote. In his essay *Concerning landscape,* the Austrian poet rejects the projective vision that sees the landscape as a reflection of the sentimental temperament of the man who contemplates it and finds in it the signs of his affective disposition, and instead sanctions the solitude of man in nature. For Rilke, the artist's task is to abandon his anthropocentric gaze on nature and confront its mystery, to become a "thing among things", to "sink into its stillness", to prefer the eternal to the ephemeral, to find his own place in its "grandiose order" (Rilke, 2009, p. 58) through art. Nature, for Rilke, is indifferent to human action, it knows its own laws and only with this premise can man approach it. And isn't it true that Llamazares lets himself be absorbed and enveloped by nature, which, if anything, *induces* in him an emotional inclination, a sentimental tone (Simmel's *Stimmung*), or rather an atmosphere that *accords* him a peculiar spiritual inclination? And still in agreement with Rilke, the author reiterates on numerous occasions that "El milagro de la naturaleza se repetía un año más [...] mientras el mundo entero contenía el aliento ante los efectos devastadores de la epidemia, nosotros asistíamos a otra primavera diferente en la que, en lugar de la muerte, era la vida la que reinaba en la tierra" [The miracle of nature repeated itself for another year [...] while the whole world was holding its breath at the devastating effects of the epidemic, we were watching a different spring where, instead of death, it was life that reigned on earth] (Llamazares, 2020a, p. 58). It is man's purpose, Llamazares seems to suggest, in tune with Rilke, to come into contact with nature, to distance from oneself and let the mind wander and wonder, to contemplate it by cultivating the senses and entering into vital communication with it, in an aesthetic and spiritual encounter that stimulates writing and instils tranquility: "Sentado en mi habitación, desde la que divisaba gran parte de la viña además del paisaje al fondo, se me iban las horas, sobre todo las de la tarde, prácticamente sin darme cuenta. Los mirlos y los ruiseñores ponían la banda sonora a mi tranquilidad" [Sitting in my room, from where I could see a large part of the vineyard as well as the landscape in the background, the hours went by, especially in the afternoon, almost without my noticing. The blackbirds and nightingales provided the soundtrack to my tranquility] (Llamazares, 2020a, p. 59). Nature awakens the author's sensibility, transmits to him that specific emotional tone, sentimentally disposes him through its elements, such as the moon that dominates the silent field and the vegetation that with its scents transports him to the faraway summers of his youth:

De repente, todo quedó iluminado, imantado por una luna gigante que de inmediato comenzó a ascender llenando el cielo de luminarias, las de las miles de estrellas que ya lo cubrían antes de que ella saliera [...] Además, el olor de la jara y de la hierba seca embriagaba. En apenas unos días, el calor las había secado y el aroma que desprendían era ya más propio del verano que de la primavera, pues evocaba el de las eras cuando todavía existían, en los veranos lejanos de mi juventud. Así que entre el olor de la jara y la hierba seca, más el silencio que cubría el monte y que aumentó al pararnos nosotros, todo se quedó en suspenso, como si bajo la luna el mundo se hubiera detenido para siempre y el tiempo dejara de discurrir [...] Costaba irse a dormir con la paz que desprendía, que quizá tardaríamos mucho tiempo en volver a ver. (Llamazares, 2020a, pp. 112-113)

[Suddenly, everything was illuminated, magnetized by a giant moon that immediately began to rise, filling the sky with lights, those of the thousands of stars that already covered it before it rose [...] In addition, the smell of the cistus and the dry grass was inebriating. In just a few days, the heat had dried them and the scent they emitted was already more typical of summer than of spring, as it evoked that of the fields when they still existed, in the distant summers of my youth. So between the smell of the cistus and the dry grass, plus the silence that covered the mountain and increased when we stopped, everything was suspended, as if under the moon the world had stopped forever and time ceased to flow [...] It was hard to go to sleep with the peace it released, which perhaps we would take a long time to see again]

The fascination with the moon, which can acquire multiple shades of meaning, can also be found in other of his works, different in genre, such as the poem *Memoria de la nieve* (1982), the novel whose very title evokes the image of the first full moon of the year *Luna de lobos* (1985) or the travelogue *El río del olvido* (1990), where the writer, doubling as the traveler who leads the narrative in third person (el *viajero*), "deslumbrado, se aleja del pueblo y, ya en campo abierto, se tumba a ver la luna en mitad de la carretera" [Dazzled, he drives away from the village and, in the open countryside, lies down in the middle of the road to look at the moon] (Llamazares, 2006, p. 97). The author treats the landscape, and not only in *Primavera extremeña*, in a way that allows us to interpret it as a *literary landscape*, i.e., not as an inert object of observation, but experienced through an active perception, which is very marked (Jakob, 2005). For this reason, we can speak of a genuine poetics of landscape, extensible to the whole of Llamazares' production, which develops a synesthetic awareness involving sight, hearing, smell and touch, and where sensory activity is correlated with the theme of memory (the scents which, as in the passage quoted and in Proust's manner, revive memories). Indeed, for the author, the landscape is memory, since it "sostiene las huellas del pasado, reconstruye recuerdos" [holds the traces of the past, reconstructs memories] (Llamazares, 2006, p. 13), while man is an element of the landscape (or a "thing among things", in Rilke's style). In this regard, we find relevant the reflection that he elaborates from the observation of a pictorial landscape by Diaz-Caneja (1905-1988) and that he collects in a short essay entitled *El espejo del alma, una meditación sobre el paisaje* [The Mirror of the Soul, a meditation on landscape], where he proposes his personal vision of the landscape and makes his own two definitions that, he claims, converge in his own literature. The first is by Nogué and reads "antes de la mirada, el paisaje era solo territorio" [before the gaze, the landscape was only territory], while the second, by Josep Pla, maintains that "lo que nos diferencia a los hombres del resto de los animales es la capacidad de sentir el paisaje, es decir, de mirar el paisaje con mirada inteligente" [what differentiates humans from other animals is the ability to sense the landscape, i.e. to look at the landscape with an intelligent eye] (Llamazares, 2012, p. 21). As Jakob states, the very concept of landscape involves man's gaze on nature: the scholar summarizes this assumption with the formula $L = S + N$, where L, S and N refer to Landscape, Subject and Nature respectively (Jakob, 2009, pp. 30-31). In other words, the subject, in this case the narrator, who alternates between the first person singular and the plural, establishes a link with nature, appropriates it and reworks it in literary representation, transforming it into landscape. A landscape that can be a source of quiet, like the one rendered by the full moon in the quoted passage, but also disturbing and threatening (a manifestation of a hostile landscape is undoubtedly the novel *La lluvia amarilla*, of 1988), like the one described in chapter 9 of the book. Here, the author resorts to Eliot's verses from *The Waste Land*, which consider April 'the cruellest month' to emphasise the cruelty of spring nature reborn from winter's death and creating a blind and unexpected turmoil (and remember that Eliot composed the poem in 1922, after the First World War, the Russian Revolution and the pandemic known as 'the Spanish flu'). The hostile character of nature, heedless of man, is associated with the element of water, which is crucial to the entire production of Llamazares, who was born, as we said, in a village then submerged, and is reflected in the rain and rivers, with which the author often identifies himself or the imaginary characters that populate his fictional universe. Water is both a source of life and death:

A comienzos de abril, además, empezó a llover y durante todo el mes no dejó de hacerlo [...] Para el campo aquella lluvia era agua bendita, pues iba a haber pasto para los animales hasta el mes de julio [...] Dos o tres noches, de madrugada, la lluvia cayó en forma de tormenta. Durante horas, los truenos retumbaban sobre la casa aislada en mitad del monte, que parecía un barco azotado por una tempestad [...] La casa del Decamerón que al principio nos pareció la nuestra se había convertido en un arca de

Noé a la deriva entre unas montañas que se confundían bajo la lluvia con unas nubes que parecía que no iban a irse tampoco nunca, como la pandemia. (Llamazares, 2020a, pp. 49-52)

[At the beginning of April, moreover, it began to rain and continued to do so throughout the month [...] For the countryside this rain was blessed water, for there would be pasture for the animals until July [...] Two or three nights, at dawn, the rain fell in the form of a storm. For hours, the thunder rumbled over the isolated house in the middle of the mountain, which looked like a ship battered by a storm [...] The house of the Decameron, which at first seemed to us to be our own, had become a Noah's ark adrift among mountains confused in the rain with clouds that seemed never to go away either, like the pandemic]

The myth of the universal deluge, which hides the spectre of the end of the world, is evoked here to illustrate, with an image belonging to the shared cultural heritage, the feeling of "shipwreck" that possesses the group confined to the *lagar*. Water, which is clement for nature, is a source of anguish for man and once again underlines the author's non-anthropomorphic vision of nature, reminiscent of Rilke, reflected in the more exquisitely diaristic pages of the book, and not only that. I mean that the landscape is the absolute protagonist of the text and the conjunction of the two genres here entwined, namely the diary (as we have seen) and the travel notebook, which connotes some chapters. If with Demetrio "nature brings you back each time, while describing it with lyrical accents, romantic emphases and rhetorical choices, to the material reality of sensory contact with it" (Demetrio, 2015, p. 262), making diaristic writing more sincere and authentic, the odeporistic component of *Primavera extremeña* corroborates the testimonial dimension of the work, which thus adds to the private one. We know that for Llamazares, travel literature "aparte de fundacional (todos los grandes libros fundacionales de todas las literaturas han sido libros de viajes, si bien a veces disfrazados de otros géneros), es la literatura en estado puro" [apart from being foundational (all the great foundational books of all literature have been travel books, albeit sometimes disguised as other genres), it is literature in its purest form] (in Hernández, 2013, p. 64) and that he devoted several books to it, the fruit of the annotations transcribed along the way in a notebook, in an activity that he considers the very essence of the journey (Llamazares, 1999, p. 4). For the author, the process of writing about a travel experience corresponds to the possibility of fixing memories and crystallizing images in the memory - landscape and memory are two constants in his work, which mingle and overlap until they become one and the same thing. Llamazares considers himself a "viajero literario" [literary traveler] who "va buscando sobre todo la poesía que los caminos guardan en cada recodo" [goes looking above all for the poetry that the roads hold at every turn], in a journey where "los caminos no se andan con las piernas, se andan con el corazón" [roads are not walked with the legs, but with the heart] (Llamazares, 2013, p. 60) and the voyage becomes a metaphor for life and an occasion to reflect on the human condition. The author's favorite landscapes are always connected to a forgotten, isolated and disappearing part of Spain, desecrated by modernity and whose memory he redeems; to rugged mountain territories, rough like the few men who inhabit them and who live in direct contact with the earth, symbols of an archaic and authentic way of life. Here, too, we discover a primitive landscape, a theatre of ruins, made up of small abandoned villages, whose culture he portrays through legends, music, anecdotes, vegetation, fauna, the products of the land and descriptions of the inhabitants, as in the pages that recount the excursions to the villages around Trujillo, which the author can make when the restrictive measures imposed by the government are relaxed, and of which the following passage is an example, encapsulating the author's typical travel narrative style:

Desde la sierra, las dehesas se adivinaban llenas de pasto y de flores, pero desde la carreterita de Herguijuela a Santa Cruz, que las cruza, su exuberancia era una constatación. La hierba se levantaba a la altura de los muros y, en medio de ella, vacas y toros pacían más flores que pasto, tal era su profusión. La paz que trasmitían y la suerte que ignoraban [...] eran las propias de un lugar arcádico sobre el que la primavera había volcado toda su generosidad, que es mucha en las dehesas extremeñas, auténticos escenarios de un primitivismo puro que las encinas y los toros representan mejor que ningún otro elemento animal y vegetal. Desde la prehistoria, estas dehesas extremeñas se conservan igual, salvedad hecha de los muros y de las alambradas que las trocean y de las carreteras que las atraviesan, ninguna de ellas muy transitada, por suerte, y el ganado que pasta en ellas es el mismo que lo hacía miles de años atrás, con la única diferencia de alguna raza de vaca importada pero adaptada ya a sus condiciones. No debe de ser difícil hacerlo, tal es la paz y la exuberancia de estas dehesas, como no lo es para las personas. Nosotros mismos, sin tener nada que ver con este paisaje, nos habíamos integrado en él sin esfuerzo, tanto como para que después de esa experiencia nos sintiéramos ya parte de él. —¿Cómo llevan la estancia aquí tanto tiempo? —me preguntó una mañana el farmacéutico de Herguijuela, un hombre con aspecto de boticario machadiano y humanista, cuya mujer, siempre sonriente, le acompaña a diario en su quehacer. —Pues muy bien —le contesté, al igual que a la panadera y al de la tienda de alimentación, que ya se habían acostumbrado a verme y también me lo habían preguntado alguna vez—. En la sierra se está muy bien. (Llamazares, 2020a, pp. 79-81)

[From the sierra, the meadows were full of grass and flowers, but from the little road from Herguijuela to Santa Cruz, which crosses them, their exuberance was evident. The grass rose up to the height of the walls and, in the middle of it, cows and bulls grazed more flowers than grass, such was their profusion. The peace they conveyed and the fate they ignored [...] were typical of an Arcadian place on which spring had poured all its generosity, which is abundant in the meadows of Extremadura, authentic scenes of pure primitivism that the oaks and bulls represent better than any other animal or plant element. Since prehistoric times, these Extremaduran meadows have remained unchanged, except for the walls and wire fences that cut them up and the roads that cross them, none of them very busy, fortunately, and the cattle that graze there are the same as they were thousands of years ago, with the only difference of a few imported breeds of cow that have already adapted to their conditions. It should not be difficult to do so, such is the peace and exuberance of these meadows, just as it is not for people. We ourselves, having nothing to do with this landscape, had integrated into it effortlessly, so much so that after this experience we already felt part of it. -How have you been staying here for so long? -asked me one morning the pharmacist of Herguijuela, a man with the appearance of a humanist apothecary, whose wife, always smiling, accompanies him daily in his work. -Well, that's very good, I replied, as I did to the baker and the grocer, who were used to seeing me and had also asked me about it a few times. In the mountains you feel good]

This passage summarizes, it seems to me, a number of aspects that have been commented on up to now and that characterize the book, which is the product of confinement and therefore of chance: the coexistence of diary and travelogue, the lyrical prose rich in intertextual references (Rilke, Eliot, Virgilio, Machado), the predilection for the mountain and uncontaminated landscape, the author's view of nature, the ancestral correspondence with the land and the subjective perspective.

CONCLUSION

Llamazares contributes to the creative production composed during the months of lockdown with a text that occupies an isolated position in that panorama, both in terms of the method of publication, which does not go through social networks or the web, and in terms of the type of testimony offered, which gathers the impressions of an epiphanic, unique and unforgettable experience. Without neglecting the collective drama that is striking the world and Spain and that darkens the author's evening hours, dedicated to listening to the news about the pandemic, the author takes refuge in the unspoiled nature of the Extremaduran countryside, where he enjoys, for the first time, the arrival and blossoming of spring, of which he absorbs smells, colors, and sounds. The sensory adventure that Llamazares experiences to the full, invites him to reflect on the meaning of existence, to remember time gone by and the homeland lost under the waters of a dam, but also simply to lives the landscape, its tranquility and to penetrate its mystery. Understood from a non-anthropomorphic perspective, the nature represented in these artistic and verbal watercolors that alternate in the pages of the book is paid homage to and sung with lyricism and emotional transport, with that sentimental inclination that Simmel called *Stimmung* and that can be found in all the author's production, especially the odeporic one, with which this text is in dialogue. *Primavera extremeña* is in fact an example of hybrid writing, in which the word-image dialectic is added to the personal diary-travelogue dialectic examined above, in a work with a lyrical tone that sanctions the therapeutic effect of writing and reading, which is valid even in times of crisis, as the author recalls: "La literatura es tiempo, tiempo que te regalan. Y tiene un efecto de consolación. Cura las heridas de la vida. Tanto al escritor como al lector" [Literature is time, time that is given to you. And it has a consoling effect. It heals the wounds of life. Both for the writer and the reader].

REFERENCES

Alba, C. (2021). *La primavera de Julio Llamazares* [The spring of Julio Llamazares]. Retrieved from https://www.rtve.es/play/audios/la-estacion-azul/primavera-julio-llamazares-31-01-2021/5775253/

Demetrio, D. (2015). *Green Autobiography. La natura è un racconto interiore* [Green Autobiography. Nature is an inner story]. Book Salad.

Freixas, L. (1996). Auge del diario ¿íntimo? en España [Rise of the intimate diary? in Spain]. *Revista de Occidente (Madrid, Spain), 182-183*, 5–14.

Hernández, D. (2013). La magia del propio andar [The magic of walking itself]. *Entrevista a Julio Llamazares Catharum, 13*, 63–65.

Jakob, M. (2005). *Paesaggio e letteratura* [Landscape and literature]. Olschki.

Jakob, M. (2009). *Il paesaggio* [The landscape]. Il Mulino.

Laguna, C. (2020). El libro que recupera la primavera robada de Extremadura en un viaje ilustrado [The book that recovers the stolen spring of Extremadura in an illustrated trip]. *Traveler*. Retrieved from https://www.traveler.es/naturaleza/articulos/julio-llamazares-primavera-extremena-libro-viaje-ilustracion/19682

Llamazares, J. (1997). *Luna de lobos* [Wolf moon]. Seix Barral.

Llamazares, J. (1998). *Trás-os-Montes. Un viaje portugués* [Back-to-back-the-hills. A Portuguese traveler]. Alfaguara.

Llamazares, J. (1999). *Cuaderno del Duero* [Duero Notebook]. Leonesas.

Llamazares, J. (2003). *Memoria de la nieve* [Memory of snow]. Amos.

Llamazares, J. (2006). *El río del olvido* [The river of oblivion]. Alfaguara.

Llamazares, J. (2008). *Las rosas de piedra* [The stone roses]. Alfaguara.

Llamazares, J. (2012). El espejo del agua. Una meditación sobre el paisaje a partir de un cuadro de Juan Manuel Díaz-Caneja [The mirror of water. A meditation on the landscape from a painting by Juan Manuel Díaz-Caneja]. *Cuadernos Hispanoamericanos*, *741*, 15–21.

Llamazares, J. (2013). El viaje como pretexto [Travel as a pretext]. *Catharum*, *13*, 59–61.

Llamazares, J. (2015a). Atlas de la España imaginaria [Atlas of imaginary Spain]. Madrid, Spain: Nórdica Libros.

Llamazares, J. (2015b). *Distintas formas de mirar el agua* [Different ways of looking at water]. Alfaguara.

Llamazares, J. (2016a). *El viaje de Don Quijote* [The journey of Don Quixote]. Alfaguara.

Llamazares, J. (2016b). *La lluvia amarilla* [The yellow rain]. Cátedra.

Llamazares, J. (2019). *Las rosas del sur* [The roses of the south]. Debolsillo.

Llamazares, J. (2020a). *Primavera extremeña. Apuntes del natural* [Extremaduran spring. Notes of the natural]. Alfaguara.

Llamazares, J. (2020b). Un canto a la vida en medio de la muerte: A song to life in the midst of death. *El País*. Retrieved from https://elpais.com/elpais/2020/11/10/eps/1605008819_369175.html

Luque Amo, Á. (2016). El diario personal en la literatura: teoría del diario literario [The personal diary in literature: literary diary theory]. *Castilla. Estudios de Literatura*, *7*, 273–306.

Rilke, R. M. (2009). Del paesaggio [Landscape]. In P. D'Angelo (Ed.), *Estetica e Paesaggio* (pp. 53–64). Il Mulino.

Simmel, G. (2009). Filosofia del paesaggio [Landscape philosophy]. In P. D'Angelo (Ed.), *Estetica e Paesaggio* (pp. 39–52). Il Mulino.

ADDITIONAL READING

Andres-Suárez, I. (2000). La prosa de Julio Llamazares [The prose of Julio Llamazares]. In F. Sevilla, M. Alvar (Eds.), *Actas del XIII Congreso de la Asociación Internacional de Hispanistas: Madrid, 6-11 de julio de 1998. Tomo II. Siglo XVIII. Siglo XIX. Siglo XX* (pp. 476-85). Madrid, Spain: Castalia.

Andres-Suárez, I. (2004). La poética viajera de *Julio Llamazares* [the travelling poetics]. In G. Champeau (Ed.), *Relatos de viajes contemporáneos por España y Portugal* (pp. 301–318). Verbum.

Blanchot, M. (1996). El diario íntimo y el relato [The intimate diary and the story]. *Revista de Occidente (Madrid, Spain), 182-183*, 47–54.

Cárcamo, S. (2006). Del aforismo a la ficción: la memoria en Julio Llamazares [From aphorism to fiction: memory in Julio Llamazares]. *Espéculo, 33*. Retrieved from http://webs.ucm.es/info/especulo/numero33/afollama.html

Caudet, F. (2002). Memoria y representación en la narrativa española contemporánea [Memory and representation in contemporary Spanish narrative]. *Sociohistórica (La Plata)*, 11–12. https://www.sociohistorica.fahce.unlp.edu.ar/article/view/SHn11-12a08

Didier, B. (1996). El diario, ¿forma abierta? [The diary, open form?]. *Revista de Occidente (Madrid, Spain), 182-183*, 39–46.

García Barrientos, J.L. (2011). ¿Teatro de viajes? Paradojas modales de un género literario [Travel theatre? Modal paradoxes of a literary genre]. *Revista de literatura, 73*(145), 35-64.

Girard, A. (1996). El diario como género literario [The diary as a literary genre]. *Revista de Occidente (Madrid, Spain), 182-183*, 31–38.

Lejeune, P. (1996). La práctica del diario personal: Una investigación (1986-1996) [The practice of the personal diary: an investigation (1986-1996)]. *Revista de Occidente (Madrid, Spain), 182-183*, 55–75.

Martín, M. R. (2011). En los límites del libro de viajes: Seducción, canonicidad y transgresión de un género [At the limits of the travel book: seduction, canonicity and transgression of a genre]. *Revista de Literatura, 73*(145), 65–90. doi:10.3989/revliteratura.2011.v73.i145.252

Milani, R. (2001). *L'arte del paesaggio* [The art of landscape]. Bologna, Italy: Il mulino.

Paleologos, K. (2017). Julio Llamazares o la historia que se borró: Julio Llamazares or the story that was removed. *Estudios Humanísticos. Filología, 39*, 39–53.

KEY TERMS AND DEFINITIONS

COVID-19 Pandemic: Pandemic of Coronavirus disease 2019, caused by severe acute respiratory syndrome coronavirus 2 (SARS-CoV-2). It was identified in December 2019 in Wuhan, China. The WHO declared the outbreak of a public health emergency of international concern in January 2020 and a pandemic in March 2020.

Diary: Form of autobiographical writing, a regularly kept record of the diarist's activities and reflections. A personal diary may include a person's experiences, thoughts, and/or feelings, excluding comments on current events outside the writer's direct experience and may provide information for a memoir, autobiography, or biography.

Landscape: The natural and physical attributes of land together with air and water which change over time and which is made known by people's evolving perceptions and associations, such as beliefs, uses, values and relationships.

Primavera extremeña. Apuntes del natural **[Extremaduran spring. Natural notes]:** Illustrated book, personal chronicle of Llamazares' lockdown, it is a poetic and intimate diary where the author sings of the beauty of nature that rises up despite the tragedy that threatens human life.

Travel Literature: The notes of a traveler, containing his impressions of the journey, descriptions of events, and observations. Travel literature seeks to communicate information about newly discovered lands or those little known to the reader. It may be the history of an imaginary journey presented as a real one but important chiefly in terms of ideological and literary content, as in adventure stories, utopias, and philosophic works.

ENDNOTE

1 The circumstances in which the author was born determine some constant thematic units in his work, such as the depopulation of rural villages and the elective subject-landscape correspondence. In particular, the exodus of the inhabitants of the villages submerged by the Porma dam, whom the author considers the new Jews of the 20th century, is the subject of the novel *Distintas formas de mirar el agua* (2015), in which the diaspora is narrated through a choral perspective. It should also be noted that the author returned to the places of his childhood on a trip along the Curueño river, to which he dedicated his travel diary *El río del olvido*, published in 1990.

Chapter 4
El tiempo que nos robaron (2021) de Rosa Huertas: Writing as a Lifeboat During COVID-19 Pandemic Confinement

Katiuscia Darici
University of Turin, Italy

ABSTRACT

The aim of this chapter is to analyse "El tiempo que nos robaron" (2021) by Rosa Huertas in the elements that can be most ascribed to pandemic writings. First of all, the author intends to underline the rise of the so called "pandemic narrative" to describe the traumatic experience during COVID-19 emergence. After presenting some theoretical considerations on journaling, the author will describe the salvific importance of writing and the primary importance of an interlocutor as an incentive for writing. The author intends to clarify to what extent the present and, in parallel, the past as it is recalled in the diary, is a stolen time. In addition, the importance of rituals must be taken into consideration. For this purpose, the author will describe the difficulty of filling the time as told by Huertas. The diary ends up being her main daily ritual. In this case, one can observe the importance of writing as a tool to objectify and distance oneself from the disease.

Revisito la idea de la literatura como resistencia. Me parece que ahora la literatura es refugio, posibilidad y certezas.

[I am revisiting the idea of literature as resistance. It seems to me that literature is now a refuge, a possibility and certainties].

Ana Pellicer Vázquez, En la covid-19, 2020.

DOI: 10.4018/978-1-6684-4735-2.ch004

INTRODUCTION

In a 1947 book entitled *La littérature et le droit à la mort*, Maurice Blanchot said: "Ce qui est étrange en elle [la littérature], c'est que, en dépît du vide –et peut-être en raison du vide–, il faut écrire" ["What is strange about it [literature] is that, in spite of emptiness – and perhaps because of emptiness – you have to write"] (quot. in Foucault 1963). Writing as the need to fill someone's personal void has interested writers and journalists throughout the lockdown during the Covid-19 pandemic, giving life to texts that can be framed in the so-called "confined" or "pandemic narrative".

[...] los pacientes, los profesionales de la salud y los reporteros que los siguieron en su travesía por los territorios de la respiración artificial constituyen una minoría de las vidas y testimonios sobre la pandemia. La gran mayoría de los ciudadanos y, por tanto, de los escritores, artistas, dramaturgos o directores audiovisuales vivimos aquellos meses en el interior de nuestros hogares. De modo que es lógico que predominen las narrativas confinadas. Muchas de ellas, en la línea de [Fang] Fang y [Andrés Felipe] Solano,[1] llegaron a nosotros en forma de diarios. Fue la opción genérica más frecuentada en las semanas más duras del año pasado. El encierro llevaba naturalmente a la introspección y a las retóricas íntimas. Pero la excepcionalidad del momento que estábamos viviendo ponía en tensión lo particular con lo universal, la experiencia concreta con las vivencias arquetípicas.

[...] patients, health professionals and the reporters who followed them on their journey through the lands of artificial respiration constitute a minority of the lives and testimonies about the pandemic. The vast majority of us and, therefore, of writers, artists, playwrights and audiovisual directors, lived inside our homes during those months. So it is natural for lockdown narratives to predominate. Many of them, as in the case of [Fang] Fang and [Andrés Felipe] Solano, have reached us in the form of diaries. This was the most common genre chosen during the toughest weeks of last year. Lockdown naturally led to introspection and intimate rhetoric. But the exceptional nature of the moment we were going through set the personal in tension with the universal, the concrete experience with archetypal experiences (Carrión, 2021).

A certain number of writers have preferred the form of autobiography (mainly diaries and journals). Among other journals, in Spain were published *La vida en suspenso. Diario del confinamiento*, by Jordi Doce (2020), *Jugar a los neandertales* (2020) and *Parte de mí* (2021), by Marta Sanz. In his *Volver a dónde* (2021), Antonio Muñoz Molina compiles diary fragments written during confinement and intertwines them with a look at and from the post-COVID-19 era.[2]

A list of the main titles published within the literary frame is given by Jorge Carrión who, in an article which came out in *La Vanguardia*, prefers to speak about "narrative on the pandemic" (2021). The traumatic pandemic experience has given life to literary products that "ha[ve] affected all areas of culture: theatre, literature, plastic arts, music, cinema, etc." (Greco 2022, p. 90). Several academic publications in the Humanities were also published (Boccuti 2020, Greco 2020, Greco 2022, Orazi 2020a, Orazi 2020b, Orazi 2022a, Orazi 2022b, Cortijo Ocaña-Martines 2022).

To some critics, the diary form seemed to be the appropriate genre to describe the day-to-day quarantined life in 2020. This literary genre also made it possible to keep track of the exceptionality of a lifestyle that has been labelled as dystopian on more than one occasion. In the case of Spanish writer Rosa María Huertas (born in Madrid in 1960) and her book *El tiempo que nos robaron* [The Time They

Stole from Us; quoted as *El tiempo* from now on] (2021), introspective writing unfolds in fifty chapters halfway between the autobiography, the diary and the epistolary novel. It is a textual strategy that allows, on the one hand, introspection and self-analysis and, on the other, retrospection. Looking back to the past has a healing function both of the present and the past, while the writer is stuck in a present situation described as an "espacio infinito de la soledad indeseada [infinite space of loneliness]" (Huertas 2021, p. 25). The past refers to Huertas's childhood and youth, which she shared with her best friend Elena, who died ten years before the pandemic.

Elena inhabits Rosa's past, and her memory is indelible (Huertas 2021, p. 74). Remembrance mainly recalls the early school days as well as the University years, although there are also parts in which the writer describes the moments when the two ladies reached adulthood, got married, gave birth to children and eventually got divorced.

Huerta's *El tiempo* is not her first experience with the autobiographical genre. Before, she also published *Mujeres que leían* (2019). In it, she tells the story of her mother, which is also the story of many post-war women who had to give up their aspirations in order to devote themselves to being wives and mothers and who "ni siquiera supieron que podían soñar [did not even know they could dream of]" a different life (Huertas 2019, p. 23). *Mujeres* partially foresees the structure of *El tiempo*, as it follows the narration in dialogue with another woman, her mother. In this case, the dialogues are inserted as fragments in italic within the first-person narration. In this way, the mother is actively involved in the construction of the past and, together with the narrator, builds up a shared memory of Rosa as a daughter and of the elder lady as a witness of a time who speaks in lieu of other women belonging to her same generation: "mamá se ha dado cuenta de que puede añadir sus propios recuerdos y parece que le agrada: no se trata solo de eliminar, de censurar, sino también de completar y eso será bueno para las dos [Mum has realised that she can add her own memories and she seems to like it: it is not just a matter of deleting, of censoring, but also of completing and that will be good for both of us]" (Huertas 2019, p. 22).

Huertas's career as a writer is almost entirely devoted to children and youth literature based on major exponents in the history of European literature, such as Miguel Hernández, Lope de Vega, Miguel de Cervantes, Cyrano de Bergerac, Mariano José de Larra and Federico García Lorca. Her books involve an accurate work of research to provide her readers with reliable stories, insofar as biographical reality and the historical environment are concerned.

THE FIRST MAJOR LITERARY DOCUMENT ON COVID-19: FANG FANG'S *WUHAN DIARY* (2020)

The first "gran documento literario sobre la Covid-19 [great literary document about Covid-19]", as Jorge Carrión defined it (2021), is Fang Fang's *Wuhan Diary* (2020). Initially intended to be a blog and only later published in book format, it inaugurates Covid-19 pandemic journaling at the epicentre of the health emergency. It is an online chronicle from the 11-million-people Chinese city of Wuhan, where the Covid-19 first appeared and spread in December 2019, after that the Chinese government declared the state of emergency and placed under lockdown the whole region on January 23, 2020.

A literary exponent of Chinese neorealism, Fang Fang entrusts the description of the pandemic, both in its trivial moments of everyday life and in its social impact, to the form of the diary, acknowledging the importance of individual memory to highlight to what extent disease, humankind and social crisis are interwoven, as well as to discuss specific issues, such as sustainability, global climate crisis, and the nature of technology, both salvific and demonic (Pesaro 2021, p. 228). From this point of view, the pandemic diaries regain the testimonial value that, historically, is specifically inherent to the intimate diary.

To fully grasp the element of intimacy but also to bring order to the multiple denominations that can designate similar forms of writing it deserves, at this point, to briefly outline the history of this form of writing from the experiences of intimate writing of the 19th century until today, after the Covid-19 pandemic. This can help to shed light on the hybrid character of Rosa Huertas's *El tiempo*, which I propose to define as an intimate, autobiographic diary of the pandemic but which, if carefully analysed, crosses the limit of the novel or the (possibly fictive) epistolary exchange, or even of diary fiction. The boundaries between all these genres are somehow blurred, which confirms the nature of the diary as an "open form" (Didier 1976, 1996) or freed from forms, as Maurice Blanchot prefers to express it:

El diario íntimo […] tan liberado de las formas, [...] y tan capaz de todas las libertades, puesto que pensamientos, sueños, ficciones, comentarios de sí mismo, acontecimientos importantes, insignificantes, todo le conviene, en el orden y en el desorden que se quiera.

[The intimate diary [...] so liberated from forms, [...] and so capable of all freedoms, since thoughts, dreams, fictions, comments about oneself, important and insignificant events, everything goes, in the order and disorder that one wishes] (Blanchot 1959, p. 229).

I propose to clarify some theoretical aspects in the next paragraph and to describe *El tiempo* in its idiosyncrasy and content.

SOME THEORETICAL CONSIDERATIONS ON JOURNALING

On a theoretical level, some scholars date the emergence of the intimate diary around 1800, just before Romanticism as a result of the influence of Rousseauian confessions and of "la ambición de los ideólogos de fundar la ciencia del hombre sobre la observación, colocando la sensación en el origen del entendimiento, de acuerdo con Locke, Helvétius y Condillac [the ideologues' ambition to found the science of man on observation, placing sensation at the origin of understanding, in accordance with Locke, Helvétius and Condillac]" (Girard 1996, p. 32). At that time the diary deals with the forms of sociological (Condorcet, Saint-Simon and Comte) or personal analyses (Stendhal) (Girard 1996, p. 33). Although initially the ambition of the first to write intimate diaries moved towards the physical and moral knowledge of man, little by little "la observación interior se transforma […] en examen de conciencia [inner observation is transformed [...] into an examination of consciousness]" (Girard 1996, p. 33) and the diary gains in intimacy.

The personal diary entered the realm of literature during the 19th century with the publication, in 1882, of Henri Fréderic Amiel's *Journal Intime*. The consequent appearance of a new public of readers "justifica su inclusión dentro de las modalidades autobiográficas [justifies its inclusion in autobiographical forms]" (Luque Amo 2016, p. 273). In parallel, a new type of writer was born: the diarist (Luque Amo 2020, p. 259). During the 20th century "el diario termina conformándose como una modalidad literaria [the diary ends up becoming a literary form]" (Luque Amo 2020, p. 259). In this period there is a gradual retrieval of experiences of the previous century (Samuel Pepys, Henri Fréderic Amiel, Stendhal, Benjamin Constant) on one hand, and as a proof that the *Journal Intime* "is not the only kind of diary"

(Raoul 1989, p. 57), the appearance of the first diaries "concebidos para ser publicados [designed to be published]" (Luque Amo 2020, p. 259). They are the so-called writer's diaries, such as those of André Gide and Julien Green published in the 1930s. With reference to Kafka's diaries, Blanchot prefers the denomination of "diaries of the creative experience", as they collect literary fragments and short drafts of books in preparation, besides descriptions of everyday life (1959, p. 224). These diaries are "not diaries as such", as they are the compilation of fragmentary texts, notes and pieces that may have been previously published in newspapers (Romera Castillo n.d., p. 7). In Spain they are thus defined as "dietarios [journals]" as per José Romera Castillo's classification of the types of diaries (n.d., p. 7). Castillo also distinguishes between "intimate diaries", written with the purpose of not being published and "public intimate diaries", which on the contrary, are written with the aim of being put in print while the author is alive or even after their death.

The origin of the diaries could be found in the captains' logs where the absence of the "I" in favor of the "we" has been attested: "es uno el que escribe, pero en nombre de todos [...]; hemos llegado, hemos zarpado, nos sobrevino una tempestad [one person writes, but in the name of everyone [...]; we arrived, we set sail, a storm came upon us" (Trapiello 1998, p. 34). Similar cases are represented by the ethnographic diaries and the expedition journals. Their aim was "fijar los pasos de una ruta [mark out the steps of a route]" and "servir de testament [serve as testimony]" (Trapiello 1998, p. 33). These two characteristics still define writer's diaries, as they are, at the same time, both "la consignación de una travesía [the record of a voyage]" and "el memorándum de una vida que fluye también hacia la Muerte [the memorandum of a life that also flows towards Death]" (Trapiello 1998, p. 34).

In Spain the intimate diary practice did not begin until the 20th century if we consider intimacy as an essential factor of the diary (Freixas 1996, p. 6). The reason surely lies in the way in which the Spanish government has been curbing freedom alongside the imposition of a climate of austerity due to the Counter-Reformation and the Inquisition (Freixas 1996, p. 7). Laura Freixas highlights nearly complete absence of women's diaries in 20th century Spain, with the sole exception of Rosa Chacel (1996, p. 8). Freixas distinguishes three stages of the intimate diary in Spain, taking as a reference point the year of the beginning of each single diary she mentions in her study. In the first stage, before the war, there are only the names of Josep Pla and Marià Manent. In the second stage, which straddles the Spanish war and the post-war periods, authors such as Manuel Azaña, Rosa Chacel, Carlo Edmundo de Ory, Carlos Barral, Jaime Gil de Biedma are included (Freixas 1996, p. 9). At this point it is interesting to underline Freixas's observation:

Todos los citados comparten una o varias de estas características: ser catalanes (ya escriban en catalán o en castellano); haber vivido gran parte de su vida fuera de España; conocer a fondo la literatura francesa o inglesa [...]. Puede decirse, pues, que, desde principios de siglo hasta la muerte de Franco, se inicia el diario íntimo en España, pero se inicia desde la periferia, cultural y geográfica; se inicia de forma paradójica: en España, pero no en español, o en español, pero fuera de España.

[All those cited share one or more of these characteristics: they are Catalan (whether they write in Catalan or Spanish); they have lived a large part of their lives outside Spain; they have a deep knowledge of French or English literature [...]. It can be said, then, that the intimate diary began in Spain between the turn of the century and Franco's death, but it began on the cultural and geographic periphery; it began paradoxically: in Spain, but not in Spanish, or in Spanish, but outside of Spain] (1996, p. 9).

Since the transition to democracy, which generated the third stage of the intimate diary in Spain according to Laura Freixas, the production of diaries has increased and

> *comprende autores de distintas generaciones: la mayoría nacidos entre los años 50 o finales de los 40 (Pere Gimferrer, José Luis García Martín, Juan Carlos Llop, Juan Antonio Masoliver, Valentí Puig, Miguel Sánchez Ostiz, Alex Susanna, Andrés Trapiello...), otros de mayor edad (Fernando Arrabal, Ramón Gaya, José Jiménez Lozano, Antonio Martínez Sarrión, José Muñoz Rojas, Rafael Sánchez Ferlosio, Antón Tovar, Francisco Umbral...), y alguno más joven (Felipe Benítez Reyes). Lo curioso es que, siendo de edades diferentes, todos ellos emprenden un diario hacia las mismas fechas (a partir de los años 70) y lo publican también en la misma época (a partir de 1980).*
>
> *[includes authors from different generations: most of them born in the 1950s or at the end of the 1940s (Pere Gimferrer, José Luis García Martín, Juan Carlos Llop, Juan Antonio Masoliver, Valentí Puig, Miguel Sánchez Ostiz, Alex Susanna, Andrés Trapiello, etc.), while others were older (Fernando Arrabal, Ramón Gaya, José Jiménez Lozano, Antonio Martínez Sarrión, José Muñoz Rojas, Rafael Sánchez Ferlosio, Antón Tovar, Francisco Umbral, etc.) and some younger (Felipe Benítez Reyes). Interestingly, despite being of different ages, all of them started writing a diary at around the same time (from the 1970s onwards) and published it in the same period (from 1980 onwards)] (Freixas 1996, p. 10).*

Not less important, this stage confirms the presence of the personal diary in Spanish critical studies carried out by Laura Freixas, Anna Caballé, Romera Castillo, Jordi Gracia, Jorge Luna Borge, Manuel Alberca, Virgilio Tortosa, Andrés Trapiello, Manuel Hierro. A broad bibliography can be found in an extensive study by Álvaro Luque Amo, *El diario literario: poética e historia* (2020, pp. 26-28).

A further stage of diary writing, which Freixas does not consider, since her essay has been written and published in 1996, includes the period starting in the late nineties up today and sees the emergence of writers' diaries, such as the ones by Miguel Sánchez-Ostiz, Andrés Trapiello, José Luis García Martín, Iñaki Uriarte and Freixas herself, as author of three diaries: *Una vida subterránea. Diario 1991-1994* (2013), *Todos llevan máscara. Diario 1995-1996* (2018), *Saber quién soy. Diario 1997-1999* (2021). The title of her second diary [*Everyone Wears a Mask*], is both an implied reference and a criticism of Spanish diarists who, in her opinion, "no construyen un verdadero texto íntimo [do not construct a truly intimate text]" (Luque Amo 2020, p. 107). Through her diaries, in fact, Freixas tries to fill the black void she condemns, that is, the lack of confessional writing. As a matter of fact, she writes with the aim of doing literature and according to the criterion of truthfulness she also includes personal failures and phobias (Luque Amo 2020, p. 108). Finally, Iñaki Uriarte's diaries stand out as "fenómeno editorial sin muchos precedentes en las letras españolas [an unprecedented publishing phenomenon in Spanish literature]": his diaries leave space to autobiographical confessions and critical-literary reflections (Luque Amo 2020, p. 108).

The interest in Rosa Huertas's diary goes beyond its autobiographical or confidential nature, since, within the group of diaries of confinement that have been published, hers constitutes a testimony of a period characterized by a state of emergency for Covid-19. In this sense, although initially conceived as an intimate diary, *El tiempo* can also be read as a source of information for the understanding of a historical period (Gracia 2004, p. 226): the 2020 pandemic, how individuals have lived their daily lives in confinement but also about the writer's past. Moreover, as I will underline in the next chapter, writing has a salvific significance to Rosa Huertas and so has the existence of an imaginary interlocutor, her best friend Elena.

THE SALVIFIC IMPORTANCE OF WRITING AND THE NECESSARY OTHER IN THE DIARY

He elegido sentirte a mi lado y escribirte como si estuvieras aquí. La literatura también nos hace libres.

[I have chosen to feel you by my side and write to you as if you were here. Literature also sets us free].

(Huertas 2021, p. 80).

Salvation, or its attempt, is an intrinsic characteristic in the diary. According to Maurice Blanchot, in fact, "escribimos para salvar la escritura, para salvar nuestra vida mediante la escritura, [...] escribimos para no perdernos en la pobreza de los días [we write to save writing, to save our life by writing, [...] we write so as not to lose ourselves in the poverty of the days]" (1959, p. 222). This element appears very clearly in *El tiempo* by Rosa Huertas, where the narrator expresses over and over again how important it is to write in order to keep track the past, defined as "lo que una vez amamos [what we once loved]" (Huertas 2021, p. 26). In the previous statement there is a clear-cut consideration that "lo que literariamente va a quedar de nuestra vida es eso que nosotros hemos rescatado de ella [what will remain of our life in literary terms is what we have rescued from it]" (Trapiello 1998, p. 30) through writing. The risk we have to take, by making our lives explicit in black on white that "nuestra vida [...] una vez escrita, *sólo* era eso[3] [our life [...] once it was written, was *only* that]" (Trapiello 1998, p. 28). It is for this reason, that is, the inability to "invent a plot" that makes our lives "evocative and appealing", that many abandon diary writing (Trapiello 1998, p. 29). In light of this, although it may seem naive, the diary represents "todo lo que de la vida queremos contar [all that we want to say about life]" (Trapiello 1998, p. 29).

Writing can also the proper medicine in order to forget the negative feelings of the confinement, as we read in *El tiempo*: "al menos he escrito una página hoy. Así he olvidado el miedo y el confinamiento durante este rato [at least I have written a page today. So, I forgot the fear and lockdown during that time]" (Huertas 2021, p. 26); "escribiendo he olvidado que no se puede salir de casa [while writing I forgot that you cannot leave the house]" (Huertas 2021, p. 39). Days look the same. Time has become "espeso, envolvente como una telaraña [thick, enveloping you like a spider's web]" (Huertas 2021, p. 43), gestures and actions are carried out notwithstanding the day of the week (Huertas 2021, p. 113). In such situation, it becomes increasingly difficult to occupy one's time in a meaningful way: "no sé qué hacer con el tiempo, solo lamentarme de lo que se me ha arrebatado, he olvidado que estoy viva [I don't know what to do with my time; I can only lament what has been taken from me; I have forgotten that I am alive]" (Huertas 2021, p. 42). In this way, writing itself becomes a perfunctory action carried out in the absence of other actions, since everyday life has been emptied out of everyday gestures. In fact, "hay en el diario como la dichosa compensación, una por la otra, de una doble nulidad. Aquel que no hace nada en su vida escribe que no hace nada y, de ese modo, no obstante, hace algo [there is something of a fortunate offsetting of one with the other in the diary, a double nullity. When you do nothing in your life but write that you are doing nothing you are, nevertheless, doing something]" (Blanchot 1959, p. 221).

In chapter 14, quite early in the flow of the narrative, precisely, Rosa compares loneliness to a shipwreck. Consequently, she realises that writing functions as a lifeboat to which Rosa has access thanks to Elena's presence and to that of an unknown woman who lives across the street. With the latter character, she exchanges eye contact during the hour of applause (given daily as a sign of thanks or health workers helping in the fight against coronavirus).[4] Rosa writes in her diary, as if she were writing to Elena, that this woman

no sabe que hablo contigo que no estás, que no respondes, aunque te cueles en mis sueños y en mis recuerdos sin pedir permiso. Ella y tú me hacéis teclear un rato cada día, me recordáis quién fui y cómo las palabras me salvaron la vida. Hoy, en este naufragio de soledad, sois vosotras quienes me rescatáis con la tabla salvavidas de la escritura. Sois como ángeles de la guarda, vigilantes para que no me ahogue en mi propio miedo.

[does not know that I am talking to you, someone who is not here and does not answer, even though you sneak into my dreams and my memories without asking permission. She and you make me type for a while every day. You remind me of who I was and how words saved my life. Today, in this shipwreck of loneliness, it is you who rescue me with the lifesaving board of writing. You are like guardian angels, watching over me so that I do not drown in my own fear] (Huertas 2021, p. 56).

According to the tradition, "diarists are supposed to write for themselves" (Porter Abbott 1984, p. 10). As briefly described above, traditionally only in logbooks "uno escribe en nombre de todos [does one write in everyone's name]" (Trapiello 1998, p. 34). Nevertheless, in some autobiographical narrations, the existence of the other as a recipient can be taken into consideration. Normally this is an ideal reader. In the case we are considering (and that is why *El tiempo* is liminal to the form of the epistolary novel) the writer's best friend is the driving force of the constant exercise of written storytelling: it is, in fact, to her (as in a series of letters) that Huertas alludes to in her daily exercise of describing the "encierro monstruoso [monstrous confinement]" (Huertas 2021, p. 29) in which she feels like a "leona enjaulada [caged lioness]" (Huertas 2021, p. 31). Elena is for Rosa a "necessary other" (Cavarero 2000) to whom to narrate one's life story: "Te llevo conmigo, como interlocutora perfecta: te hablo y siento que me escuchas [I take you with me, as a perfect interlocutor: I speak to you and I feel that you listen to me]" (Huertas 2021, p. 175). While filling her diary and telling the story of her present and of a shared past with Elena, in fact, the writer establishes an imaginary dialogue that she refuses to call monologue (Huertas 2021, p. 176), and that helps her to free from anxieties (Huertas 2021, p. 107) and loneliness (Huertas 2021, p. 93).

The woman from across the street is a necessary other, too. In the beginning they are only two strangers. Like most of people in Spain during confinement they go out to the balcony or look out of the window at 8 p.m. and applause. As time goes by, Rosa wants to know more about the lady, and meet her in person, if possible. So, one day, when going back home from a quick visit to the pharmacy, she makes an attempt.

Regresaba a casa con mi caja de pastillas [...] cuando pasé por delante del portal de la mujer que me saluda cada tarde a las ocho y sentí la tentación de preguntar por ella. Elegí el 4.° A, pues las ventanas son las del extremo de la casa, y llamé. Respondió la voz de un hombre mayor, desabrido, que me trató con resquemor y antipatía. Le conté la historia completa, nuestros saludos diarios, el afecto, la condición de mujeres solitarias, pero no logré conmoverlo.

[I was going home with my box of pills [...] when I passed the doorway of the woman who greets me every evening at eight o'clock and was tempted to ask for her. I chose flat 4A, as the windows are at the end of the building and pressed the buzzer. The voice of a gruff elderly man replied who treated me with suspicion and antipathy. I told him the whole story, of our daily greetings, the affection, the condition of solitary women, but I did not manage to move him] (Huertas 2021, p. 76).

At this point Rosa invents a parallel reality made of memories of the past, in which the woman in front of her would be none other than Elena. This strategy helps the protagonist feel stronger and more accompanied.

Eres tú la mujer que me saluda cada tarde. El hombre no mintió, el 4.° A se encuentra vacío desde hace meses. Ahora lo habita tu sombra, tu recuerdo. Me vigilas tras las cortinas para asegurarte que sigo aquí, escribiendo. Ves la mesa, mi rostro que se asoma por encima de la pantalla del ordenador, me espías, me das un motivo para levantarme cada mañana, para esperar a que lleguen las ocho y saludemos con la mano a lo lejos, como hacíamos de niñas en el balcón de la casa de tus padres.

[You are the woman who greets me every evening. The man did not lie, 4A has been empty for months. Now it is inhabited by your shadow, your memory. You watch me behind the curtains to make sure I am still here, writing. You see the desk, my face peeking out over the computer screen. You spy on me, you give me a reason to get up every morning, to wait for eight o'clock to come and wave to each other in the distance, like children on the balcony of their parents' home] (Huertas 2021, p. 76).

Later, at the end of the same chapter, she reinforces the idea of feeling accompanied: "Me gusta sentir que me observas con los ojos de la vecina y también a mi espalda [I like to feel that you are watching me with the neighbour's eyes and also behind my back]" (Huertas 2021, p. 78). Rosa does not give up. After the first unsuccessful attempt to meet the woman across the street, she tries again, one day, after food shopping:

el día soleado me ha empujado a subir la calle hasta la plaza, a cruzar la acera contraria y a plantarme delante del edificio donde vive la vecina que me abraza en la distancia. Antes de llamar al 4.° D he respirado hondo. Enseguida ha respondido una voz femenina y he contado mi historia.

[the sunny day has pushed me to walk up the street to the square, to cross to the other side and stand in front of the building where the neighbour who hugs me from a distance lives. I took a deep breath before buzzing 4D. A female voice answered immediately and I told her my story] (Huertas 2021, p. 107).

Talking on the intercom, the two ladies introduce themselves to each other and Rosa is invited upstairs. At last, the woman across the street is no longer a nameless stranger.

Se llama Ana. Ya no es una señora anónima que me saluda desde lejos, ni siquiera es tu sombra agazapada tras las cortinas, es mi amiga Ana que tiene una voz cálida y un rostro agradable.

[Her name is Ana. She is no longer an anonymous lady who greets me from afar. She is not even your shadow hiding behind the curtains. She is my friend Ana who has a warm voice and a pleasant face] (Huertas 2021, p. 108).

This timid social gathering, together with another one, with a neighbour who is a doctor and helps Rosa giving her "unos pares de guantes de latex y unas mascarillas que no encontraba en ninguna farmacia ni supermercado [a pair of latex gloves and some masks that [she] could not find in any pharmacy or supermarket]" (Huertas 2021, p. 100), helps the writer to feeling more confident about solidarity. It also confirms her belief that, as human beings, "somos pasajeros en el mismo barco a la deriva [we are passengers on the same drifting ship]" (Huertas 2021, p. 100).

RITUALS OF DAILY LIFE DURING CONFINEMENT

What makes the case of the 2020 lockdown peculiar is the feeling that the whole world has been affected by the pandemic (Žižek 2020). Humans were sharing the experience of a disease that was and still is considered an "amenaza invisible [invisible threat]" (Huertas 2021, p. 41) that can potentially reach each and everyone. For this reason, it leaves the floor to a common sense of fear, panic, and melancholy (Huertas 2021, pp. 15, 17, 111) that must be worked through in total loneliness by social distancing. People reacted in different ways such as by getting grip on cooking. As a matter of fact, it has not been uncommon for supermarkets to run out of flour since everyone decided to bake cakes or pies for their beloved ones, as Huertas herself remarks: "Se agotó la harina porque todos hacen tartas con los hijos. [They have sold out of flour because everyone is making cakes with their children." (Huertas 2021, p. 158). Every week she prepares "cocido [stew]", in order to make her home smell "a sopa y a hogar, a vida cotidiana y a normalidad [of soup and home, of everyday life and normality]" (2021, p. 62). The house is like a "refugio [refuge]" (Huertas 2021, p. 84), in which her friend Elena is always there, although in her imagination. People are scared to go out and face reality as if there was a war (Huertas 2021, p. 83). And it could be worse than a war since "ninguna sirena te avisa del bombardeo porque se trata de una amenaza invisible, imposible de detectar, es inútil huir de ella, solo sirve esconderse[5] [no siren warns you of the bombing because it is an invisible threat, impossible to detect; it is useless to run away from it, the only thing you can do is hide]" (Huertas 2021, p. 84).

As Žižek posits, in the confinement "the main thing is to structure your daily life in a stable and meaningful way" (2020). Rosa expresses her difficulty by filling her time. Initially, she does not know what to do and feels that her own body and house are like a prison to her, although she is aware that her daily routine can calm her thoughts (Huertas 2021, p. 93). The virus "occupies a space within us, limiting our possibilities of action" (Monti 2012, p. 8)[6]. In her diary, Huertas recounts her day-to-day little accomplishments, which include: sitting by the window as a "refuge" (2021, p. 63) and a way to escape with the imagination. She creates (literally "invents") a daily routine:

invento rutinas, sigo limpiando con lejía, cocino, disfruto un rato del sol cuando las nubes no lo impiden, corrijo cientos de ejercicios de mis alumnos, leo después de comer hasta que me duermo, sigo contestando correos, hago videollamadas con los amigos y con mi hermana, llamo por teléfono a mi madre varias veces, intento dormir ante el televisor con una película aburrida

[I invent routines, I keep cleaning with bleach, I cook, I enjoy the sun for a while when the clouds are not in the way, I mark hundreds of my students' exercises, I read after lunch until I fall asleep, I keep answering e-mails, I make video calls with friends and my sister, I phone my mother several times, I try to sleep in front of the TV with a boring film] (Huertas 2021, p. 93).

She also finds reassuring the eight o'clock outdoor clapping perceiving it as a choral way of dealing with the confinement, in which she happens to make eye contact with a woman who lives across the street.

Enfrente está la mujer mayor sola, como yo, la única sin compañía de toda la calle. Ambas lo sabemos, salgo a asomarme por ella. Antes de aplaudir nos miramos y nos saludamos, aquí seguimos, otro día más.

[Across the road is the old woman, alone like me, the only one without company in the whole street. We both know it. I go outside to show myself to her. Before applauding we look at each other and greet each other. We are still here, yet another day] (Huertas 2021, p. 43).

There is an uncommon silence (Huertas 2021, p. 56) if compared to pre-Covid time, when "el mundo existía, llegaba el bullicio de la gente que se encaminaba hacia el Rastro, de los coches y autobuses [the world existed; I heard the hustle and bustle of people heading to El Rastro flea market, crowded buses and cars]" (Huertas 2021, p. 83). Huertas considers this silence to be untrue, as

detrás de cada ventana hay gente que llora, que grita, que intenta vivir dentro de la pesadilla. El silencio traga las quejas, las palabras, las risas que desaparecieron, los sueños que perdimos. Por la acera asoman quienes van a la compra, arrastran el carrito con desgana, se tapan, se alejan de los demás, se convierten en zombis

[behind every window there are people crying, screaming, trying to live inside the nightmare. Silence swallows the complaints, the words, the laughter that disappeared, the dreams we lost. People going shopping appear on the pavement, reluctantly dragging their trolleys, covering themselves, moving away from others, turning into zombies] (Huertas 2021, p. 83).

Rosa's experience is equally distressing, and, in fact, she confesses to taking anti-anxiety medication (Huertas 2021, p. 75-76). Lastly, life in confinement is a life "sin caricias [without caresses]" (Huertas 2021, p. 63) and "la ausencia de contacto humano, tan necesario, nos corroe y nos congela [the absence of human contact, so necessary, corrodes and freezes us]" (Huertas 2021, p. 64).

Women's Diaries and the Action of Writing from the Inside

Could we state that there is feminine component of the diary? The narration coming from a female point of view, as a distinctive characteristic, has been studied, among others, by Béatrice Didier (1976; 1981), Valerie Raoul (1989), Nora Catelli (1996) and Laura Freixas (1996). Historically,

the lack of an imposed form and of rules to follow has been part of the diary's attraction for women writers. [...] The predilection of women for the intimate diary coincides for modern women writers with the search of a feminine voice, for a mode or style which can include what has been excluded from the dominant male discourse (Raoul 1989, p. 62).

At the same time, we should not forget the big number of women that used to keep a diary, as it was the main kind of writing they practiced during a long time in the past centuries (Didier 1976, p. 106). In the 19th century, for instance, "women were discouraged from writing for the public" (Raoul 1989, p. 58).

More recently, in her extensive analysis of the *Wuhan Diary*, Nicoletta Pesaro underlines the fact that the narrative is more subtle and oblique in describing the complexity of the disease and its implications in the social and human fabric, precisely because it has been told by a woman (2021, pp. 228-229).

If there is a key factor that can distinguish feminine writing (intended as presenting a woman's point of view) from one that is not, it is to be seen in Huertas's writing, which tries to convey through narratorial techniques, the time that was stolen from her during adolescence, when, together with her friend Elena, she studied at a convent school. They were taught that "casi todo era pecado [almost everything was a sin]" (Huertas 2021, p. 18) and, for that reason, men were not allowed to enter the building and the girls used to hide their bodies due to a sort of shame they were taught to feel (Huertas 2021, p. 18).

When Béatrice Didier observes that "l'écriture féminine est une écriture du Dedans: l'interieur du corps, l'interieur de la maison" (1981, p. 37), it is particularly appropriate when reading the beginning of chapter 10 of *El tiempo*: "El encierro me obliga a mirar hacia dentro [Lockdown forces me to look inwards]", (Huertas 2021, p. 42). Looking inwards, "encogerme en la frontera de mi cuerpo [to shrink within the borders of my body]" (Huertas 2021, p. 43), as we read in *El tiempo* is precisely the level of introspection we find most typically in women's writing. It goes without saying that self-contemplation is also a condition that is facilitated by forced confinement within four walls. This book is also a celebration of a friendship between two women and of sorority: "las amigas crean un vínculo eterno, irrompible, como el nuestro, más allá de la muerte, como se dice del amor en los sonetos de Quevedo [female friends create an eternal, unbreakable bond, like ours, beyond death, as Quevedo's sonnets say of love]" (Huertas 2021, p. 151).

A STOLEN TIME: PRESENT AND PAST

Time plays an important role in the act of writing a diary. According to Blanchot, the only condition to which the diary must be subject to is the one of the calendars: "el calendario es su demonio, el inspirador, el compositor, el provocador y el guardian [the calendar is [the] demons inspirer, composer, provocateur and guardian]" of the diary (1959, p. 219). However, the diarist often skips this condition (Trapiello 1998, p. 35). An example could be found in *El tiempo* which, in its liminal position between different autobiographical genres, also touches the form of diary fiction, as it is divided into fifty numbered chapters and not into dated diary entries. Fifty is an ambiguous number in this case, as it may refer to the approximate recount of days under quarantine. For that reason, chapter numbers may not allude to chapters *per se* but to the specific day of confinement. Huertas does not clearly declare what her intention is. She leaves this detail to the reader's interpretation, and it may be part of a strategy to stress the uncertainty felt during the pandemic.

The treatment of time is also a parameter to distinguish the diary from the memoirs. The latter keeps a greater temporal distance with the narrated events: in fact, contrary to what happens in the diary, memoirs are usually written considerably after the events and acquire a historical dimension (Didier 1976, p. 9).

As Antonio Muñoz Molina observes in the prologue to the Spanish translation of the *Wuhan Diary*, the diary is, along with the chronicle, "el lugar de la escritura en presente [the place of writing in the present tense]" (2020), also because the writer cannot see his entire life as a whole (Piccone Stella 2008, p. 15) and the distance from the narrated events is inevitably reduced (Didier 1976, p. 9).

The sequence of dates on which the diarist writes give the narrative its temporal continuity. This present-tense progression tends to dominate the subject matter, so that the diarist usually writes about events of the immediate past – events that occur between one entry and the next – or records his momentary ideas, reflections, or emotions (Martens 1985, p. 5).

The ordinary represents the frame and limit within which "lo que se escribe se enraiza, [...] se quiera o no" [what is written takes root, [...] whether you want it to or not]" (Blanchot 1959, p. 219): el presente aparece "sin futuro" [the present appears "without future"] (Huertas 2021, p. 13). The empty time of the confinement, as Huertas defines it, establishes in the writer's mind a parallel feeling with the past.

Pienso hoy en la vida que perdimos, en la infancia gris, en la adolescencia que me robaron. Tantos años, frente a estos pocos meses de vida desperdiciada. Ya nunca retornará la edad dorada para otros, ni la alegría de la que no gozamos. Este tiempo vacío me recuerda a los años de espera, entonces me preguntaba cuándo llegaría la felicidad, cuándo la persona amada, cuándo la libertad de hablar y decidir.

[I think today of the life we have lost, of grey childhood, of the adolescence that was stolen from me. So many years, compared with these few months of wasted life. The golden age will never return for others, nor the happiness we are not enjoying. This empty time reminds me of the years of waiting, when I wondered when happiness would come, when my beloved would come, when the freedom to speak and decide would come (Huertas 2021, p. 92).

If life, as in Huertas's *El tiempo*, is perceived as stolen, the diary allows its material preservation in a book (Raoul 1989, p. 61) through remembrance.

The present is stolen from the possibility of being happy (Huertas 2021, p. 41) due to confinement. The past was also stolen, and the writer refers in particular to her adolescence (Huertas 2021, p. 89) and youth (Huertas 2021, pp. 57, 110):

Aterrizamos en la adolescencia ignorantes y asustadas. Nos robaron también la juventud: nos la abarrotaron de normas, de represión absurda, de mentiras nada piadosas, de sueños prestados que creíamos nuestros

[We landed in adolescence ignorant and frightened. They also robbed us of our youth: they stuffed it with rules, with absurd repression, with unpitying lies, with borrowed dreams that we thought were ours] (Huertas 2021, p. 56).

The past is hurtful and so are the memories of a youth that was limited by the "convencionalismos absurdos [absurd conventions]" (Huertas 2021, p. 88) of a school for only girls, a place described as "obscure" (Huertas 2021, p. 89), which constrained individuality and students' free will, in particular with reference to a narrow-minded sentimental education, that obliged the young ladies to *fingir, a aparentar frialdad, a no expresar de verdad nuestros sentimientos hacia ellos [los hombres], a no tomar la iniciativa, a esperar, a callar, a reprimir los deseos. Ambas pagamos el precio de aquella mala educación.*

[to pretend, to feign coldness, not to truly express our feelings towards them [men], not to take the initiative, to wait, to keep silent, to repress our desires. We both paid the price for that bad education] (Huertas 2021, p. 88).

Rosa and Elena's youth bear a strong resemblance to that of their mothers "que vivieron en la dictadura [who lived under the dictatorship]" (Huertas 2021, p. 106).

The book reveals a constant disillusionment with the past and an awareness that the lost time will not return. The presence of Elena during a long-shared period life, until her death, alleviated the burden of the lack of experiences, as Rosa explains. This is why she is so important during the confinement: Elena was in the past, and still is, even in her memory, the anchor of life to Rosa.

CONCLUSION

A todos nos robaron el tiempo alguna vez.

[We were all robbed of our time at some point].

(Huertas, 2021, p. 142)

The intimate diary was traditionally characterized, among other things, by a lack of coherence and global unity (Raoul 1989, p. 62), which contributed to its exclusion from the literary canon for a long time. The same thing cannot be said of a diary of confinement. Its overall concept, coherence, argument, in short, its *raison d'être*, is to be found over the time of confinement. The days spent at home, the daily routine and the rituals shared with her neighbours (such as the applause), all this, gives form and containment to the writing, as it is in describing the confinement itself that the diary acquires coherence and global unity. Another difference between any diary and a diary of confinement is that generally diaries, by their very nature, usually do not require conclusions (Mildonian 2001, p. 131), while a diary of confinement tends to find its conclusion in the ending of the quarantine, as in the case of *El tiempo*.

As H. Porter Abbott posits, "the term diary evokes an intensity of privacy, cloistering, isolation" (1984, p. 11). Nevertheless, a distinction should be made between intimate diaries and the ones that Enric Bou has defined as "external diaries", with reference to diaries that approach the form of the chronicle with a historian's perspective (1996, p. 129). Huertas's attitude in this book is not –strictu sensu– that of a historian, nor is her declared intention to leave testimony of a vital moment characterized by confinement. Nevertheless, the result is that she leaves a record of a period lived indoors: her diary, in fact, will increase its value when being read retrospectively by future generations of readers. Thanks to the importance of her friendship with Elena (who prematurely died and therefore cannot be physically there), and the metaphorical confinement with her, something that drives the writer to the constant exercise of storytelling, writing and, for that reason, literature, becomes the lifeboat used by the narrator to survive the confinement within the walls of her house. In this daily exercise of remembrance of the past and of description of the present, the diary of the pandemic is a testimony of a peculiar historical time but also a way not to forget "que existe la belleza en medio de la incertidumbre [that there is beauty in the midst of uncertainty]" (Huertas 2021, p. 108).

El *tiempo* highlights that rituals in general during confinement are salvific (Huertas 2021, p. 114), mainly because "aplacan los malos pensamientos [they placate bad thoughts]" (Huertas 2021, p. 93) The diary ends up being Rosa main daily ritual. In this case, we can observe the importance of writing as a tool to objectify and distance oneself from the disease. The long period of introspection also leads the writer to the conviction of personal change (Huertas 2021, p. 169) as well as a reconciliation with the past. After all, "ninguna persona concreta nos robó la adolescencia, hoy tampoco puedo reclamar que me devuelvan estos meses perdidos [no specific person stole our adolescence; but today I cannot reclaim these lost months]" (Huerta 2021, p. 180).

REFERENCES

Asmundson, J. G., & Taylor, S. (2020, December). Coronaphobia revisted: A state-of-the-art on pandemic-related fear, anxiety, and stress. *Journal of Anxiety Disorders*, *76*, 102326. Advance online publication. doi:10.1016/j.janxdis.2020.102326 PMID:33142124

Ávila, R., & Horvat, S. (Eds.). (2021). *Todo debe cambiar! El mundo después de la Covid-19* [Everything must change! The world after Covid-19]. Rayo Verde.

Blanchot, M. (1959). El diario íntimo y el relato [The intimate diary and the story]. *El libro por venir. Madrid. Trotta*, *2005*, 219–224.

Boccuti, A. (2020). Pandemia y literatura: variaciones erótico-sentimentales en la imaginación distópica [Pandemic and literature: erotic-sentimental variations in the dystopian imagination]. In *COVID19 – LiTraPan. Literary Training via ICT for Higher Education Improvement, Behavioral Coaching and Discomfort Management during the Coronavirus Pandemic [Branch: UniTo]. II International Symposium "Forbidden Delights: Sex, Eroticism, Beauty, Aesthetics, Pleasure, Law, Sin and Prohibition"*. Retrieved from https://www.youtube.com/watch?v=kQRss0sXAk8, 19

Bou, E. (1996). El diario: Periferia y literatura [The Journal: Periphery and literature]. Revista de Occidente, (102-103), 121-135.

Carrión, J. (2021). Narrativas de la pandemia [Narratives of the pandemic]. *La Vanguardia, Suplemento Culturals*. Retrieved from https://www.lavanguardia.com/cultura/culturas/20211127/7883333/narrativas-pandemia-libros-covid.html#foto-1

Catelli, N. (1996). El diario íntimo. Una posición femenina [The intimate diary. A female position]. Revista de Occidente, (102-103), 87-98.

Cavarero, A. (2000). Relating narratives. Storytelling and selfhood (P. A. Kottman, Trans.). Routledge.

Cortijo Ocaña, A., & Martines, V. (Eds.). (2022). Handbook of Research on Historical Pandemic Analysis and the Social Implications of COVID-19. IGI Global.

Didier, B. (1976). *Le journal intime* [The diary]. Presses Universitaires de France.

Didier, B. (1981). *L'écriture-femme* [Women's writing]. Presses Universitaires de France.

Didier, B. (1996). El diario ¿forma abierta? [The diary, open form?]. Revista de Occidente, (102-103), 39-46.

Fang, F. (2020). *Wuhan Diary. Dispatches from a Quarantined City* (M. Berry, Trans.). Ebook.

Fernández Prieto, C. (2004). Enunciación y comunicación en la autobiografía [Enunciation and communication in autobiography]. In C. Fernández Prieto & Ma Á. Hermosilla Álvarez (Eds.), Con la colaboración de A. Caballé. Autobiografía en España: un balance. Actas del Congreso Internacional celebrado en La Facultad de Filosofía y Letras de Córdoba del 25 al 27 de octubre de 2001 (pp. 417-432). Madrid: Visor.

Foucault, M. (1963). Le langage à l'infini [Language to infinity]. *Tel quel*, *15*, 44-53. Retrieved from https://www.idixa.net/Pixa/pagixa-1607121915.html

Freixas, L. (1996). Auge del diario ¿íntimo? [Rise of the intimate diary?]. Revista de Occidente, (102-103), 6-14.

Girard, A. (1996). El diario como género literario [The diary as a literary genre]. Revista de Occidente, (102-103), 31-38.

Greco, B. (2020). Amor y cuarentena en la narrativa breve de confinamiento [Love and quarantine in the short narrative of confinement]. In *COVID19 – LiTraPan. Literary Training via ICT for Higher Education Improvement, Behavioral Coaching and Discomfort Management during the Coronavirus Pandemic [Branch: UniTo], II International Symposium Forbidden Delights: Sex, Eroticism, Beauty, Aesthetics, Pleasure, Law, Sin and Prohibition. 19-20/06/2020.* Retrieved from https://www.youtube.com/watch?v=ki5DktWtYoA&feature=youtu.be

Greco, B. (2022). Pandemic and Literary Creativity. The Spanish Case of Relatos de confinamiento. In A. Cortijo Ocaña & V. Martines (Eds.), Handbook of Research on Historical Pandemic Analysis and the Social Implications of COVID-19 (pp. 80-93). IGI Global. doi:10.4018/978-1-7998-7987-9.ch007

Huertas, R. (2019). *Mujeres que leían* [Women who read]. Barcelona: Tres hermanas.

Huertas, R. (2021). *El tiempo que nos robaron* [The time they stole from us]. Barcelona: Tres hermanas.

Luque Amo, Á. (2016). *El diario personal en la literatura: teoría del diario literario* [The personal diary in literature: literary diary theory] (Vol. 7). Castilla. Estudios de Literatura., Retrieved from https://revistas.uva.es/index.php/castilla/article/view/315

Luque Amo, Á. (2020). *El diario literario. Poética e historia* [The Literary Journal. Poetics and history]. Peter Lang. doi:10.3726/b17261

Martens, L. (1985). *The Diary Novel.* Cambridge University Press. https://www.merriam-webster.com/dictionary/narrative

Mesa Gancedo, D. (2014). Diario y autoficción en la narrativa hispanoamericana contemporánea [Diary and autofiction in contemporary Latin American narrative]. In A. Casas (Ed.), *El yo fabulado* (pp. 191–206). Iberoamericana-Vervuert.

Mildonian, P. (2001). *Alterego. Racconti in forma di diario tra Otto e Novecento* [Alterego. Stories in diary form between the nineteenth and twentieth centuries]. Marsilio.

Monti, S. (Ed.). (2012). *Malattia e scrittura. Saperi medici, malattie e cure nelle letterature iberiche* [Illness and writing. Medical knowledge, diseases and cures in Iberian literature]. Cierre Grafica.

Muñoz Molina, A. (2020). Dar testimonio. Prólogo [Bear witness. Prologue]. In F. Fang (Ed.), *Diario de Wuhan. Sesenta días desde una ciudad en cuarentena*. Seix Barral. Trad. de Cheng L. Ning, Aurora Echevarría y Lorenzo Luego.

Orazi, V. (2020a). COVID19 – Literatura, interculturalitat, TIC, entrenament conductal i gestió de l'estrès durant la pandèmia per Coronavirus [Literature, Interculturality, ICT, behavioral training and stress management during the Covid-19 Pandemic]. In *Coneixement en temps de pandèmia*. Universitat d'Alacant. Seu Universitària de La Nucia. Retrieved from https://www.youtube.com/watch?v=PqVAi9-E2ro&fbclid=IwAR3dbgxgJylCSYOqTbn-BBv80WdVT0XdC-s8KYRHhgy7VRYnbex9PTZc_fQ

Orazi, V. (2020b). Sex and the Pandemic in *#Coronavirusplays*. In *COVID19 – LiTraPan. Literary Training via ICT for Higher Education Improvement, Behavioral Coaching and Discomfort Management during the Coronavirus Pandemic [Branch: UniTo], II International Symposium Forbidden Delights: Sex, Eroticism, Beauty, Aesthetics, Pleasure, Law, Sin and Prohibition*. Retrieved from https://www.youtube.com/watch?v=lp6jOx0EExY&feature=youtu.be

Orazi, V. (2022a). Jordi Casanovas' #Coronavirusplays: Spanish and Catalan microtheatre in the framework of the Project COVID-19 LiTraPan. In A. Cortijo Ocaña & V. Martines (Eds.), Handbook of Research on Historical Pandemic Analysis and the Social Implications of COVID-19 (pp. 175-194). IGI Global.

Orazi, V. (2022b). *Microteatro spagnolo e catalano al tempo della pandemia* [Spanish and Catalan microtheatre at the time of the pandemic]. Torino: Università di Torino. QuadRi – Quaderni di RiCOGNIZIONI XII.

Pellicer Vázquez, A. (2020). En *la* covid-19 [In covid-19]. In P. del Collado Lobatón, G. Nettel & Y. Weiss (Coords.), *Diario de la pandemia*. CulturaUNAM, Revista de la Universidad de México. Retrieved from https://www.revistadelauniversidad.mx/articles/40d935fa-99ad-4d1d-ac3e-2047e0a01421/en-la-covid19

Pesaro, N. (2021). Fang Fang e le altre: la narrazione femminile del virus in Cina [Fang Fang and the others: the female narrative of the virus in China]. *DEP. Deportate, Esuli, Profughe*, *45*, 227-251. Retrieved from https://www.unive.it/pag/fileadmin/user_upload/dipartimenti/DSLCC/documenti/DEP/numeri/n45/24_Pesaro.pdf

Piccone Stella, S. (2008). *In prima persona. Scrivere un diario* [Firsthand. Write a journal]. Il Mulino.

Porter Abbott, H. (1984). *Diary fiction. Writing as action*. Cornell University Press.

Raoul, V. (1989). Women and Diaries: Gender and Genre. *Mosaic: A Journal for the Interdisciplinary Study of Literature*, *22*(3), 57-65. Retrieved from https://www.jstor.org/stable/24780526

Romera Castillo, J. (n.d.). *Literatura y vida en la España actual* [Literature and life in today's Spain]. SELITEN@T. Retrieved from https://www2.uned.es/centro-investigacion-SELITEN@T/pdf/autobio/I2.pdf

Sabucedo, J.M., Alzate, M., & Hur, D. (2020). COVID-19 y la metáfora de la guerra [COVID-19 and the metaphor of war]. *International Journal of Social Psychology, 35*(3), 618-624. doi:10.1080/02134748.2020.1783840

Sánchez-Villena, A. R. & V. de La Fuente-Figuerola (2020). COVID-19: Quarantine, isolation, social distancing and lockdown: Are they the same? *Anales de Pediatría, 93*(1), 73-74. doi:10.1016/j.anpedi.2020.05.001

SELITEN@T: A bibliographic guide on (auto)biographical writing. (n.d.). Retrieved from https://www2.uned.es/centro-investigacion-SELITEN@T/escritura_autobio.html

Trapiello, A. (1998). *El escritor de diarios. Historia de un desplazamiento* [The diary writer. History of a displacement]. Península.

Žižek, S. (2020). *Pandemic! COVID-19 Shakes the World*. Polity.

ADDITIONAL READING

Alberca, M. (2000). *La escritura invisible. Testimonios sobre el diario íntimo* [Invisible writing. Testimonies about the intimate diary]. Oyarzun: Sendoa.

Baricco, A. (2021). *Lo que estábamos buscando. De la pandemia como creatura mítica* [What we were looking for. Of the pandemic as a mythical creature]. Anagrama.

Bou, E. (2018). Teorías del diario. A propósito de Iñaki Uriarte y Pere Rovira [Theories of the diary. About Iñaki Uriarte and Pere Rovira]. In G. Laín Corona & R. Santiago Nogales (Eds.), *Cartografía literaria en homenaje al Profesor José Romera Castillo* (pp. 375–390). Visor Libros.

Caballé, A. (1995). *Narcisos de tinta: ensayos sobre la literatura autobiográfica en lenguaje castellano (siglos XIX y XX)* [Ink Daffodils: Essay on Autobiographical Literature in Spanish Language (centuries XIX and XX)]. Megazul.

Dahl, L. (2021). Loneliness during the COVID-19 pandemic. Aging & Mental Health, 25(7), 1161–1164. doi:10.1080/13607863.2021.1875195

Darici, K. (2022). Sherezade en el búnker, un cuento pandémico de Marta Sanz [Sherezade in the bunker, a pandemic tale by Marta Sanz]. *eHumanista/IVITRA*, 21. https://www.ehumanista.ucsb.edu/ivitra/volume/21

Ferrús Antón, B. (2004). Escribirse como mujer: autobiografía y género [Writing as a woman: autobiography and gender]. In C. Fernández Prieto & Ma Á. Hermosilla Álvarez (Eds.), In cooperation with A. Caballé. Autobiografía en España: un balance. Actas del Congreso Internacional celebrado en La Facultad de Filosofía y Letras de Córdoba del 25 al 27 de octubre de 2001 (pp. 433-443). Madrid: Visor.

Freixas, L. (2013). Prólogo [Prologue]. In A. Gide (Ed.), *Diario* (pp. 9–30). Alba.

Giordano, P. (2020). En tiempos de contagio [In times of contagion]. *Salamandra (Frankfurt)*.

Girard, A. (1963). *Le journal intime* [The diary]. PUF.

Gracia, J. (2004). La voz literaria y la materia del dietarista [The literary voice and the matter of the dietitarian]. In C. Fernández Prieto & Ma Á. Hermosilla Álvarez (Eds.), Con la colaboración de A. Caballé. Autobiografía en España: un balance. Actas del Congreso Internacional celebrado en La Facultad de Filosofía y Letras de Córdoba del 25 al 27 de octubre de 2001 (pp. 223-233). Madrid: Visor.

Hierro, M. (1999). La comunicación callada de la literatura: Reflexión teórica sobre el diario íntimo [The quiet communication of literature: theoretical reflection on the intimate diary]. *Mediatika, 7*, 103–127.

Lejeune, P. (1994). *El pacto autobiográfico* [The autobiographical pact]. Megazul.

Lejeune, P. (2009). *On Diary*. University of Hawai'i Press. doi:10.1515/9780824863784

Macip, S. (2021). *Lecciones de una pandemia. Ideas para enfrentarse a los retos de salud planetaria* [Lessons from a pandemic. Ideas to face the challenges of planetary health]. Anagrama.

Pardo, J. L. (1996). *La intimidad* [Intimacy]. Pre-Textos.

Quintana Trias, L. (2020). La literatura confinada [Confined literature]. *L'Avenç, 467*.

Rodríguez Ferrándiz, R. (2020). Magias de la ficción [Magics of fiction]. *Devenir*.

Romera Castillo, J. (2004). Algo más sobre el estudio de la escritura diarística en España [Something more about the study of diaristic writing in Spain]. In C. Fernández Prieto & Ma Á. Hermosilla Álvarez (Eds.), In cooperation with A. Caballé. Autobiografía en España: un balance. Actas del Congreso Internacional celebrado en La Facultad de Filosofía y Letras de Córdoba del 25 al 27 de octubre de 2001 (pp. 223-233). Madrid: Visor.

KEY TERMS AND DEFINITIONS

Diary Fiction: Fictive diary; fiction in the form of a journal.

Confined or Pandemic Narrative: Narrative on pandemic produced during COVID-19 lockdown.

Coronaphobia: Fear of the coronavirus, SARS-CoV-2.

National Applause for Coronavirus Health Workers (Aplauso por los trabajadores de la salud): It was an applause given by the population as a sign of recognition and gratitude to health professionals in tribute to their work during the COVID-19 (SARS-CoV-2) pandemic. It was an activity that emerged mainly in January 2020 in the Chinese city of Wuhan, the origin of the pandemic, and then spread to several countries around the world during the quarantines (among others Spain, Italy, Great Britain). Particularly in Spain 8 p.m. was the time set for the national applause.

Post-COVID-19 Era: The world after COVID-19 Pandemic.

ENDNOTES

1 Andrés Felipe Solano (born in Bogotá, 1977) is a Colombian novelist, author of *Los días de la fiebre* (2020), a literary account of the pandemic as he experiences it while living in Seoul.

2 "Pese a sus orígenes antitéticos –Sanz compila sus publicaciones en Instagram y Muñoz Molina, que escribe a mano con pluma estilográfica, parte de anotaciones cotidianas para acabar firmando un libro de memorias–, ambos libros tienen otros llamativos puntos en común, además de haber sido escritos y vividos en Madrid durante y después de la cuarentena. Los dos autores utilizan el presente pandémico para explorar la dimensión más emocional de sus recuerdos; hablan con calidez de parejas, familia o amigos; leen más que nunca; y coinciden en destacar la importancia de sus casas, sus plantas y sus animales de compañía. La gata Calabardina en el caso Sanz y, en el de Muñoz Molina, la perra Lolita". ["Despite their antithetical origins —Sanz compiles her publications on Instagram and Muñoz Molina writes by hand with a fountain pen, starting with everyday notes and ending up with a book of memoirs— both books have striking points in common other than having been written and experienced in Madrid during and after the quarantine. Both authors use the pandemic present to explore the more emotional dimension of their memories; they speak warmly of partners and their family or friends; they read more than ever; and they both highlight the importance of their homes, plants and pets. Calabardina, a cat, in Sanz's case and Lolita, a dog, in the case of Muñoz Molina"] (Carrión 2021: n.p.).

3 Italics in the original. Also: original orthography of the word "sólo".

4 "Aplaudimos mucho, con los vecinos, a los autobuses, a los bomberos que dan vueltas por la plaza haciendo sonar las sirenas, a quienes trabajan para todos, a los que se quedan en casa, a los que resisten". ["Together with the neighbours we do a lot of applauding the buses, the firemen who go around the square sounding their sirens, the people who work for everyone, those who stay at home, those who resist"] (Huertas 2021: 43)

5 The use of war metaphors to refer to the pandemic and their normalisation in the lexicon of governments and ordinary people is not uncommon. According to Sabucedo *et. al.*, the metaphor serves as a "rhetorical device" capable of converting the unexpected and extraordinary situation (such as the pandemic), that is, the unknown, into something known and somehow acceptable (2020: 618-619).

6 My translation.

Chapter 5
August Bover, "El contagi" (2021):
Pandemic, Isolation, and the Therapeutic Power of Poetry

Veronica Orazi
Università degli Studi di Torino, Italy

ABSTRACT

In November 2021, August Bover (Barcelona 1949) published the collection of poems El Contagi. His previous poetic works include En pèlag d'amor (1999); L'hivern sota el Cadí (2001); Mojave (2006); the bilingual anthology Vicino al mare (2006); Terres de llicorella. Imatges del Priorat (2008); the trilogy Cloc! (2011), Beabà (2014), and Tornaveu (2018); and the collection of poetry and prose Blau marí (2018). El Contagi contains 41 poems which, with the exception of the last one ("Senyal?"), were composed between March and June 2020, during the lockdown that was decreed in an attempt to contain contagions in the first phase of the pandemic. This contribution synthesises the results of the study of the text, according to the methodology based on the objectivisation, problematisation, and literarisation of the experience of the pandemic and its psychological consequences. This kind of investigation focuses on the use of literature as a therapeutic tool, in order to face, process, and progressively overcome the trauma caused by this impactful experience.

INTRODUCTION

In November 2021 August Bover (Barcelona, 1949) published the collection of poems *El Contagi* [The Contagion]. In it, the author expresses his experience of the pandemic and isolation through the filter of poetry. In this way, the act of poetic composition and the resulting verses make it possible to express and convey thoughts, sensations, and feelings, both positive and negative, but also acquire a therapeutic function. Al this turns into a therapy of the self, which becomes a collective therapy through sharing a common experience, even and especially in a dramatic moment like the one from which these verses are inspired. Thus, poetry becomes a space of freedom, a self-managed perimeter, in which to allow

DOI: 10.4018/978-1-6684-4735-2.ch005

joys and fears, hopes and frustrations to emerge and flow, to shape and communicate to oneself and to readers an unprecedented, unimaginable experience, to objectify and observe it from the outside, and to transform it into a starting point for reflection on known and unknown aspects from a subjective and collective perspective. This double vision, individual and shared, derives from a common experience, from thoughts and states of mind that have affected each individual as well as the entire global community, which was (and still is) sharing an epochal and difficult phase in the history of the planet and of mankind.

August Bover gives form to all this through the poetic word, which becomes the instrument for (self-) therapy, a reflection so profound that it seems to be a process of self-analysis. This is the way to start dealing with the unknown and the unimaginable: how to live through and survive an epoch-making event such as the one the planet is experiencing from the early 2020s, and to do so through writing. Literature, in this case poetry, reveals this component, that at first glance might be surprising, but that constitutes its essence: its cathartic and curative, therapeutic and almost thaumaturgical power, which emanates from the balm of the writer's (narrator, poet, playwright) words.

These pages summarize the results of the *El Contagi* [The Contagion] study from this perspective: how literature, more specifically poetry, proves to be a therapeutic tool for the author and the reader. This happens thanks to a mechanism of objectification, problematization and literalization of the trauma, of what strikes and upsets in the depths and nevertheless, and precisely for this reason, needs to be addressed. This collection of poems also fulfils this function, as do other works of other genres (fiction, drama, graphic novels, etc.), that have been written since the first phase of the pandemic and have sometimes been published online and then in print or have appeared directly in print. The results confirm the assumptions of this type of research and recognize the added value of these texts, in addition to their artistic-literary and aesthetic relevance, the poignancy of the themes dealt with, and the peculiar strength of this artistic individuality, the expression of a voice that is always powerful and always different.

AUGUST BOVER AND HIS POETRY

The author is a Professor Emeritus of Catalan Philology at the University of Barcelona, member of the Secció Filològica of the Institut d'Estudis Catalans, scholar, essayist, writer and poet. His previous books of poetry include *En pèlag d'amor* [In Pelagic of Love] (1999), *L'hivern sota el Cadí* [The Winter under the Cadí] (2001), *Mojave* [Mojave] (2006), the bilingual anthology –in Catalan and Italian– *Vicino al mare* [Near the Sea] (2006), *Terres de llicorella. Imatges del Priorat* [Liquorice Lands. Images of the Priorat] (2008) and the trilogy *Cloc!* [Cloc!] (2011, re-edited in 2014), *Beabà* [Spelling Book] (2014) and *Tornaveu* [Echo] (2018), and the collection of poetry and prose *Blau marí* [Navy Blue] (2018). His poems have been translated into English, French, German, Spanish, Italian, Occitan, Finnish, Korean and Japanese. Together with the soprano and cellist Eulàlia Ara, he created the Taller de Vora Mar, and produce poetic and musical performances based on his poems and on the music of the compositor Manuel Garcia Morante. His prose works include the diary of his stay in Canada (1976-1977), *Dotze llunes a Saskatchewan. Impressions des de la Gran Pradeia canadenca* [Twelve Moons in Saskatchewan. Impressions from the Canadian Great Prairie] (re-edition 2013), and the very recent collection of anecdotes *Tutti frutti* [Tutti Frutti] (2021). August Bover has always developed a solid and profound production, supported by impeccable writing, great vivacity, surprising naturalness and a solid knowledge of poetry, nourished by reading, studying and developing a personal aesthetic. This is a process that starts from the classical and popular tradition, from rhetoric to themes, authors and currents, both foreign and Catalan, to reach a highly original and personal aesthetic within Catalan lyric production, which the poet has enriched with his own work.

In order to present, albeit in extreme synthesis, the fundamental aspects of August Bover's writing, some works are, in my opinion, especially significant: *Blau marí* [Navy Blue] and the trilogy inspired by the OULIPO poetry.

The title of the collection *Blau marí* [Navy Blue] derives from the colour of the Mediterranean, which links all the texts in the collection. It is an intense blue, which should not only be seen as a chromatic reference but also as a reference to the sea and the culture that flourishes on its shores, a transnational heritage that recalls Greece, Naples, Alghero, Menorca and Barcelona. The first, Greece, is the radiating point of this shared essence, which spreads through a route made up of ports of call and stops in the Mediterranean basin. Along this poetic journey emerges a rich variety of tones and accents, metrical and formal choices, alternating between haiku, poetic prose, sonnets, ballads and songs. Cohesion is ensured precisely by the perspective of the sentimental, moral, aesthetic and cultural journey that starts with classical Greece, passes through the Florentine Renaissance, the Neapolitan Baroque and arrives at Jacint Verdaguer's *Renaixença*, Joan Maragall's *Modernisme* and Josep Carner.

The reading of *Blau marí* [Navy Blue] traces a peculiar geography, with its images linked to the author's journey and stay in those places, its great capacity for evocation which, together with personal experiences, identifies its essence. The poet, however, goes beyond the topicality of Mediterranean poetry: in the stopovers of this journey, he skirts the Mediterranean basin, passing through different cities and places, in an itinerary that reflects the author's writing, who stops, lives, writes and remembers these places. *Blau marí* [Navy Blue], therefore, embodies a Mediterranean poetics made up of experience, memory and evocations, as the poet illustrates in the *Nota de l'autor* [Author's Note], entitled *La vida a riba mar* [Life by the Sea] (Bover, 2018b, pp. 95-101).

The work is divided into three sections, *Garraf* [Garraf], *Els estudis dels nois de casa* [The Studies of the Boys of the House] and *De Grècia a Barcelona, amb escales a Nàpols, l'Alguer i Menorca* [From Greece to Barcelona, with Stops in Naples, Alghero and Menorca]. All of them are expressions of lived geographies linked to personal and collective roots, in which local elements are projected towards universal aspects.

The first section, *Garraf* [Garraf], refers to the living environment and to the origins of the poet. This part is a tribute to Sitges, the author's adopted country. In it, he uses the mythical landscape to evoke the beauty of the rural dimension and to criticise the degradation caused by human action. The second section, *Els estudis dels nois de casa* [The Studies of the Boys of the House], contains five poems. Here, the father-son relationship takes shape and becomes a poetic and narrative presence, expressed with restrained tenderness and irony. In this second part, the importance of the domestic sphere also emerges, together with a reflection on the relativity of individual, personal and human history. The third section, *De Grècia a Barcelona, amb escales a Nàpols, l'Alguer i Menorca* [From Greece to Barcelona, with Stops in Naples, Alghero and Menorca], is inspired by the poet's journeys from East to West. The verses echo the Catalan tradition and describe Delphos, Athens, Aegina and Sunio, linking past and present, myth, history and personal experience. The stay in Naples refers to the experience of the author and other writers and artists who preceded him in the city. The vision is sometimes deliberately circumscribed, otherwise it unfolds generously across the city. All of this constitutes the preparation for the poems and poetic prose that close the collection, dedicated to Barcelona, the poet's native city, which represents his homeland, childhood, lost paradise, militant youth and a disturbing, conflicting, traumatic and yet hopeful present. These poems speak of the desire to embrace life in all its complexity and contradictions.

In Bover's production, *Blau marí* [Navy Blue] represents the contribution of a rich literary background, of an important cultural legacy, that of his origins and belonging. In the book, the word expresses with profound intensity a free, passionate, committed and tender vision, which reaches its absolute fullness.

Bover's Oulipian poetry trilogy offers a different but equally suggestive perspective. With the publication of the collection *Tornaveu* [Echo] (2018), the poet completes a poetic triptych including *Cloc!* [Cloc!] (2011, then 2014) and *Beabà* [Spelling Book] (2014). The publication of the third volume of the trilogy marks a significant moment in the author's lyrical trajectory, characterised by intensity and depth of expression and a series of variations on themes and modes that have always made his voice unique. Again, Bover's poetry blends with the work of another artist, in this case, the painter Pere Capellà Simó, who illustrates the trilogy.

The prologue to *Cloc!* [Cloc!], by Màrius Serra, with the significant title *Boverisme* [Boverism], describes the phenomenon alluded to in the definition he coined to introduce the collection: the state of mind that the reader is about to activate, and which will enable him to approach the author and share his vision. This "boverisme" ["boverism"] is fed by the verbal inventiveness an in it order and chaos, sign and verb, converge. In *Cloc!* [Cloc!], the author dialogues with the tradition of potential literature, initiated by the French mathematicians and poets of the Oulipo group. The collection opens up new perspectives on potential literature in Catalan language, through the concepts of constraint and obstacle, which are the conditions for writing. This results in the self-imposition of restrictions that complicate the flow of writing and at the same time stimulate it, directing it towards new paths. In these verses, Bover confines himself in a labyrinth full of difficulties, which leads him to the creation of magnificent verses: poems with echoes, gentiles and ethnicities, monovocalic and monosyllabic lipograms, and tautograms. However, the poet also creates new compositional mechanisms or renews others that have already been tried out, and the result is a creative vortex in which the poet captivates the reader.

The second collection of the trilogy, *Beabà* [Spelling Book], continues the Oulipian experimentation. In this case, the *contrainte* at the basis of the Oulipian poetic mechanism is renewed even more profoundly or is the result of an original creation. If in *Cloc!* [Cloc!] the constraint varied from poem to poem, in *Beabà* [Spelling Book] every poem is a tautogram, in which the initial letter of all words is always the same. The collection reflects the structure of a primer, and the poems are arranged alphabetically. This evocative poetic syllabary reinterprets this concept and its basic compositional mechanism in a surprising way: an entire poem is dedicated to each letter, created through a series of complex procedures, made even more challenging by a further self-imposed metric constraint. So, the text makes sublime use of Catalan's lexical richness, and the collection ends up being a syllabary of national culture, rooted in the historical past and projected into the future. This aspect is reinforced by the almost total absence of the poetic first person, of memory and subjective experience.

Tornaveu [Echo], as mentioned, closes the trilogy dedicated to potential poetry. One of the main aspects of the work is the strong impulse to spread the Oulipo movement and its techniques in the Catalan context and to overcome the naive vision of this subgenre. The collection emphasizes the poetic research on the language and the possibilities of renewing it. It takes its everyday and conventional uses to extremes, enhances the playful potential of speech, creates daring ludo-linguistic inventions and stresses the process of morphological purification.

In short, this trilogy constitutes another challenge oriented towards poetic research and experimentation, characteristic of the author's entire lyrical trajectory.

THE CONTEXT: THE COVID-19 PANDEMIC

The worldwide diffusion of the Covid-19 disease had and is still having a huge impact on the world's population and radically transformed the life of the planet's inhabitants (Sohrabi et al., 2020; Pengfei et al., 2020). This is an epochal event and consequently everybody had to face with limitations in everyday life, such as isolation. As to be expected, the pandemic had also psychological and behavioral implications, such as typical acute stress responses, because it suddenly and unpredictably created a rapid and diffuse uncertainty and undermined the conviction of both personal and societal sense of safety. The negative psychological impact of a pandemic, of the consequent isolation, quarantine and of other measures to cope with it is well-known, due to its consequences for subjective as well as collective psychological health. Although, this type of relapse is less visible than others (Brooks et al., 2020) and that is why psychological health is probably the most neglected aspect of the actual situation (Schimmenti, Billieux, and Starcevic 2020, p. 41; Marazziti 2020, pp. 39-40).

From a psychological and behavioral point of view, the present pandemic needs also attention and interventions in supporting people in isolation to face the consequences of quarantine, as reclusion and other restrictions (Brooks et al., 2020). It also must be taken into consideration the unavoidable long-term psychological disorders and how to prevent them (Xiang et al., 2020; Srivatsa and Stewart, 2020; Marazziti and Stahl, 2020) as well as the psychologically negative impact of the resulting economic crisis (Marazziti et al., 2020).

One of the most relevant consequences of the Coronavirus pandemic and the resulting lockdown and isolation is the change of the perception of space and time. Whereas previously existed an outdoor space and an indoor space, during quarantine the individual found himself isolated in a single space, i.e., the place where he spent the lockdown. In the same way, the distinction between the idea and perception of a public space and a private space has therefore disappeared. Similarly, the temporal dimension has also been altered: whereas previously existed a public-professional time and a private-leisure time, now in the single place in which the individual is confined, public and private time also coexist and end up overlapping each other. Thus, in the scenario generated by the pandemic and lockdown, existence in isolation flows in a mono-time within the mono-space in which one is confined.

With regard to psychological reactions to this situation, the most evident one was the emergence of fear and anxiety (Schimmenti, Billieux, and Starcevic, 2020): facing them is critical on the individual level, but effective coping them can also help the entire community to manage in a better way the situation, because the resilience of a society dealing with a pandemic also depends on how its members endure their anxiety and fear of loneliness, contagion and death (Schimmenti, Billieux, and Starcevic, 2020, pp. 41-43).

PILOT METHODOLOGY AND STUDIES

This abnormal context brought out strongly the need to express and share the experience that all individuals were having. From the very beginning of the pandemic, the field of artistic creation powerfully manifested the overwhelming drive to elaborate the impactful experience of the pandemic and the isolation. This specific response has given rise to an abundant and very interesting production concerning different types of artistic expression (literature, plastic and figurative arts, photography, music, etc.) and more specifically various literary genres (short story, drama, graphic novel, etc.) (Orazi 2022a, pp.

179-180). This artistic and, in particular, literary production is of great interest and inspired the planning of an international project starting in March 2020: COVID19 LiTraPan – Literary Training via ICT for Higher Education Improvement, Behavioral Coaching and Discomfort Management (Orazi, 2022a). One of the research lines of the project consists of studying the literalization of the individual and collective reactions to the pandemic, initially disseminated through the Internet and social networks and subsequently, in some cases, in paper format or as an electronic edition. The project fits in with the lines of research that characterize the present situation and the progressive approximation to the new reality. Indeed, already in early 2020 appeared some key studies that reoriented teaching/learning and research/dissemination as well as the promotion of innovation (*The COVID-19 Outbreak* 2020; or the materials published by the UNESCO member International Association of Universities, https://www.iau-aiu.net/Covid-19-Higher-Education-challenges-and-responses). These contributions study the alteration of space-time perception, isolation and its consequences, the change in interpersonal dynamics and the resulting behavioral responses, the need to manage stress and consolidate resilience.

The initial phase of the project included the creation of corpora to collect cases of literalization of the pandemic. So, the census and collection of disciplinary content inspired by the pandemic, created and disseminated via the web during the emergency began, in order to feed corpora for use in disciplinary teaching, individual and group research, discomfort management and resilience building. The first phase results were presented in May and June 2020 within a cycle of videoconferences (*Coneixement en temps de pandèmia* [Knowledge in Times of Pandemic], from 22 May to 22 June 2020) and an International Virtual Symposium (*Forbidden Delights*, 19 and 20 June 2020) organized by the University of Alicante (Seu Universitària de la Nucia).

Regarding the corpora, microplays, plays, tales and short stories, comics and graphic novels have been collected. All these works use literary expression (utopian or dystopian, fantastic and neo-fantastic, comic-humoristic and parodic, absurd and non-sense, catastrophic, apocalyptic, horror, science fiction, etc.) to reflect the individual and collective response to the experience of the pandemic and can work as a tool to elaborate stress/trauma and overcome the present crisis.

The most interesting aspect was to note how these literary transpositions of the pandemic experience fit in with the findings of the psychological and neuropsychiatric studies conducted since the beginning of the virus outbreak. The most evident individual and societal reaction to this situation was the emergence of different fear and anxieties. At a psychological level, they are manifested in four domains: corporal, interpersonal, cognitive and behavioral (Schimmenti, Billieux, and Starcevic, 2020, p. 41). The classification of the four fear domains can be summarized as follows:

- **Corporal domain:** fear OF the body / fear FOR the body
  the subject perceives her/his body as a potential source of danger via infection, as a threat; or as a treasure that may be lost and that s/he must protect.
- **Interpersonal domain:** fear OF others / fear FOR others
  the subject perceives that the others could infect her/him; or that her/his beloved ones could be infected by others.
- **Cognitive domain:** fear OF knowing / fear of NOT knowing
  the subject avoids knowing what s/he thinks is better left unknown; or s/he wants to know, due to the impression of partial and therefore unsettling knowledge.
- **Behavioral domain:** fear OF acting / fear of NOT acting

the subject is afraid to take actions that could put her/him at risk of becoming infected; or s/he is afraid to be unable to act, even to guarantee her/his safety.

Based on the close correspondence between the results of scientific research and the literatization of lived experience, it was possible to identify the constitutive structure of these literary transpositions, whatever genre they belong to. This showed that certain psychological-behavioral responses are precisely reflected in the literary work. This should not come as a surprise, because artistic creation expresses mechanisms of signification connected with what can be described as collective archetypes, which can turn in a source of inspiration for artistic creation.

On the basis of an inductive study of the attestations collected in the corpora, it was possible to outline the constitutive structure of these literary manifestations, regardless of the literary genre to which they are to be ascribed. The shared macrostructure presents certain fundamental elements, that are enriched by other constituent and accessory elements, depending on the literary genre to which every work refers and on its peculiar structural and signification characteristics.

This has made it possible to develop a methodological model (Orazi, 2022a, pp. 183-186; Orazi 2022b, p. 23) for the study of such artistic production, which results have been published recently or are currently in press (Boccuti, 2020, 2022; Cortijo Ocaña-Martines, 2022; Cortijo Ocaña, Martines-Orazi, 2022, Darici 2022a, 2022b, Greco, 2020, 2022a, 2022b, 2022c; Orazi 2020a, 2020b, 2022a, 2022b, 2022c; Vacalebri 2020, 2022a, 2022b).

As the results of the study show, it is possible to outline the constitutive macrostructure shared by the different attestations collected in the corpora as follows:

- **Locutor:** delivers a Soliloquy-Monologue / establishes a Dialogue
- Locutor > Recipient (the Locutor himself / a present or absent character)
- Direct or Mediated communication (the latter can be live or deferred)
- **Topic/s:** issues related with the COVID-19 pandemic
- Literary frame/features/references: dramatic, tragic, sentimental, comic, humoristic, parodic, absurd and non-sense, catastrophic, apocalyptic, horror, science fiction, utopian, dystopian, (neo-) fantastic, etc.
- (Possible) Final twist that subverts the situation
- Open / Closed ending
- **Fear Domain:** Corporal, Interpersonal, Cognitive, Behavioral

Using this model and the illustrated methodology, Bover's last collection of poems dedicated to the experience of the pandemic was analyzed. It was found that it presents elements that are shared with the other works collected in the corpora, at the level of macrostructure, of constituent features, and even of more nuanced ones, concerning both the text and its message. The results of the study carried out on this Bover's poetic work demonstrate its compliance with the model identified. At the same time, they underline the peculiarities of his poems, which constitute a kind of variation on the theme of isolation, a central one to the author's experience and sensitivity. These variations are due both to the uniqueness of the author's voice and to the literary genre to which the work refers and, precisely for this reason, offer suggestive evidence of the manifestation of these themes through poetic expression.

EL CONTAGI [THE CONTAGION] (2021)

As mentioned, the collection is the result of the isolation to which the author, like everyone else, was forced in the early months of 2020, when the initial phase of the rapid spread of the virus forced the governments of many countries around the world to declare a state of alert and impose a lockdown. The book is complemented by several paratexts: a prologue by the epidemiologist Antoni Trilla; eight epigraphs, taken from different works of different periods, referred to epidemics and pandemics of the past; and a final note by August Bover, written a few months after the period of composition of the verses. The collection consists of 41 poems, which, with the exception of the last one –*Senyal?* [Signal?]–, were composed between March and June 2020, during the lockdown that was decreed in an attempt to contain contagions during the first period of the Coronavirus pandemic. The titles of the poems, which are also key paratextual elements, are always significant and hint very effectively at the content of the poems, sometimes metaphorically or by exploiting contrast and oxymoron.

The poems are illustrated by Alba Gàmiz and also offer an interesting hybridization of text and image. The graphic artist created the drawings that accompany every single poem and gave them to the author as a gift to celebrate the feast day of Sant Jordi (the *Diada de Sant Jordi*), which could not be celebrated in 2020 due to the pandemic. The inspiration for the drawings, therefore, stems from one of the subthemes dealt with in the collection, as in other works composed at the time on the theme of the pandemic, namely that of uncelebrated festivities, both personal (birthdays, anniversaries) and moments of collective gathering (civil and religious festivities and feasts).

Bover's poems reflect the experience of those dramatic days, when an unknown and terrible phase began for the whole humanity, which duration and evolution were unknown. In each of them, the poet captures with immediacy, capacity for synthesis and uncommon sensitivity the feelings and conflicting sensations that we have all experienced during the pandemic. With his usual formal rigor and verses ranging from tetrasyllabic to decasyllabic, in varied strophic forms, such as *dècimes* and sonnets, Bover leads the reader through an anomalous time, made of observing the outside world from inside our homes and of holidays cancelled, due to isolation and distancing measures.

The poems were written in Sitges, where the poet has lived for many years. They develop some themes that undoubtedly have a therapeutic effect: they offer the reader the possibility of satisfying the need for balance through a poetic pause, whose topics we share as the result of a global experience. It will make it possible to start expressing, objectifying and processing the trauma, both individual and collective, that this hard and unprecedented time represents for everyone.

The Paratexts: The prologue

The book opens with a Prologue by Antoni Trilla, epidemiologist at the Hospital Clínic in Barcelona and Professor of Salut Pública at the University of Barcelona. He defined these verses as "poemes de la pandèmia. Poemes pandèmics" [poems of the pandemic. Pandemic poems] (Trilla, 2021, p. 13) and pointed out that

> *la pandemia de la Covid-19 ha alterat i trasbalsat el món, ha dut els sistemes sanitaris propers a límits que no ens podíem imaginar, ha danyat greument l'economia, ha canviat la nostra forma de vida, ha restringit el moviment de persones i mercaderies i, en resum, ha incidit negativament en tota la nostra societat (Trilla, 2021, p. 13).*

[the Covid-19 pandemic has altered and upended the world, it has pushed healthcare systems to limits we could not imagine, it has seriously damaged the economy, it has changed our way of life, it has restricted the movement of people and goods and, in short, has had a negative impact on our entire society]

Trilla therefore summarizes in a few pages the description of an impactful and tremendous era and does so from the perspective of the doctor. Once again, from his words as well as from reading the neuropsychiatric and psychological studies consulted, there is a striking correspondence between what science has found and the key aspects of the works composed during the pandemic to express this anomalous experience, including the one under analysis. As mentioned above, the artistic and literary production created since March 2020 that revolves around this theme has a number of basic elements that return systematically in each of them. These shared elements represent the constitutive structure of a thematic nucleus articulated in subthemes, variously declined from work to work, but still an expression of the same matrix. Such common matrix derives from a psychological experience, from the response of body and mind to the health emergency that united the entire mankind in the scenario of an incredible and destabilizing dystopia that suddenly seemed to have turned into reality. Trilla's dense prologue refers precisely to this: to a reality, our reality, made up of science and *humanitas*, in which the two elements, apparently independent and even perceived as antithetical, turn out to be two inseparable components of human nature. This is why he writes, talking about the content of the book, "els seus poemes, les seves reflexions, són també curative" [his poems, his reflections, are also healing] (Trilla, 2021, p. 15). The therapeutic power of poetry reaffirms itself, helping us to deal with the discomfort produced by the isolation to which the pandemic has forced us.

The Paratexts: The Epigraphs

Paratexts play a key role, orienting the reader and creating a precise horizon of expectation. The title, for example, is quite transparent and focuses the reader's attention on what was perhaps the greatest fear experienced globally, namely, the fear of contagion, of disease, of consequences that could be fatal. It also indirectly emphasizes the body, our body and the body of others, an ambivalent element, to be taken care of and at the same time a vehicle for the virus. From the very title, the focus is on this key aspect, that underpins the entire collection and every single poem in it, as will be seen below.

Epigraphs, likewise, are especially significant:

En aquell temps, es va declarar una epidèmia que de poc no acaba amb tot el gènere humà (…). Aquells dies semblava que no era gens fàcil veure ningú als llocs públics, almenys a Bisanci, sinó tots els que resultava que estaven sans es quedaven a casa

(Procopi, Història de les guerres [History of Wars], II, 22-23, sec. VI).

[At that time, an epidemic was declared that almost did not end the entire human race (…). In those days it seemed that it was not at all easy to see anyone in public places, at least in Byzantium, but everyone who happened to be healthy stayed at home]

Experiència mostre cascun jorn que can foch se pren en alcun alberch, que tots los vehins n'an temor, e.ls qui pus prop li son major deven haver pahor. Per què, com aja ohit dir a persones dignes de fe que epidímia ho pestilència e mortaldats de gents regnen e han regnat en algunes partides e regions a nos vehines, si n'é dupte ni pahor, no s'és maraveylla

(Jacme d'Agramont, Regiment de preservació a epidímia o pestilència e mortaldats [Epidemic or pestilence and mortality regiment], 1348).

[Experience shows every day that when a fire takes place in a building, all the neighbors are afraid of it, and those who are near it must be afraid. Because, as I have heard from people trustworthy who say that epidemics, pestilence, and deaths of people reign and have reigned in some parts and regions in our neighbors, if there is doubt or fear, it is not surprising]

(…) encara és universalment en memòria de cascuns, la pestilencial mortaldat que poch ha és pasada, la qual cascuns avem vista e per aquella avem lançades innumerables làgremes, les quals portam encara scrites en los nostres fronts

(Giovanni Boccaccio, Decameron [Decameron], 1350-1353).

[(…) it is still universally in the memory of everyone, the pestilential mortality that has just passed, which everyone has seen and for which we have cried countless tears, which we still carry written in our frontheads]

XVII. Ítem, se mane que ninguna persona de casa sospitosa puga ixir de aquella y anar per la ciutat sots graves penes, per no ne succehir inconvenients y danys, y que las guàrdies li haien de servir y dar tot lo recapte necessari

(Quinto Tiberio Angelerio, Instructions dal matés auctor dades axí al principi com en tot lo progrés de la sobredita pesta als magnífichs señors jurats del regiment de la ciutat de l'Alguer, l'any MDLXXXII y MDLXXXIII [Instructions of the same author, both at the beginning and throughout the progress of the above-mentioned plague, to the magnificent gentlemen of the regiment of the city of Alghero, years MDLXXXII and MDLXXXIII], 1588).

[XVII. Item, it is ordered that no person of a suspicious house may leave that house and go through the city under severe penalties, so that inconvenience and damage do no occur, and that the guards should serve him and give him all the necessary revenue]

Diumenja, als 8 de janer de dit any [1651], en una casa del carrer Nou, que.s deya Martín de Langa, que era sego, s'i morí una donzella, parenta de sa muller; y, de prompte, se enmaltí sa muller, la qual també va morir; y algunes persones que avíen entrevingut en ditas malaltias també se enmaltiren. Sabut assó per los consellés, anaren dit dia, en la nit – per no enmalaltir la gent ho no espantar-los –: feren aportar los malalts de dites cases als Àngels Vells, y tots los que estaven bons y eren entrats en dites cases, los aportaren a la torra de Sant Pau y torra de Sant Sever, per traure'ls de la comunicatió dels altros; y les dites cases del carrer Nou les feren molt perfumar y netejar, y cremaren molta roba

(Miquel Parets, De molts sucsesos que han sucseÿt dins Barselona y en molts altros llochs de Catalunya, dignes de memòria… [Of the many events that have happened in Barcelona and in many other places in Catalonia, worthy of memory], 1626-1660).

[On Sundaym January 8th of that year [1651], in a house in Carrer Nou, called Martín de Langa, who was second, a maiden, a relative of his wife, died; and, immediately, his wife fell ill, who also died; and some people who had experienced these diseases aldo fell ill. Knowing this by the council, they went during that day, at night -so as not to make people sick or scare them-: they brought the sick from those houses to the Àngels Vells, and all those who were well and had entered those houses, they brought them to the tower of Sant Pau and the tower of Sant Sever, to remove them from the communication of others; and the mentioned houses of the Carrer Nou were perfumed and cleaned a lot, and they burned a lot of cloths]

Entrado el mes de Otubre era en Valencia el duelo y sentimiento universal, por ser tan grande la mortaldad que no podían los cuerpos enterrarse a braços de sepultureros. Proveyó la Ciudad a las Parroquias de unos carros, los quales ivan recogiendo por las calles los cuerpos que por las ventanas descolgavan, embueltos algunos con unas sávanas y otros aun sin esta

(Francesc Gavaldà, Memoria de los sucessos particulares de Valencia y su Reino en los años mil seiscientos quarenta y siete y quarenta y ocho, tiempo de peste [Memory of the peculiar successes of Valencia and its kingdom in the years one thousand six hundred and forty-seven and forty-eight, time of plague], 1651).

[At the beginning of the month of October, there was a universal mourning and feeling in Valencia, because the mortality was so great that the bodies could not be buried by the gravediggers. The city provided the parishes with carts, which went around the streets collecting the bodies that were hanging from the windows, some wrapped in sheets and others without]

En este any 1749 hagué en Mallorca unas pèssimas malaltias y pensaren que eren ocasionades del mal menjar del any antecedent; y hagué casa que no romangué ningú

(Tomàs Amorós, Relació de algunas curiositats escritas, comensant lo any 1740 y prosehint cada any, per a que el lector tenga present lo que, si olvida la memòria, se tròpia en los papers, que algunas vegades servex o, per millor dir, és necessari per alguns casos [Report on some written curiosities, beginning in 1740 and continuing every year, so that the reader can keep in mind his memory, found in the papers, which is sometimes useful or, better said, is necessary for some cases], 1740-1800).

[In this year 1749 there were terrible illnesses in Mallorca and they thought they were caused by the bad food of the previous year; and there was a house where no one survived]

Com que hi ha tanta grip, han hagut de clausurar la Universitat

(Josep Pla, El quadern gris [The gray notebook], 1918).

[Because there is so much ill, they have had to close the University]

Eight epigraphs therefore precede the work: a large number of references, considering the size of the collection (41 poems). This abundance underlines the author's need to reconnect with texts and authors that recall analogous experiences. Similarly, the wide chronological span of the epigraphs refers to even remote contexts and eras, embracing a mental panorama made up of testimonies of diverse geographical and temporal origins. However, these quotations refer to epidemics of the past, except for the last one, from Josep Pla's *Quadern gris* [The gray notebook], which concerns the outbreak and spread of Spanish flu in the years 1918-1920. This fact is significant: in the experience of past centuries, transmitted by the texts that Bover recalls in the epigraphs, the reality described refers to a number of epidemics that have followed one another over the centuries, except for the last example, which concerns a pandemic. The current situation is even worse and can only be linked to the Spanish flu mentioned by Pla in his work (last epigraph): this aspect radically changes the lived experience, which this time is on a global scale and has affected the entire planet. The practical, psychological and behavioral consequences of the actual situation are therefore amplified by the sheer magnitude of the phenomenon, the speed of its development, its suddenness and unpredictability and its huge impact on the perception and therefore the concept of personal and social security at transnational level. What was experienced on this occasion undermined our certainty and sense of security, and gave rise to a profound sense of vulnerability, fragility and crisis.

The Paratexts: The Author's Endnote

The collection closes with a final note by the author, written for the publication of the collection; thus, after the poems that compose it, even after the last one –*Senyal?* [Signal?]–, written in July 2020, and consequently after the first phase of the spread of the virus:

Llevat del darer, que va ser escrit el mes de juliol –quan es va fer visible el pas del cometa Neowise–, aquests poemes foren compostos a Sirges (Garraf) entre els mesos de març i juny de 2020, durant l'estricte confinement que va decretar-se amb la intenció d'aturar els contagis en el primer embat de la pandèmia de coronavirus que s'estenia, imparable, pel nostre país com a arreu del món. Tot i viure-ho des de la posició afortunada de qui no va patir de prop cap urpada dramàtica aquests textos reflecteixen sensacions i sentiments que hom experimentava aquells dies de malaltia i de mort, en què per a la humanitat s'iniciava una etapa desconeguda i terrible, de la qual no es veia la fi.

[Except for the last one, which was written in the month of July -when the passage of the comet Neowise became visible-, these poems were composed in Sitges (Garraf) between the months of March and June 2020, during the strict confinement that was decreed with the intention of stopping contagions in the first phase of the coronavirus pandemic that was spreading, unstoppable, throughout our country as well as throughout the world. Despite experiencing it from the fortunate position of those who did not suffer from any dramatic attack, these texts reflect sensations and feelings that people experienced in those days of illness ans death, in which for humanity an unknown and terrible stage began, of which there was no end in sight]

As was to be expected, the note presents a different perspective, far from the terrible scenario that inspired the 41 poems, and reflects a vision that had already evolved, in part comforted by the possibility of vaccination, and a panorama that was evolving, still in a complicated way and, however, less tragic than the first three months of the health emergency.

The Poems

The analysis of the 41 poems of the collection makes it possible to identify their constituent structure, their main and secondary features, the themes and subthemes dealt with and expressed as variations on certain key topics, due to the tone, perspective and emotional note of each of them. These verses express a poetic self which I characterized by different connotations each time, which we will call Locutor. This voice can pronounce a soliloquy; or address an Interlocutor, that can also be represented by the split poetic self, which addresses itself using the second person singular ('you'), and pronounces a monologue of the split self; or alternate different verbal persons, in a monologue of the multiple self (Sanchis Sinisterra, 2009; Orazi 2014, 2022b, pp. 21-23):

- Locutor: delivers a Soliloquy-Monologue or establishes a Dialogue
- Locutor > Interlocutor (the Locutor himself or a present/absent-real/ideal/imaginary Interlocutor)

The main constituent element is, therefore, the poetic voice, which changes with some frequency from poem to poem and takes on different roles. The predominant voice in these verses is definitely 'we'. It strongly confirms the sense of sharing a common experience. Indeed, there is only one poem in the collection in which the poetic self expresses itself in the first person singular, focusing on subjectivity. This is what happens in *Ciutat deserta* [Deserted town] (Bover, 2021, p. 51), where the desolate vision of the empty city is evoked through the personal perspective.

Otherwise, it is 'we' that prevails, as in *El contagi* [The contagion] (Bover, 2021, pp. 17-18) that opens the collection and in which the use of the first person plural expresses at the level of collective experience the reaction to the rapid spread of the virus in the first phase of the pandemic and the subsequent confinement; in *Aplec* [Gathering] (Bover, 2021, p. 21), reflecting the only kind of contact possible, mediated –in this case– by a computer screen; in *Res no serà com abans* [Nothing will be like before] (Bover, 2021, p. 22), with a reflection that involves the whole of mankind; in *El so de la gratitud* [The sound of gratitude] (Bover, 2021, p. 27), an expression of gratitude towards doctors and health workers; in *Primavera confinada* [Confined spring] (Bover, 2021, p. 28), where the beginning of spring is experienced by everyone in isolation; in *Basarda* [Fear] (Bover, 2021, p. 29) which, like the first poem in the collection, expresses the generalized fear produced by the spread of the pandemic and the sudden and profound disorientation it has caused; in *Signes del temps* [Signs of the time] (Bover, 2021, p. 33), on the sense of temporal suspension that isolation aroused in the whole population; in *El retorn* [The return] (Bover, 2021, p. 37), in which confined humanity sees improbable fauna (wild boar, foxes, roe deer) reappearing in urban space; in *Pluja amarga* [Bitter rain] (Bover, 2021, p. 41), about a nature that has become distant for everyone, due to isolation; in *Només ulls* [Only eyes] (Bover, 2021, p. 53), on the psychological impact of the use of the mask; and in *Senyal?* [Signal?] (Bover, 2021, p. 61), which contains a hesitant final hope.

The 'we' is sometimes contaminated with a 'you', second person singular, that expresses an impersonal perspective, as in *Resiliència* [Resilience] (Bover, 2021, p. 54), in which the need for a resilient attitude is insinuated in order to reach the desirable response of the whole community ("has d'afrontar" [you have to face]).

This 'we' can be opposed to a 'you', second person plural, as categories that face each other. This is what we find in *Metròpolis* [Metropolis] (Bover, 2021, p. 48), where the second person plural refers to the political class criticised for its choices, actions and dispositions.

Otherwise, the 'you', second person singular, appears and play different roles: sometimes it is an impersonal 'you', that the poet uses to express general concepts or situations; as in *El terrat* [The roof] (Bover, 2021, pp. 23-24) on the possibility of enjoying a domestic but at the same time outwardly projected space; in *Whatsapp* [Whatsapp] (Bover, 2021, p. 34), on mediated communication with the other, often via mobile phone; in *Xiuxiueig* [Whispering] (Bover, 2021, p. 47), that through a contrast refers to a conversation now only aloud, from the confined space (window or balcony) outwards (other windows and balconies or towards the street); in *Paisatge enfinestrat* [Windowed landscape] (Bover, 2021, pp. 38-39), a description of the view of an outside world that isolation has deprived mankind of and that is cut out of the window pane; in *Represa* [Recovery] (Bover, 2021, p. 43), a general reflection on the uncertain improvement of the situation and a consequent cautious reopening; and in *Enemic invisible* [Invisible enemy] (Bover, 2021, p. 57) on the dangerousness of the virus. In these cases, this generic and impersonal 'you' is closely linked to the 'we' and fulfils the same function: to emphasize a commonality, a vision and an experience shared by all.

This 'you', however, can also occupy the entire poetic space and thus materialize a monologue of the split 'I', when the poetic 'I' doubles up and addresses itself: as in *El calendari* [The calendar] (Bover, 2021, p. 26), in which the 'you' the poet addresses is a split self, meditating on the alteration of time and its perception; and in *Rutes obertes* [Open routes] (Bover 2021: 44), that reflects with an oxymoron the opening onto the world offered by reading during confinement.

In other cases, it is a real or ideal (reflection of a category), even imaginary 'you', second person singular; as in *Ventafocs* [Cinderella] (Bover, 2021, p. 45), which heralds the liberation of an imaginary figure from isolation; and in *Elevació* [Elevation] (Bover, 2021, p. 46), on elderly and/or frail subjects supported by a (distanced and) friendly presence.

The 'you', second person singular, can be accompanied by other voices, such as the second person plural: for example in *Enmascarats* [Masked] (Bover, 2021, p. 25), where 'you' refers to anyone who encounters another hurried passer-by on her/his way, in a dramatically surreal encounter, emphasized by the use of masks that make everyone unrecognizable; and in *La solitud de l'àgora* [The solitude of the agora] (Bover, 2021, p. 32), where the presence of 'you', second person singular, and second person plural gives the impression that the poet is observing the empty solitude of urban space from an external perspective.

Otherwise, the poetic voices involved can be 'you', second person singular, and 'we', as in *Anacoreta* [Anchoret] (Bover, 2021, p. 31), where the generic 'you' that appears in the first part of the poem is included in the second part in an all-encompassing 'we'.

Sometimes, however, the perspective changes several times within the same composition, as in *Sense agenda* [Without agenda] (Bover, 2021, p. 30), where the poetic 'I' addresses at first a 'you', second person singular, and then a second person plural, and finally a 'we' that encompasses everyone; or in *Sota l'amenaça del drac* [Under the threat of the dragon] (Bover, 2021, p. 42), in which the 'we' of the global perspective, the 'you', second person plural, to whom the poet ideally addresses himself, and a 'they' referring to the observed subjects alternate; or again in *Rumors* [Rumors] (Bover, 2021, p. 49), that presents the alternation of 'they' (the bearers of news from outside), an impersonal 'you', second person singular, and a 'we' that refers to the whole confined population.

More rarely, a 'you', second person plural, appears, referring to precise categories, as in *Entre la pell i el guant* [Between the skin and the glove] (Bover, 2021, p. 40), a composition referring to doctors and health workers; in *Corpus sitgetà* [Sitgetan Corpus] (Bover, 2021, p. 59) and in *Comiat* [Farewell] (Bover, 2021, p. 60), which describes a dramatic call for a last farewell mediated by a screen, due to the isolation and restrictive measures adopted during the health emergency, that made any direct contact impossible, even in the most extreme circumstances.

Sometimes, the verses take the form of a soliloquy, which can be used to describe the scenario of the time, as in *País reclós* [Secluded country] (Bover, 2021, p. 20), where no defined poetic voice appears, emphasizing the desolation of the deserted streets, orphaned by human presence; in *A corrua feta* [Lined up] (Bover, 2021, p. 55), that describes the queue ("trista i desesperada" [sad and desperate]) of those waiting for a plate of food; in *El nen del davant* [The boy in front] (Bover, 2021, pp. 35-36), depersonalized observation of the behavior of a child in isolation; and in *Al darrere* [Behind] (Bover 2021: 56), which contrasts the ineffectiveness of the government apparatus with those –doctors and healthcare staff– 'behind' them, in the backstage, working tirelessly.

In other cases of soliloquy, the poetic self expresses its reflections, as in *El mar de lluny* [The see in the distance] (Bover, 2021, p. 19); however, from the stream of consciousness, a different perspective can also emerge, which is linked to 'us', a collective reflection (as in the last verse: "I ens cal bregar per l'anhelat retorn" [and we must fight for the longed-for return]); and in *Esperit viatger* [Traveller spirit] (Bover, 2021, p. 50), an oxymoronic daydream from within the confinement, which is overlooked, again in the last verse, by the omnicomprehensive poetic 'we' ("per creure que podem tornar a volar" [to believe we can fly again]).

Or it may happen that other categories are involved in the soliloquy: a 'you', second person singular, as in *Desitjos extraordinaris* [Extraordinary desires] (Bover, 2021, p. 52), about the joys of which isolation has deprived us, involving a 'you', second person singular, who turns out to be the companion of a denied experience; or a 'you', second person plural, as in *Corpus Christi a Barcelona* [Corpus Christi in Barcelona] (Bover, 2021, p. 58), about uncelebrated festivities, in which the local population, to whom the poet addresses himself for a moment, appears.

- Topic/s: issues related with the COVID-19 pandemic

The themes and subthemes dealt with in the poems offer a suggestive overview of those aspects that have affected the entire world population and have been developed in the literary production (but not only) that has flourished since the beginning of the pandemic. It is impressive to note that they are the precise literary reflection of what neuropsychiatrists and psychologists have pointed out in their scientific studies.

Among the themes and subthemes dealt with in the collection, contagion stands out, starting with *El contagi* [El contagi] (Bover, 2021, pp. 17-18), the piece that opens the book and gives the volume its title. In it the other themes and subthemes are hinted at, declining in various ways in the subsequent poems: the spread of the virus and its consequences, isolation, quarantine, restrictions, lack of personal and physical contact, fear, deaths, the need/obligation to carry out any professional or leisure activity via the network, the complex management of children, the commitment and sacrifice of healthcare staff, etc. The virus is referred to as "nova pesta" [new plague], in an attempt to somehow describe the insidiousness to be faced and to give it a name, linking it to the epidemics of past centuries. Otherwise, the disease is called *Enemic invisible* [Invisible enemy] (Bover, 2021, p. 57) and is perceived as extremely insidious because it is intangible and therefore difficult to identify. In addition, the text also has another shared characteristic, namely, the type of language and vocabulary used at all levels to refer to the pandemic and the need to progressively contain it, such as war metaphors and vocabulary. The virus is perceived as an enemy, even more insidious because it is invisible, creeping, making us feel totally defenseless. A positive reaction is represented by the drive to organize oneself, to adapt to the situation, to protect oneself but also to move forward psychologically, as summarized in *Sota la amenaça del drac* [Under the threat of the dragon] (Bover, 2021, p. 42).

Fear is the other central element of the collection, which runs through all the poems. *Basarda* [Fear] (Bover 2021: 29) focuses on this aspect in an emotional and dramatic way: these verses speak of "ai al cor" [painful premonition], "malson" [nightmare], "tristor" [sadness], "solitud" [loneliness], describing a scenario that seems to concretise the worst dystopia, "arrecerats al fons de les trintxeres" [sheltered at the bottom of the trenches], using a term from the semantic field of war to refer to home, the place where one has been confined. One is fully aware that the worst can happen, as summarised in *Comiat* [Farewell] (Bover, 2021, p. 60), where several subthemes converge: death due to the disease, isolation and the impossibility of direct contact which makes the last farewell even more heartbreaking, with a tremendous "darrer adeu / a la pantalla" [last farewell / on the screen] of a mobile phone.

From the outset, isolation plays a central role in the perspective offered by these poems: due to it, mankind has been relegated to a mono-space and suspended in a mono-time, in the place where everyone has spent their confinement. Because of the quarantine, the outside world, be it natural or urban, is now unreachable, something to be observed from inside the house, through the window. It therefore becomes a forbidden place, to which access is prohibited, in an opposition that sees an 'inside' and an 'outside' facing each other, like two watertight compartments that radically changed the existence of the world's population during those months. So, some compositions focus on the foreclosure of natural or urban space for individuals: *El mar de lluny* [The see in the distance] (Bover, 2021, p. 19), *Primavera confinada* [Confined spring] (Bover, 2021, p. 28) and *Pluja amarga* [Bitter rain] (Bover, 2021, p. 41) treat the theme from the perspective of the loss of the possibility of enjoying nature, to be watched in the distance, in its unstoppable rebirth, with a note of bitterness. Other poems offer the same reflection but from the point of view of urban reality: *Paisatge enfinestrat* [Windowed landscape] (Bover, 2021, pp. 38-39) describes the activities of a neighbourhood that is confined to the inside of houses or, at best, take advantage of balconies. On the other hand, *País reclós* [Secluded country] (Bover, 2021, p. 20), *La solitud de l'àgora* [The solitude of the agora] (Bover, 2021, p. 32) and *Ciutat deserta* [Deserted town] (Bover, 2021 p. 51) describe a disturbing urban scenario, emptied of human presence: the subtheme consists of the desolation produced by the absence of man, intensified also through the surreal contrast between the memory of the city's former bustle and the current emptiness. The two perspectives converge in *El terrat* [The roof] (Bover, 2021, pp. 23-24), a hybrid space, an extension of the domestic perimeter, the 'licit' space, projected towards outer space, an area of escape that, however, is the privilege of a few. The only exception to this condition is the rapid incursions into the deserted city for basic needs. At this point, another subtheme emerges, that of personal protective equipment, such as the use of mask and gloves, and the psychological effects of this practice. This can be seen in poems such as *Enmascarats* [Masked] (Bover 2021: 25), which alludes to the measures taken against the virus using the metaphor of 'camouflage', and in *Només ulls* [Only eyes] (Bover, 2021, p. 53), which sadly emphasises the impossibility of recognising people behind the mask. However, the confinement of human beings and the emptying out of urban space have brought animals back, having been kept away from the noise and bustle of built-up areas. In the outer space from which man is banished, nature now reappears and in some way takes possession of it through a 'return': *El retorn* [The return] (Bover 2021: 37) hints to the incursions of wild animals (wild boars, foxes, roe deers) into the urban environment; *Rutes obertes* [Open roads] (Bover, 2021, p. 44) and *Esperit viatger* [Traveller spirit] (Bover, 2021, p. 50), on the other hand, are totally introjected into the single space of confinement and, as a result, open up an entirely interior dimension, made up of imagination and propitiated by reading, capable of opening up new worlds, and helping to sustain the precarious balance of a subject "empresonat entre quatre parets" [imprisoned between four walls].

The cancellation of any kind of face-to-face contact, including physical contact, from a simple handshake to a hug, is another key subtheme. It emerges strongly and emotionally in *Xiuxiueig* [Whispering] (Bover, 2021, p. 47), in which the title produces a strong contrast between loud conversations, exchanged now from a window, from balcony to balcony or from house to street; they have replaced low-key conversation, between acquaintances, neighbours, and passers-by, because physical proximity has been definitively banned. Similarly, *Aplec* [Gathering] (Bover, 2021, p. 21) draws attention to the only type of contact possible, an indirect one, at a distance, necessarily mediated by the telephone or the video call, with the sad reference to relationships maintained through the computer screen. This is also the case in extreme cases, such as waiting for happy or fatal news to arrive via a mobile phone message, as *Whatsapp* [Whatsapp] bitterly illustrates (Bover, 2021, p. 34). This subtheme combines with the theme of isolation, when it reflects the harsh reality of those who have experienced quarantine in solitude. This can be seen in *Anacoreta* [Anachoret] (Bover, 2021, p. 31), where the poetic self identifies itself and the entire mankind with the figure of the hermit. However, for the latter the decision to live in solitude in order to devote himself to contemplation and prayer is the result of a free choice; on the contrary, in the case of isolation imposed by governments all over the world to protect individual and collective health, this was a forced choice. In *Elevació* [Elevation] (Bover, 2021, p. 46), for example, there is a reference to the help of a friend, defined as "un bri de llum per a desfer la tenebra" [a ray of light to dispel the darkness], an image that highlights the negativity of the confinement during quarantine. Finally, *El nen del davant* [The boy in front] (Bover, 2021, pp. 35-36) describes the anomalous experience of a child segregated at home and deprived of his affections (grandparents, uncles, cousins, friends and teacher).

Like for space, perception and conception of time have also been altered: the anomaly represented by isolation, by the sharp contraction or even elimination of personal contacts, by an existence confined to a single space in what has become a single time, has given rise to a sense of suspension, altering the rhythm, the scanning of the day and of existence itself. This radical change constitutes the other key element of the isolation experience. The result is a suspended time, which seems no longer to flow and to have come to a standstill, as illustrated in *El calendar* [The calendar] (Bover, 2021, p. 26), a time that has lost its future perspective and the feeling of being able to identify the end of this abnormal time. *Signes del temps* [Signs of the times] (Bover, 2021, p. 33) emphasizes the same concept through the metaphor of punctuation, using the imagery of brackets to convey the impression produced by the sense of temporal suspension. Another subtheme linked to the chronological dimension is connected with the concept of cancellation: in this timeless time everything has deleted, all outdoor activities have been cancelled and with them a part of professional and private commitments, at best reconverted through smart working and the possibility of enjoying some leisure activities through the Internet. In *Sense agenda* [Without agenda] (Bover, 2021, p. 30) all this is expressed through the emptiness left by the disappearance of appointments, meetings and commitments. In this time reflected metaphorically in the emptied agenda, the "dies bessons" [twin days] follow one another in the same way. This aspect is also expressed in another peculiar way: altered time, also perceived as lost time, is also the time of feasts and festivities, that like everything else has been suppressed. It was therefore no longer possible to experience the festive moments that marked the year, i.e., the festivities and anniversaries that were not celebrated: a wealth of common traditions and family and social cohesion that was swept away, as the poems *Corpus Christi a Barcelona* [Corpus Christi in Barcelona] (Bover, 2021, p. 58) and *Corpus sitgetà* [Sitgetan Corpus] (Bover, 2021, p. 59) testify.

However, the collection also criticises the action of the government, accused of having "proferit només absurdes ordres / rere un mur de condecoracions" [uttered only absurd orders / behind a wall of decorations], as stated in *Metròpolis* [Metropolis] (Bover, 2021, p. 48), that refers to the overly centralised management of the state of emergency. Nevertheless, behind the parade of official figures broadcast on television, behind the state apparatuses parading on the screens, there are those who work tirelessly to contain the emergency: the reference to doctors and medical staff is transparent, as in *Al darrere* [Behind] (Bover, 2021, p. 56), or quite explicit, as in *Entre la pell i el guant* [Between the skin and the glove] (Bover, 2021, p. 40), dedicated to the recognition of their work and gratitude towards them, which also emphasises the human support offered by these figures to sick people. Or again in *El so de la gratitud* [The sound of gratitude] (Bover, 2021, p. 27), which recalls the collective ritual of daily applause from windows and balconies, a symbolic act of hope and venting at the same time that has united everyone. This is an ideal tribute to those who have made a personal effort to contain the spread of the virus and manage an unmanageable situation, risking their physical integrity and their very lives, as has unfortunately often happened.

Bover does not forget the dramatic issue of the economic crisis caused by the pandemic and its heavy repercussions, reflected in *A corrua feta* [Lined up] (Bover, 2021, p. 55): in these verses, the people standing in line are not simply waiting to get into a supermarket or a pharmacy, but form a "trista i despesperada" "cua de la fam" [sad and desperate hunger queue], impoverished, if not reduced to misery by the tremendous situation.

The longed-for conclusion of this total blockade (of time, activities, access to outer space) is expressed through *Desitjos extraordinari* [Extraordinary desires] (Bover, 2021, p. 52). They actually represent actions and gestures that were common in the previous normality, whose absence is felt, highlighted by the contrast produced by the juxtaposition of title and content: it is about the little everyday things that were denied to us at the time, deleted by isolation. The hope for the recovery of 'normality' is cautiously formulated in *Rumors* [Rumors] (Bover, 2021, p. 49), where the possible solution to the situation is presented, precisely, as a rumor. These cautious voices, however, announce in some way the *Represa* [Recovery] (Bover, 2021, p. 43), described in a hesitant way and with a note of fear, for its actual arrival is still uncertain. It will however come and will have the fearful face of the suffering experienced and of the losses incurred. From an imaginative perspective, *Ventafocs* [Cindarella] (Bover, 2021, p. 45) offer an ideal projection towards a natural space defined "món de meravelles" [world of wonders], finally recovered once the emergency is over. All this will be realised through the effort of each individual, that will then become collective, to build the *Resiliència* [Resilience] (Bover, 2021, p. 54) necessary to overcome the situation. The last composition, written in July 2020, is *Senyal?* [Signal?] (Bover, 2021, p. 61): it questions, once again with extreme caution, the end of this terrible epochal and global experience. In the text, the poet wonders, "tal com feien els antics" [just like the ancients did], whether the appearance of the comet Neowise in the days of the writing of this final text can be interpreted as a good omen, giving concrete form to a hope that is still almost hard to formulate, for fear of being disappointed and forced to face a new phase of crisis. However, that question mark, although it still expresses the sense of uncertainty that has pervaded everyone during this difficult period, also insinuates a note of hope, which even in the most cautious hesitation reveals a willingness to look ahead to the future.

CONCLUSION

The analysis of August Bover's *El Contagi* [The contagion] reveals the prevalence of the theme of isolation, which is taken up with a number of variations in most of the poems. Some of them, starting with *El contagi* [The contagion], which opens the collection and gives it its title, provide an overview of the general situation, focusing on the initial spread of the virus and the diffusion of COVID-19. Other texts, in particular *Resiliència* [Resilience], refer to the need for a behavioral and psychological response in order to manage and contain the fallout from a dramatic situation. Indeed, the necessary condition for this to happen is the elaboration and progressive consolidation of resilience, both on a subjective and collective level: as mentioned at the beginning, the capability of the individual and the community to strengthen this kind of response is an indispensable element for the ability of society as a whole to cope with the crisis. Other poems focus on the gradual conclusion of the emergency, on the definitive containment of the virus in order to eradicate the disease once and for all. In these cases, the tone is one of cautious hope, because it was not yet possible to see the light at the end of the tunnel and to assume that the pandemic had finally been overcome. This is what emerges from the poems *Rumors* [Rumors] and *Represa* [Recovery], for example. In this scenario, the function of artistic creation and, in particular, of literary production, is a powerful tool for conceptualizing and problematizing the lived experience and the trauma that results from it. They constitute a curative and therapeutic tool for beginning to process this dramatic and epochal experience and gradually overcoming it, as Trilla states in the prologue to Bover's collection.

The results of the study on August Bover's collection *El Contagi* [The contagion], on the specific context in which it was created, the themes it develops, and the peculiarities with which it shapes a series of suggestive variations on themes shared with other works produced during the period of the Coronavirus pandemic, demonstrate the therapeutic function and healing power of literature, a highly effective tool for managing and processing distress and, in this case, the shocking experience of a pandemic. It does finally highlight the therapeutic power of poetry.

This research received no specific grant from any funding agency in the public, commercial, or not-for-profit sectors.

REFERENCES

Boccuti, A. (2020). Pandemia y literatura: variaciones erótico-sentimentales en la imaginación distópica [Pandemic and literature: erotic-sentimental variations in the dystopian imagination]. In *COVID19 – LiTraPan. Literary Training via ICT for Higher Education Improvement, Behavioral Coaching and Discomfort Management during the Coronavirus Pandemic [Branch: UniTo]. II International Symposium "Forbidden Delights: Sex, Eroticism, Beauty, Aesthetics, Pleasure, Law, Sin and Prohibition". 19-20/06/2020*. Retrieved from https://www.youtube.com/watch?v=kQRss0sXAk8, 19

Boccuti, A. (2022). Contagios narrativos: crónicas y diarios del coronavirus desde América Latina [Narrative infections: chronicles and diaries of the coronavirus from Latin America]. *eHumanista/IVITRA*, 21.

Bover, A. (2014). *Beabà*, prefaci de Denise Boyer i Eliseu Trenc [*Beaba*, preface by Denise Boyer and Elisha Trenc]. *Tarragona*. Arola Editors.

Bover, A. (2018a). *Tornaveu*. Pròleg de Vicent Pitarch i Almela [*Come back*. Foreword by Vicent Pitarch i Almela]. Tarragona: Arola Editors.

Bover, A. (2018b) Blau marí. Poemes i proses [Navy blue. Poems and prose]. Vilanova i la Geltrú: El Cep i la Nansa Edicions.

Bover, A. (2021). El contagi [Contagion]. Barcelona: Edicions Saldonar.

Bover, A. (2022). Cloc! Pròleg de Màrius Serra [Stop! Prologue by Màrius Serra]. Tarragona: Arola Editors (2nd ed.). Academic Press.

Brooks, S. K., Webster, R. K., Smith, L. E., Woodland, L., Wessley, S., Greenberg, N., & Rubin, G. J. (2020). The psychological impact of quarantine and how to reduce it: Rapid review of the evidence. *Lancet*, *395*(10227), 912–920. doi:10.1016/S0140-6736(20)30460-8 PMID:32112714

Coneixement en temps de pandèmia, Coneixement en temps de pandèmia. (n.d.). Universitat d'Alacant. Seu Universitària de La Nucia. Retrieved from https://web.ua.es/es/seus/lanucia/documentos/actividades-culturales/2019-2020/cicle-pandemia.pdf

Cortijo Ocaña, A., & Martines, V. (Eds.). (2022). Handbook of Research on Historical Pandemic Analysis and the Social Implications of COVID-19. IGI Global.

Cortijo Ocaña, A., Orazi, V., & Martines, V. (Eds.). (2022). Managing Pandemic Isolation with Literature as Therapy. IGI Global.

Costa-Gramunt, T. (2021). Poemes de la pandèmia [Poems from the pandemic]. *Eix Diari*. Retrieved from https://www.eixdiari.cat/opinio/doc/98425/poemes-de-la-pandemia.html

Darici, K. (2022a). Marta Sanz, *Parte de mí* (2021) [Marta Sanz, *Part of Me* (2021)]. *eHumanista/IVITRA, 21*.

Darici, K. (2022b). El tiempo que nos robaron (2021) [The Time They Stole From Us (2021)]. In A. Cortijo Ocaña, V. Orazi, & V. Martines (Eds.), Managing Pandemic Isolation with Literature as Therapy. IGI Global.

Greco, B. (2020). Amor y cuarentena en la narrativa breve de confinamiento [Love and quarantine in the short narrative of confinement]. In *COVID19 – LiTraPan. Literary Training via ICT for Higher Education Improvement, Behavioral Coaching and Discomfort Management during the Coronavirus Pandemic [Branch: UniTo], II International Symposium Forbidden Delights: Sex, Eroticism, Beauty, Aesthetics, Pleasure, Law, Sin and Prohibition*. Retrieved from https://www.youtube.com/watch?v=ki5DktWtYoA&feature=youtu.be

Greco, B. (2022a). Pandemic and Literary Creativity. The Spanish Case of Relatos de confinamiento. In A. Cortijo Ocaña & V. Martines (Eds.), Handbook of Research on Historical Pandemic Analysis and the Social Implications of COVID-19 (pp. 80-93). IGI Global. doi:10.4018/978-1-7998-7987-9.ch007

Greco, B. (2022b). Cómic y Covid: *COnVIvienDo 19 días* de David Ramírez [Comics and Covid: *COnVIvienDo 19 days* of David Ramírez]. *eHumanista/IVITRA, 21*.

Greco, B. (2022c). A song to life in pandemic times: *Primavera extremeña* by Julio Llamazares. In A. Cortijo Ocaña, V. Orazi, & V. Martines (Eds.), Managing Pandemic Isolation with Literature as Therapy. *Hershey*. IGI Global.

Marazziti, D. (2020). The COVID-19 Outbreak: The Latest Challenge to Psychological and Psychiatric Intervention. *Clinical Neuropsychiatry, 17*(2), 39–40. doi:10.36131/clinicalnpsych20200201 PMID:34908965

Marazziti, D., Avella M. T., Mucci, N., Della Vecchia, A., Ivaldi, T., Palermo, S., & Mucci, F. (2020). Impact of economic crisis on mental health: a ten-year challenge. *CNS Spectrums*, 1-7. doi:10.1017/S1092852920000140

Marazziti, D., & Stahl, S. M. (2020). The relevance of COVID-19 to Psychiatry. *World Psychiatry, 19*(2), 261. doi:10.1002/wps.20764

Orazi, V. (2014). El monólogo en el teatro de Max Aub [The monologue in the theater of Max Aub]. *RiCOGNIZIONI, 1*(2), 151–160.

Orazi, V. (2020a). COVID19 – Literatura, interculturalitat, TIC, entrenament conductal i gestió de l'estrés durant la pandèmia per Coronavirus [COVID19 – Literature, interculturality, ICT, behavioral training and stress management during the Coronavirus pandemic]. In *Coneixement en temps de pandèmia*. Universitat d'Alacant. Seu Universitària de La Nucia. Retrieved from https://www.youtube.com/watch?v=PqVAi9-E2ro&fbclid=IwAR3dbgxgJylCSYOqTbn-BBv80WdVT0XdC-s8KYRHhgy7VRYnbex9PTZc_fQ

Orazi, V. (2020b). Sex and the Pandemic in *#Coronavirusplays*. In *COVID19 – LiTraPan. Literary Training via ICT for Higher Education Improvement, Behavioral Coaching and Discomfort Management during the Coronavirus Pandemic [Branch: UniTo], II International Symposium Forbidden Delights: Sex, Eroticism, Beauty, Aesthetics, Pleasure, Law, Sin and Prohibition*. Retrieved from https://www.youtube.com/watch?v=lp6jOx0EExY&feature=youtu.be

Orazi, V. (2022). Drammatizzare la pandemia. Microteatro spagnolo e catalano attuale [Dramatize the pandemic. Current Spanish and Catalan microtheatre]. *EHUMANISTA, 21*, 22–42.

Orazi, V. (2022a). Jordi Casanovas' #Coronavirusplays: Spanish and Catalan microtheatre in the framework of the Project COVID-19 LiTraPan. In A. Cortijo Ocaña & V. Martines (Eds.), Handbook of Research on Historical Pandemic Analysis and the Social Implications of COVID-19 (pp. 175-194). IGI Global.

Orazi, V. (2022b). *Microteatro spagnolo e catalano al tempo della pandemia* [Spanish and Catalan microtheatre at the time of the pandemic]. Torino: Università di Torino. QuadRi – Quaderni di RiCOGNIZIONI XII.

Pengfei, S., Xiaosheng, L., Chao, X., Wenjuan, S., & Bo, P. (2020). Understanding of COVID-19 based on current evidence. *Journal of Medical Virology, 92(6)*, 548–551. https://doi:10.1002/jmv.25722

Sanchis Sinisterra, J. (2009). El arte del monólogo [The art of monologue]. *Revista Teatro CELCIT, 35-36*, 162–170.

Schimmenti, A., Billieux, J., & Starcevic, V. (2020). The Four Horsemen of Fear: An Integrated Model of Understanding Fear Experiences during the COVID-19 Pandemic. *Clinical Neuropsychiatry, 17*(2), 41-45. doi:10.36131/CN20200202

Sohrabi, C., Alsafi, Z., O'Neill, N., Khan, M., Kerwan, A., Al-Jabir, A., Iosofidis, C., & Agha, R. (2020). World Health Organization declares global emergency: A review of the 2019 novel coronavirus (COVID-19). *International Journal of Surgery, 76*, 71–76. doi:10.1016/j.ijsu.2020.02.034 PMID:32112977

Srivatsa, S., & Stewart, K. A. (2020). How should clinicians integrate mental health into epidemic responses. *AMA Journal of Ethics, 22*(1), 10–15. doi:10.1001/amajethics.2020.10 PMID:31958385

The COVID-19 Outbreak. (2020). *Clinical Neuropsychiatry, 17*(2).

Trilla, A. (2021). Pròleg [Prologue]. In A. Bover (Ed.), El contagi (pp. 13-15). Barcelona: Saldonar.

Vacalebri Lloret, Ú. (2020). Gestió emocional i ensenyament de Català com a Llengua Estrangera en temps de pandèmia: els tàndems lingüístics en línia UniTo-UA [Emotional management and teaching of Catalan as a Foreign Language in times of pandemic: UniTo-UA online language tandems]. In *COVID19 – LiTraPan. Literary Training via ICT for Higher Education Improvement, Behavioral Coaching and Discomfort Management during the Coronavirus Pandemic [Branch: UniTo], II International Symposium Forbidden Delights: Sex, Eroticism, Beauty, Aesthetics, Pleasure, Law, Sin and Prohibition*. Retrieved from https://www.youtube.com/watch?v=nSH4pT5vpRg&feature=youtu.be

Vacalebri Lloret, Ú. (2022a). Emotional and Psychological Effects of the COVID-19 Pandemic in College Students: A Language Exchange Project as a Tool to Manage Psychological Disorders Related to the COVID-19 Pandemic. In A. Cortijo Ocaña & V. Martines (Eds.), Handbook of Research on Historical Pandemic Analysis and the Social Implications of COVID-19 (pp. 274-287). IGI Global.

Vacalebri Lloret, Ú. (2022b). Les metàfores conceptuals I la pandemia de la COVID-19: una guerra sense bales [Conceptual metaphors and the COVID-19 pandemic: a war without bullets]. *eHumanista/IVITRA, 21*.

Xiang, Y.-T., Yang, Y., Li, W., Zhang, L., Zhang, Q., Cheung, T., & Ng, C. H. (2020). Timely mental health care for the 2019 novel coronavirus outbreak is urgently needed. *Lancet, 7*(3), 228–229. doi:10.1016/S2215-0366(20)30046-8 PMID:32032543

ADDITIONAL READING

Polo Bettonica, T. (2020). Una radiografía de la cuarentena en clave teatral [An x-ray of quarantine in a theatrical key]. *El País*, Cataluña. https://elpais.com/espana/catalunya/2020-04-13/una-radiografia-de-la-cuarentena-en-clave-teatral.html

KEY TERMS AND DEFINITIONS

Bibliotherapy: Also referred to as book therapy, poetry therapy or therapeutic storytelling, it is a creative arts therapy modality that involves storytelling or the reading of specific texts with the purpose of healing. It uses an individual's relationship to the content of book as therapy.

COVID-19 Pandemic: Pandemic of Coronavirus disease 2019, caused by severe acute respiratory syndrome coronavirus 2 (SARS-CoV-2). It was identified in December 2019 in Wuhan, China. The WHO declared the outbreak of a public health emergency of international concern in January 2020 and a pandemic in March 2020.

ICT in Education: ICT enables the use of innovative educational resources and the renewal of learning methods, establishing a more active collaboration of students and the simultaneous acquisition of technological knowledge. ICT can complement, enrich, and transform *education* for the better.

Isolation During COVID-19 Pandemic: The COVID-19 pandemic is assumed to have caused an increase in the number of socially isolated people. Social Isolation was defined as less frequent contact with people other than co-residing family members. Mental health outcomes of such situation include psychological distress, suicidal ideation, loneliness, and fear of COVID-19.

PPE – Personal Protective Equipment: The COVID-19 pandemic has touched almost every continent. PPE is the final line of protection. There is variation as well as controversy of infection control recommendation with regards to the use of PPE between institutions. PPE is part of the measure within a package of prevention and control of pandemic.

Reader Involvement: The process of actively involving the Reader in the communication act, in order to increase their engagement with the message. Its aim is to inspire awareness (and dissent), stance and even action.

Soliloquy: An act of speaking one's thoughts mentally or even aloud when by oneself or regardless of any hearers. Expression of the self in which the subject expresses his thoughts or feelings mentally or aloud while either alone or with others keeping silent.

Chapter 6
About Some Spanish Graphic Novels in Times of COVID-19 Pandemic:
Cathartic Panels for the End of the World

Eduard Baile-López
https://orcid.org/0000-0001-7685-6487
Universitat d'Alacant, Spain

ABSTRACT

The purpose of this chapter is to attend to comics produced during COVID-19 pandemic, especially those referring to the hardest moments of confinement and which may allow to observe the use of comics as a tool to analyze reality, both from a psychological point of view and from a sociopolitical one. Being such a recent phenomenon, corpus selection is introduced as temporary since new items continue to emerge, and furthermore, it is still early to assess its significance. As a pragmatic criterion, two vectors will be used: on the one hand, focus will be stressed on works belonging to the Spanish comics market in order to portray a particular cultural environment; on the other hand, four items will be selected to establish a coherent story which may adapt the stages of the hero's journey into a new paradigm (1. Fear, 2. Anger, 3. Humor, and 4. Healing).

INTRODUCTION: COMICS ARTISTS ARE THE NEW HUMANISTS IN TIMES OF CRISIS

This chapter aims to analyze a corpus of comics produced in Spain as a result of the COVID-19 pandemic and which show, as their central plot, the representation of the consequences derived from the spread of the virus and, especially, from confinement. In this sense, the contributor's goal is to observe various factors ranging from psychological aspects to sociopolitical reflections (how this confinement situation has affected citizens, in short). It is, therefore, a consideration which adheres to the analysis of fiction as an instrument to understand contemporary reality (Yrigoyen, 2020), that is, art as a humanistic tool

DOI: 10.4018/978-1-6684-4735-2.ch006

which highlights uncertainties and social changes; in a way, it means using art to identify *zeitgeist*. More specifically, it is based on a selection of comics aimed at an adult audience and which, hence, follows the postulates of the *Graphic Novel* movement (García, 2010), which defines comics characterised by marked author-centered traits and which are oriented to cross-sectional readers who are not necessarily specialised in comics. However, this fact does not prevent that, at the same time, works to be analysed may contain usual elements of industrial comics, because they are twisted so that creator's voice is pre-eminent (more meditations on this author-centered/mainstream hybridisation will be adressed for each graphic novel subsection).

Concerning the choice of a communicative and artistic medium which is different from conventional ones in an academic environment (essentially, literature), it should be noted that the language of comics refers to a multimodal and interdisciplinary component and that it is fully connected with the leading intermedial and transmedia panorama in early 21st century (Jenkins, 2003; Scolari, 2013). In other words: current cultural consumers have before them a panoply of referents whose raw material is no longer based unequivocally on the power of words but it is implemented on an integrating mold which adds image and sound, among other elements, to the literary factor (therefore, reading canon parameters are widened, as explained in Rovira-Collado, 2017). For this reason, the chapter's author would like to suggest that it is necessary, with regard to an effective analysis of surrounding reality, to attend to the historical changes occurring about reading paradigm, a process in which comics, especially by means of *Graphic Novel* current movement, must assume a prominent position. Likewise, assimilation of content through an alternative communicative medium involves a different decoding process as specific instruments are used. Particularly, comics-based semantic and semiotic decipherment is linked with a narrative interpretation which, at the same time, is centered on the page layout, often dependent on sequential storytelling and in accordance with a reading process which tends to verge on intuition and on sensoriality, usually following a premise of a simultaneous visual impact (Cohn, 2013), mediated by *functionality* in turn (Matly, 2020). Hence, mimicking some reflections by Roland Barthes (1973) regarding the completion of the final meaning of a text by readers, it may be established that, precisely, the language of comics is ideal to create an open debate between creators and users (Yus, 1997) since decoding visual items offers a greater margin in favour of metaphors and symbolisms, even allegories (this action would be, without a doubt, a specific application of *opera aperta* concept by Umberto Eco, 1962). In a certain way, there is something about this peculiar medium language which acquires some sort of a mystical patina, that is, what is hinted but cannot be reliably explained. Then again, this chapter's author does not consider that it should be understood that the language of comics cancels literary values, but it provides complementary elements since, obviously, relations between both media may give rise to a fruitful study of formal tangentialities (Pizzino, 2016), especially if a new *reading intertext* iteration is adressed (Mendoza Fillola, 2001). Not surprisingly, comics are a modern medium due to their industrial origins but, at the same time, they connect with almost innate human processes of understanding the world (Bartual, 2014), such as the use of panels to structure knowledge (Carrión & Sagar, 2018), an operation which seems to be very similar to the terminological categorizations scientific methodology delimits reality with.

Because of this potential for mirroring reality comics possess by means of its complex language, this chapter's author believes it will provide resources for scholars to explain (or, rather, to try to explain) a credible critical account about the emotional and social consequences of confinement. Specifically, as it will be later specified, in order to signify the corpus as a reflection of its surrounding reality, a kind of chronicle based on four phases has been forged: fear, that is, the bewilderment before *status quo* is changed; anger, a feeling tied in with stupefaction and the sensation of inability to find solutions (and which allows personal aspects to connect with political ones); humour as a defensive weapon or an antidote to cope with misfortune; and healing, a light at the end of the tunnel. Somehow, these guidelines emulate the hero's journey, but they do it in a resignified way through an everyday point of view so a *post-heroic* label is followed (Bröckling, 2021), meaning how normal people (the everyday hero) confront progressively what is perceived as an unwanted unforeseen event which, by breaking daily banalities, has called traditional values and system into question. This phases scheme, pragmatically presented under a correlative structure for an orderly analysis but which, in truth, functions in synchronicity, will be discussed within four Spanish graphic novels. These items, whose description will be fleshed out in the 'Background' section of this chapter, have been chosen, as a matter of fact, because of their ability to convey a symbolic account. This selection does not mean that they are the only works which could have been chosen out of Spanish comics production, but the author believes that they are the most suitable ones to convey the methodological approach which has just been alluded to.

Moreover, it may be be said that this decision about centering works selection basing it only on the Spanish publishing market responds to the intention of establishing a set of items which is homogeneous enough to allow the precise conformation of the aforementioned account, which is founded according to four phases or stages refering to an emotional hero's journey. Additionally, it may be considered that this chapter's author will analyse and understand this graphic novels collection in a more effective way since it relates to his own sociocultural reality. However, as it is discussed in another chapter section, more specifically throughout 'Future Research Directions' part, this corpus of comics will be expanded as well as its thematic variety for further academic investigations which will extend what may be accomplished thanks to this very contribution.

BACKGROUND: POST-HEROISM FACING THE UNPROPHESIED APOCALYPSE

Undoubtedly, psychological consequences caused by the pandemic, both in terms of interpersonal contact absence due to the isolation derived from confinement and the loss of family and friends (often without being able to say goodbye to them) have been around the media all the way through (WHO. Regional Office for Europe, 2021). For this reason, analysis of representation in fiction of both uncertainty and confusion generated on most of the population may be extremely interesting for scholars to reveal inadvertent aspects regarding the social psyche, and also to conceive art from a cathartic perspective, an approach which is undertaken beautifully by the *Graphic Medicine* movement, that is, the vindication of comics for adressing health issues (González Cabeza, 2017). In this process of psychological affectation, it is important to observe some various adaptation processes in order to not fall into depression or to overcome it, if that should be the case. Thus, fear or anxiety are logical derivations from confinement stress, a situation which possibly will persist over time (Brooks et al., 2020). On the other hand, the pshychological side of the pandemic is inextricably linked to the inevitability of social change (Giordano, 2020; Žižek, 2020), an intellectual landscape which may be resignified as a chance to overcome previous deficiencies and, since a new normality is expected to take shape sooner or later, to get morally and ethically better than before (Bringel & Pleyers, 2020; De Sousa Santos, 2020).

To carry out this analytical operation, as it has already been indicated in previous section, a critical comment is proposed on four graphic novels through which a passage or a stage for each one may be symbolized for developing a new hero's journey, now following a resignification filtered by an emotional premise. Thus, these items will refer, respectively, to fear (*Conviviendo 19 días* by David Ramírez, Norma Editorial, 2020); anger (*Días de alarma* by Víctor Coyote, Salamandra Ediciones, 2020); humour (*El murciélago sale a por birras* by Álvaro Ortiz, Astiberri, 2020); and, finally, healing (*El superpoder más importante. Una historia de Superman, Krypto y su vecina*, by David Rubín, ECC, 2020), although these are not watertight traits and, therefore, they may get mixed.

This renewed hero's journey, because it focuses on starring-characters who mirror everyday life through the common individual (even if, as it will be exposed, traditional heroic archetypes are used for some examples), puts scholars on the track of *post-heroism* (Featherstone, 1992). Under this paradigm assumption, an intervention is accomplished to dismantle the archetypal hero, who is constructed as an imperfect individual, gripped by doubts and moral relapses as any human being suffers, but who overcomes through affection and civic conscience. To this operation, an ethical stimulus which, *mutatis mutandis*, refers to a Christian perspective (Román Maestre, 2021) or even a Judeo-Christian one taking the superheroic paradigm into account for some of the selected works (Saunders, 2011), is added. They are, hence, characters whose heroism is not based on battles but on compassion (although these factors are not, in any case, discriminatory between them), since they do not appeal to the epic paradigm but to empathy. This re-enactment, however, does not imply that the notion of sacrifice gets lost; on the contrary, it is not filtered through a narrative in search of glory and honour, but it is built on the will to love. In this sense, what is essential about the behavior these post-heroes show, whether they are anonymous individuals or resignifications of archetypes filtered through *mainstream* franchises, is the uninterrupted journey towards freedom of thought through affection: their Holy Grail, in short, is to participate in the construction of a community of free human beings whose spur is love as an end in itself.

MAIN FOCUS OF THE CHAPTER: THE SPANISH GRAPHIC NOVEL MOVEMENT CONFRONTING THE SCOURGE OF THE PANDEMIC

Fear (or the Horror of the Sentimental Intimate Wound): *Conviviendo 19 días*, by David Ramírez

Regarding the representation of fear, *Conviviendo 19 días* by David Ramírez (Norma Editorial, 2020) is a graphic novel which allows to focus on love and on the anguish of loss. It is an autobiographical sentimental chronicle (a *slice of life* or a *tranche de vie*, if specialized terminology should be used) which, through a naive mood, narrates a forced separation from the loved one to avoid contagion. Ramírez does not reject the use of humour, but he uses it as a tool to filter the anguish of living with an inffected lover (his husband, so an LGTBIQ+ perspective is also introduced subtly). Likewise, the fact that the infected person is a medical assistant offers some civic remarks about social conscience, an operation which naturally connects with anger (see next subsection), though not as harshly.

This work, which was originally published through digital format, follows a similar structure to a personal diary (as the selected work for the next subsection also does) and shows an artistic style which is reminiscent of the *Valencian School* of comics (Porcel, 2002). This way, thanks to soft colors and cartoonish graphics based on rounded shapes with a high metaphorical load, a situation of profound emotional disorder is presented in a far from dramatic way. Thus, inadvertently for the reader, various thematic interests are introduced to denote an authorial resignification of Spanish classic comics, an operation which also signals an evident connection with the so-called *New Valencian School* (Porcel &

Pons, 2007). Among these contents alluding to personal concerns coming from the creator (and which mirror social concerns which are based on a leftist ideology), a progressive meditation on the value of public health stands out, a factor which is not insignificant at all when it takes place at the same time that a health emergency has highlighted the dangers posed by a hospital management progressive neo-liberalization. Through this framework, the one refering to the need to care for each other, it is when allusions to the *post-heroic* factor come into play (Bröckling, 2021; Featherstone, 1992), since it focuses on the courage of showing afection by means of simple actions.

Another interest core, also already alluded to, refers to the vindication of *affective-sexual diversity* (overcoming, therefore, the predominance of heteronormative relationships in mainstream fiction), an issue which sneaks through several passages in which Ramírez exposes himself being terrified that he may lose his partner: thus, the long hours he spends contemplating him in silence while he sleeps, constantly anguished in case he stops breathing (day 4 during confinement). Likewise, taking advantage of the specific characteristics of the language of comics, page structure often forms a visual metaphor, for example, when, through a double *splash page*, Ramírez imagines himself as a puzzle missing a piece, who is none other than his very husband (days 19 and 20). This graphic resource will be, again, activated to symbolize the confinement on day 49, when Ramírez's husband is also visualized as a puzzle, but now the metaphor refers to the bars of a prison, which becomes equivalent to the separation between panels.

Figure 1. The capability of art to refer to the symbolic and the universal depends on the accurate description of what is close and familiar. © Norma Editorial, 2020.

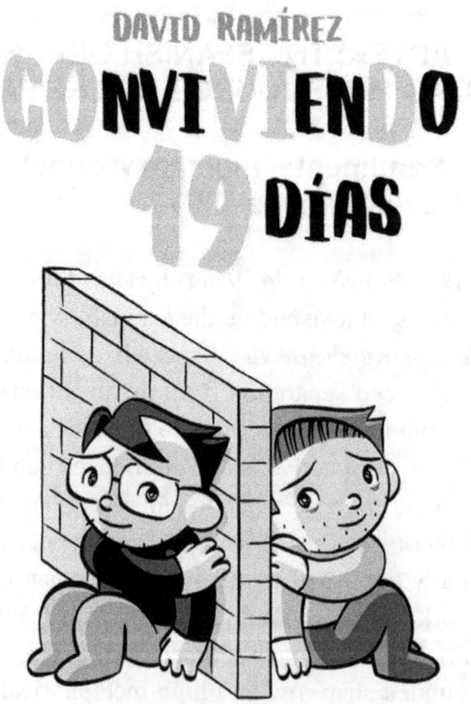

In addition to this brilliant recurrence to concretize abstraction, it is also worth noting Ramírez's use of iconicity degree, something which may get associated with symbolic graphics: by simplifying optical representations, this work sometimes becomes a kind of pictograms-based instruction manual to satisfactorily explain various hygienic measures to combat contagion wave. This intervention helps, of course, to show that comics' multimodal possibilities allow creators to convey complex reflections through a format which facilitates information transmission. On the other hand, despite the fact that humour is not the most prominent contributor to the tone of the story, which is closer to sentimentality without being strident, the truth is that it is also present in a subtle way as it successfully underlines that sarcastic modulation can convey any kind of of narration (Adanti, 2017). It is, precisely, this humorous aura which definitively makes this graphic novel leap from a personal scope to a collective range by avoiding a tragedy depending on sensationalism.

Anger (or Sociopolitical Awareness): *Días de alarma*, by Víctor Coyote

Anger is brilliantly reflected in *Días de alarma* by Víctor Coyote (Ediciones Salamandra, 2020), particularly because it focus on sociopolitical vindication in a way which is, at the same time and not paradoxically, propagandist and meditated. By distilling content in little instalments through newspaper strip format or political graphic humour (it was first released online on an almost daily basis, before being compiled into a book), which emphasizes the astonishment and outrage at the ineffectiveness of politicians, press manipulation or lack of solidarity between citizens, it offers an approach which, ultimately, rises from an apparently autobiographical perspective to transmute into a collective voice against social injustices (such as joblessness) derived from the economic halt, without the Government fulfilling its social duty.

Despite the fact that a few hints of caustic humour are introduced, sociopolitical anger is what, undoubtedly, drives the tone of this story. It is, therefore, a cry of protest coming from bewilderment, a situation to which people initially do not know how to respond (they are frightened); however, once the initial shock is assimilated, anger arises. Thus, this work, which is not exempt from irrational populism, hits against political class through a somewhat dirty pencil graphic style (it transmits roughness and ferocity) and some spotted colors, apparently, by means of ink crossing the page, a trope which mirrors citizen's weariness. Starting, then, from a day-by-day structure as a diary, Coyote establishes a series of social demands as if he was speaking through a megaphone to make himself be heard loudly and clearly: however, unlike David Ramírez's graphic novel, who transcends intimacy by symbolically evoking his vital anguish, in this case the diary format acquires, from the very beginning, a pamphleteering nuance, close to a political manifesto. On the other hand, readers feel stired to go out into the streets to express their right to complain, a consequence which underlines the capacity for ideological mobilization fiction can transmit, a facet of art which scares authorities as it shows its potential to induce citizens to question system values (Gopegui, 2008; Bordería, Martínez Gallego, & Gómez Mompart, 2015).

Figure 2. As daily references show, Días de alarma is developed as a daily logbook in order to report sociopolitical reality. © Ediciones Salamandra, 2020.

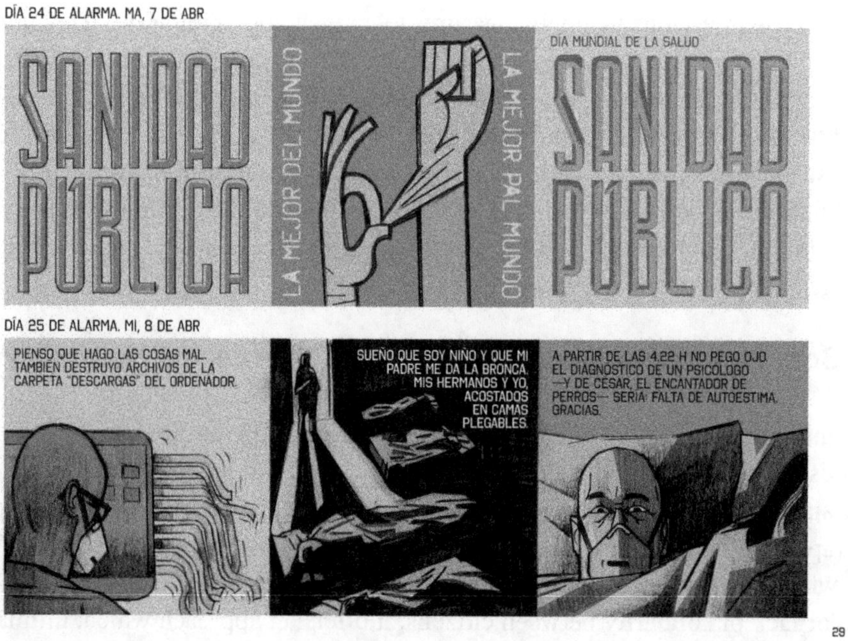
DÍA 24 DE ALARMA. MA, 7 DE ABR
SANIDAD PÚBLICA
LA MEJOR DEL MUNDO
LA MEJOR PAL MUNDO
DÍA MUNDIAL DE LA SALUD
SANIDAD PÚBLICA
DÍA 25 DE ALARMA. MI, 8 DE ABR
PIENSO QUE HAGO LAS COSAS MAL. TAMBIÉN DESTRUYO ARCHIVOS DE LA CARPETA "DESCARGAS" DEL ORDENADOR.
SUEÑO QUE SOY NIÑO Y QUE MI PADRE ME DA LA BRONCA. MIS HERMANOS Y YO, ACOSTADOS EN CAMAS PLEGABLES.
A PARTIR DE LAS 4.22 H NO PEGO OJO. EL DIAGNÓSTICO DE UN PSICÓLOGO —Y DE CÉSAR, EL ENCANTADOR DE PERROS— SERÍA: FALTA DE AUTOESTIMA. GRACIAS.
29

Via this description, it could be argued that this graphic novel only appeals to propaganda but, as it has been pointed out before, it is an item which is also introspective. In this sense, it should be noted that this balance is achieved through a mechanism of progressive intellectualization: initial protests consisting on a cry of daily despair are followed by a process of reflection halfway between essay and opinion column, which relates this item to *comics journalism* (Matos, 2017), though not establishing an identification strictly. On the other hand, as the diary goes on, protests mix with personal yearnings refering to Coyote's cultural tastes (jazz or pop culture, in general), which allows him to be humanized in reader's eyes and, therefore, more complex.

Humour (or Only Parody Will Save Humanity): *El murciélago sale a por birras*, by Álvaro Ortiz

El murciélago sale a por birras (Astiberri, 2020) by Álvaro Ortiz filters classic superhero traits with a graphic style borrowed from classic Spanish funny comics, from both *Bruguera School* (Moix, 1968) and, like David Ramírez before, *Valencian School* and *New Valencian School* trends (Porcel, 2002; Porcel & Pons, 2007), to elaborate an insanely amusing and sacrilegious discourse which fuels emotional overcoming (strictily speaking, it is not a superhero *comic book*, but rather it takes this thematic mold and then deconstructs it). Thus, against fear, anger leads to survival but, ultimately, human beings cannot survive through uninterrupted anger, so ways of escape through laughing are much needed to reduce tension and to avoid, therefore, mental health collapse: humans need to joke against misfortune as the optimal defense mechanism.

Across this work, also initially released as a digital newspaper strip, the superhero genre is, thus, subverted through a parody tone which gets so extreme that it constitutes both a tribute and a desecration at the same time. Certainly, its vulgarizing slang dialogues and the unrestrained sexual desires showed by the inhabitants of Batman's universe, refering to both his rogues gallery and his allies (perhaps only Comissioner Gordon remains relatively close to the original source through a *straight man* archetype against the rest of the characters, depicted as frenzied *clowns*), denote that Ortiz uses genre *clichés* to build his own ideological microcosm, to which an improvised graphic design, close to rough-draft, contributes. In this sense, *the Caped Crusader* becomes just another citizen, equally harassed by the pandemic development as anyone and, therefore, he does not stray far from the figure of the everyday hero. On the other hand, as an apparent paradox, this parody operation unequivocally transmits love for the genre: there is no doubt, it should be noted, that Ortiz knows all character's runs in depth (the television series starring Adam West in the 60s; the *hard-boiled* conversion by Frank Miller and David Mazzucchelli in the mid-1980s, etc.) and that this irreverent expression is also a love letter to what is truly a model of contemporary mythologization (American pop culture is the equivalent of European folklore).

Figure 3. Parody goes wild as an antidote when human minds wander in the dark. © Astiberri, 2020

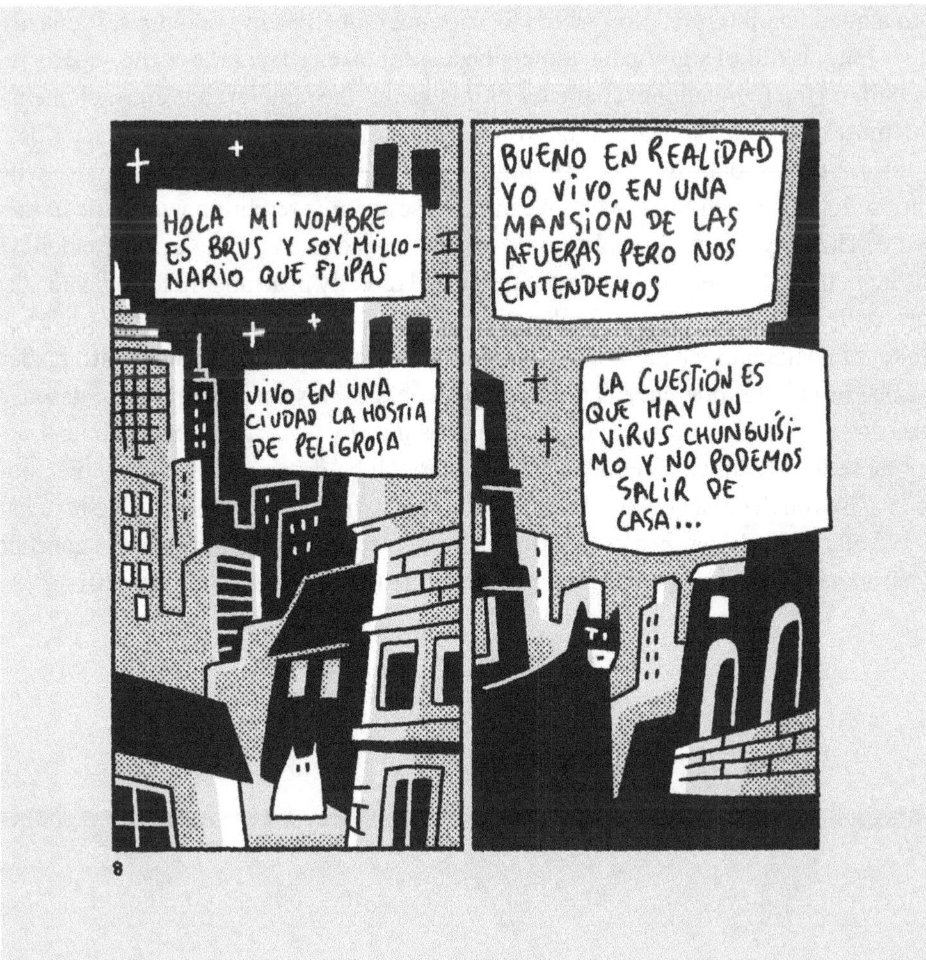
HOLA MI NOMBRE ES BRUS Y SOY MILLONARIO QUE FLIPAS
VIVO EN UNA CIUDAD LA HOSTIA DE PELIGROSA
BUENO EN REALIDAD YO VIVO, EN UNA MANSIÓN DE LAS AFUERAS PERO NOS ENTENDEMOS
LA CUESTIÓN ES QUE HAY UN VIRUS CHUNGUÍSIMO Y NO PODEMOS SALIR DE CASA...
8

Through this sacrilegious maneuver, Ortiz devises an escapist way to combat both fear and rage. Undoubtedly, human beings need to balance transcendental situations by means of small joys, and through this harmonization process humour assumes a preponderant role. In this sense, parody is extremely effective because it immediately appeals to laughter as it presupposes a shared knowledge between creator and readers. On the other hand, this supposed lightness is not as it seems to be, maybe just superficially, as, in its own way, its exaggerated ridicule scale also functions as an alert and it ensures that anger does not lead, sooner or later, to boredom and conformism: in part, laughter keeps citizens attentive and ready to be in the thick of it. In addition to this camouflage in terms of humour's critical potential, a *post-humorous* component is evidently glimpsed (Costa, 2018) which, through contemporary intermedial framework, when judging comedians has become usual, leads to reflect on the limits of humour, if there are any limits indeed (Adanti, 2017; Fontdevila, 2013).

Healing (or the Everyday Redefinition of the Hero's Journey): *El superpoder más importante. Una historia de Superman, Krypto y su vecina*, by David Rubín

Finally, healing is crucial to *El superpoder más importante. Una historia de Superman, Krypto y su vecina* (ECC, 2020) by David Rubín, which, as it has been already alluded to, redefines hero's journey last stage by refering to a quotidian interpretation which focuses not on battles but on ethics. It consists just on a four-page story but it is full of significant content because it takes advantage of the superhero archetype (narration is built on the foundational character of this genre: the simplest and most elemental one and, therefore, the most malleable one). Although this item is based on a franchise character owned by DC Comics, its release corresponds to a specific initiative of the Spanish publishing house which has the pertinent edition rights in Spain, so that Rubín can exercise an *indie* rendition within the framework of an industrial genre. This way, what originally would have been told as an epic tale, it is rendered intimately.

Thus, this item, the only one which has been published directly in an analog format and, also, the only one based on *comic book* format (very similar to magazine form), makes use of the superheroic archetype as a model of contemporary mythology through which a space for dialogue with readers is easily established since its cultural reference is universally shared. In this case, Rubín activates an alternative process to the one Álvaro Ortiz activated, since he does not shy away from the canonical postulates of the genre but he rather sublimates them: certainly, although he does not resort to depict any battle, he precisely emphasises on the essential elements of the genre, which become even more revelant as Superman is the mold all other *mistery men* derive from, an intervention which refers to the conceptualization of the superhero archetype as an aspirational role model (Embid, 2018; Saunders, 2011).

Figure 4. The universal metaphor of the superheroic archetype allows, as an apparent paradox, to formulate reflections which encompass the entire moral and ethical spectrum. © ECC, 2020.

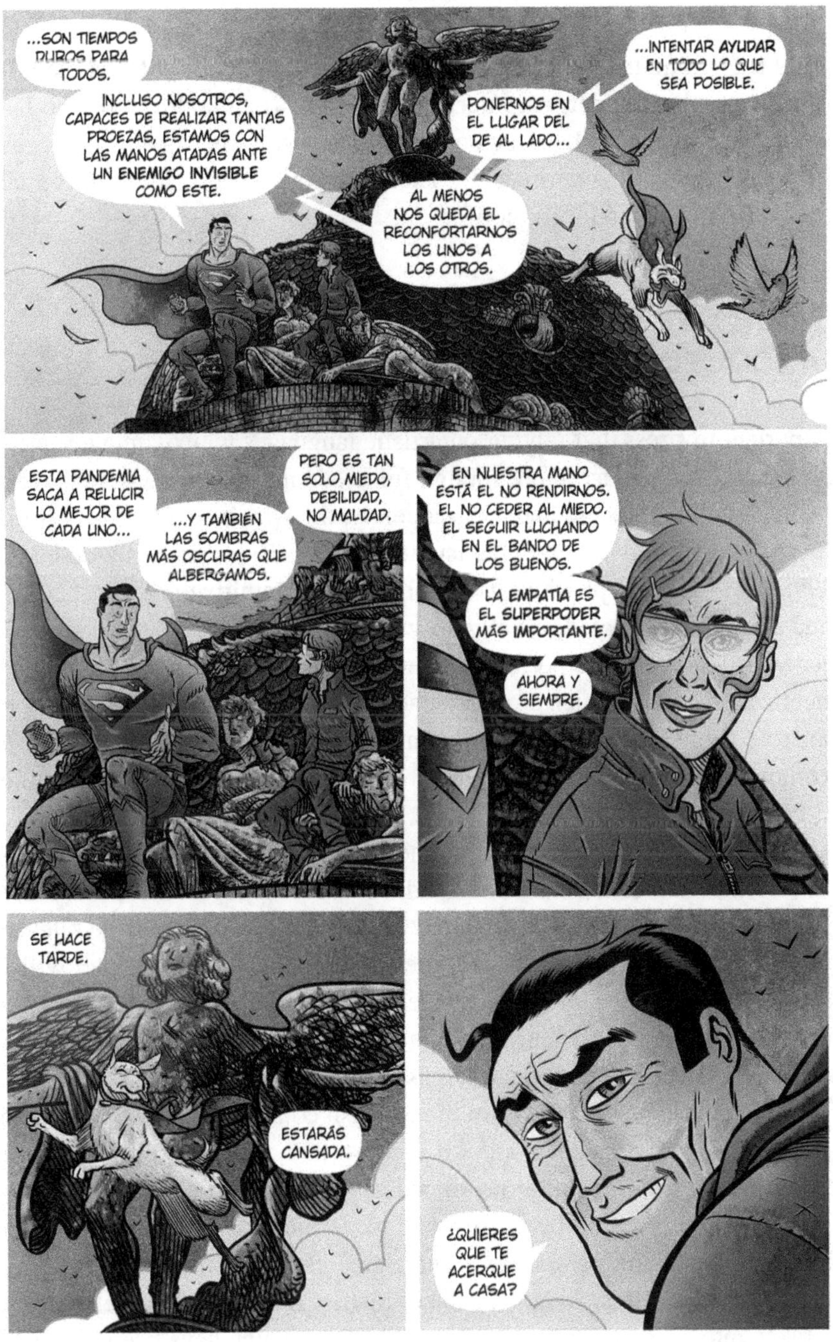
...SON TIEMPOS DUROS PARA TODOS.
INCLUSO NOSOTROS, CAPACES DE REALIZAR TANTAS PROEZAS, ESTAMOS CON LAS MANOS ATADAS ANTE UN ENEMIGO INVISIBLE COMO ESTE.
AL MENOS NOS QUEDA EL RECONFORTARNOS LOS UNOS A LOS OTROS.
PONERNOS EN EL LUGAR DEL DE AL LADO...
...INTENTAR AYUDAR EN TODO LO QUE SEA POSIBLE.
ESTA PANDEMIA SACA A RELUCIR LO MEJOR DE CADA UNO...
...Y TAMBIÉN LAS SOMBRAS MÁS OSCURAS QUE ALBERGAMOS.
PERO ES TAN SOLO MIEDO, DEBILIDAD, NO MALDAD.
EN NUESTRA MANO ESTÁ EL NO RENDIRNOS. EL NO CEDER AL MIEDO. EL SEGUIR LUCHANDO EN EL BANDO DE LOS BUENOS.
LA EMPATÍA ES EL SUPERPODER MÁS IMPORTANTE.
AHORA Y SIEMPRE.
SE HACE TARDE.
ESTARÁS CANSADA.
¿QUIERES QUE TE ACERQUE A CASA?

Through this operation, Rubín implicitly shows that the epic component of the genre only works if there is previously an ethical foundation appealing to affection and tolerance, to respect for human rights and empathy (Román Maestre, 2021). Thus, a vicissitude takes place for which Superman stands as the last resource for an anonymous ordinary citizen who, because of her job in a supermarket, is rejected by her neighbors as they believe she is a source of contagion. Certainly, reliance on a messianic metaphor is tangible (it is, in fact, behind the original foundation of the character) but it is reconfigured through a conversational scene in which Superman intervenes, simply, as a good friend who listens to, a good friend who does not abandon anyone because he knows that love is the way. Not surprisingly, the most beautiful leitmotif associated with Superman is: "There's always a way", so it may be said that *the Last Son of Krypton* is, himself, a metaphor for hope.

FUTURE RESEARCH DIRECTIONS: THE LANGUAGE OF COMICS AS A TOOL FOR CRYTICAL ANALYSIS

It is extremely important to stress that relying on artistic languages which are alternative to traditional ones increase the chances to produce more thoughtful academic meditations since each medium determines a particular decoding process and, consequently, the way its content is assimilated by users-readers (Sousanis, 2015, p. 54). In this case, the language of comics, which is based on *iconic solidarity* (Groensteen, 1999, p. 82), a concept which is connected with intuitive and sensorial elements rather than to textual and linear ones (related, usually, to words-based media), and whose reading rhythm is dependent on readers' choice, offers a potentially remarkable interpretative margin, since it involves a complex hermeneutical process in which an open space is generated (Ahmed, 2016) for the reader, who acquires a creator role about final meaning decoding, to intervene (*intentio lectoris*) in tension with the artist's will (*intentio auctoris*). This perspective, in summary, would empower scholars to describe comics as the art of the ineffable.

As the pandemic is still a recent event, though, the corpus of selected works is not constituted to be a canonical list but a temporary one: on the one hand, because it is foreseeable that more comics about this situation will emerge in the future (Tebeosfera, 2020), some of which may be relevant; on the other hand, because it is too early to reliably assure that the chosen items for this chapter will endure as basic references over time. However, *hic et nunc* these selected works have been notably disseminated in the Spanish comic industry and, therefore, analysing them allows to build a coherent account to understand the society in which they have been created. Likewise, as it has been said, the fact that this corpus has been limited to graphic novels produced within the Spanish comics market is justified on the grounds that they represent an homogeneous sociocultural context, and, morover, they offer overviews which may be contrasted with the chapter's author personal knowledge.

In any case, in the future it would be appropriate to develop a study based on a broader body of works, even comprehensive if uniting various researchers' efforts was possible, to produce a kind of graphic novels canon regarding this chapter's subject matter. In fact, comics selection for this chapter itself could have taken into account other contemporary items which have been discarded just because those which have finally been chosen represent, as far as the author is concerned, more complete visions with respect to the pandemic and, besides, they serve a convenient purpose for constructing a coherent story. In this sense, it would be worth keeping in mind, to broaden analysis framework for further papers, some other graphic novels such as: *Beti Berdin Taberna. En tiempos del coronavirus* by Asier Iturralde

(Gaston Ediciones, 2021), a funny collective-starring series set in a local bar and which is modulated through a story based on short and poignant scenes about loneliness and, above all, sociological and sentimental confusion affecting regular customers; *Algo extraño me pasó camino de casa* by Miguel Gallardo (Astiberri, 2021), which is connected with literary diaries template and which, therefore, collects autobiographical impressions which, thanks to a subtle comical touch and a rough draft-based style of graphics, allows readers to internally identify with the intimate narrative voice (Gallardo, a key creator since the so-called first Spanish adult comics *boom* in the early 1980s, is highly influenced by the *carnets de voyage* genre, typical of *Bande Dessinée* tradition, consisting on spontaneous sketches); *Mi novio, un virus y la madre que me parió* by Sebas Martín (La Cúpula, 2021), which describes, through an approach whose analysis could be arranged according to a *queer studies* perspective, the romantic unease facing, apparently, the end of times, despite the fact that, once again, melodramatic load is reduced by laughter and sillyness; or *Efectos secundarios. 19 historietas del Covid* (Astiberri, 2021), a collective-authorship work which, sponsored by Fundación Cultura en Vena following the aforementioned *GraphicMedicine* postulates (González Cabeza, 2017), is linked with the power of comics to shake consciences in relation to topics such as, among other areas of interest, care for the elderly and climate change (in fact, a traveling exhibition was held in parallel for hospitals and rural locations). Further expanding the hermeneutic spectrum, it would be even possible to add hybrid items such as *A casa. Diari gràfic del confinament* by Goyo Rodríguez (Onada, 2020), a reinterpretation of instruction manuals by virtue of the pictographic paradigm to which comics can be ascribed to and which refers, fundamentally, to how to deal with confinement at home; or *La muerte rosa* by Jaume Pallardó (Contrabando, 2018 and 2019), a work wich seems to deserve to be initially discarded because it is prior to the COVID-19 pandemic but which, considering the predictive power that sometimes manifests throughout tales, is configured as a dystopian science fiction graphic novel which captures a post-pandemic landscape which ends up being very similar to the real one.

On the other hand, the expansion of the vanishing point for future papers could not only be implemented focusing on specific works, but, alternatively, it could be outlined through a series of varied topics which would put scholars on the track of items which do not deal strictly with the pandemic phenomenon but which, following a more elusive way, would empower them to establish interrelationships by means of allegories or parables (in addition, this operation would lead to a comparison between various local industries' approaches to comics storytelling so that a universal corpus may become real). Thus, how catastrophism is dealt with in mainstream comics (settings, routes, archetypes...), a kind of subgenre mirroring apocalyptic cinema; contagion as a resignification of segregation; the use of viruses as a weapon for villains in the superhero genre, etc.

Come what may, comics' potential to act as an ideological disseminator and as a communicative tool for empathy seems to be obviously clear. In this sense, as John Berger (2015) highlighted about photography, comics medium, through its multimodal language, activates very effective mechanisms to capture any specific moment destined to last. Also, cathartic results dealing with impending reality concerns should be an added bonus.

CONCLUSION: COMICS MEDIUM IS A VACCINE LOADED FOR THE FUTURE

Ursula K. Le Guin, in her novel *A Wizard of Earthsea* (1968), pointed out that those who deny the existence of dragons are often, as a matter of fact, devoured by them. These words may serve as a metaphor to highlight the unforeseen blow, therefore even more painful, brought to population by this pandemic, both from a point of view which is linked to mental health and from a sociological perspective. For good measure, it could be said that the world, as it has been known until now, will surely not return. Undoubtedly, human interrelationships (friendships, romantic partnerships, neighborhood communities, workplaces, national groups, governments...) have been severely wounded and now, unfortunately, an atmosphere of mistrust and resentment prevails, a difficult situation to overcome since it is not clear who is guilty of what and which other more effective ways could have been embraced on time. Likewise, as confinement has not only caused a fierce emotional confusion and an evident disenchantment about the desire for sociability, but also an economic crisis, a breeding ground has been created for the consolidation of conservative ideologies which attempt or intend to attack those basic norms which society, at least the Western one, had given to itself since the conclusion of Second World War, all nuances notwithstanding, of course (this authoritarian drift has been already present for some time before but now it has grown exponentially as a result of the pandemic, since the history of the 21st century is probably about a welfare state collapse due to a manifest inability of capitalism renewing itself). No one was prepared, after all, for this kind of of surreptitious apocalypse, so that, as a result, people have been deprived of instruments with which to react against.

In this sense, obviously fiction works not only do not represent any panacea or magic antidote to the world's problems but, in fact, this chapter's author declares himself to be skeptical of the naive thought by which art, music, literature, etc. the intellectual factor, in short, may function pragmatically as a solution. Culture, then, is not a guarantee by itself for facing real problems: books do not magically solve crises (Brottman, 2018). However, it can be argued that culture does have an essential value for an early detection of such problems; in other words: it does empower citizens to be alert in a critical and documented way (Christopher, Wendt, Marecek, & Goodman, 2014), by whose virtue a cathartic value also may follow. On this matter, this chapter bets, lowering the shamanic value of culture, a naive expectation indeed, to highlight its potential as a hermeneutic instrument to analyse events, that is, it recovers an idea which has been already alluded to at the very beginning and which asserts that fiction may be conceived as a first-order decoding weapon (Zurita, 2020). Another issue, for sure, would be about subsequent implementations, an operation which requires political and, mostly, economic power, which determines the former aspect across the neoliberal framework: large corporations have long been shaping the true national mosaic around the planet and, therefore, they are the ones who control the geostrategic game, so it may well be pointed out that certain science fiction dystopias which describe states substitution (*res publica* substitution) by means of large industrial emporiums have ceased to be predictions to become into a tangible reality, but news control by media makes this event goes unnoticed.

Delving into this instrumental consideration about fiction (*instrumental* does not denote any pejorative claim), this author would like to recommend adopting comics, especially through *Graphic Novel* movement precepts (García, 2010), as an ideal medium, precisely, for reflecting critically on our environment and, if it would be possible, to stimulate proposals for actions againts a crisis situation, despite the fact that, as it has been insisted upon, art by itself will not get far successfully if economic and political resources are not available in order to allow putting any postulates suggested narratively into practice. Comics, as it has been shown throughout this chapter, present an integrative language which is absolutely connected with multimodal and interdisciplinary reality in tune with current cultural consumer landscape, that is, with transmedia narrative paradigm. For this reason, the author considers that selecting items belonging to this communicative field empowers researchers to carry out satisfactory explorations around the analysis of surrounding reality insofar as they adress, from a narrative staging point of view, the spectrum multisensory setting in which citizens live nowadays. In any case, it must be said that this chapter has been written with the intention of drawing attention to the fact that, concerning the critical academic field, attending to literary texts is no longer enough and, consequently, it is necessary to promote a renewal of reading process conceptualization in favour of an idea of enriched reading which, ultimately, will expand the margins of canon (Rovira-Collado, 2017).

ACKNOWLEDGMENT

This research was supported by a COST Action which must be refered as *Investigation on Comics and Graphic Novels in the Iberian Cultural Area - iCOn-MICS* [CA19119]; a university teaching network which must be refered as *América Latina a través del cómic y del álbum ilustrado: nuevas experiencias educativas y lectoras para ampliar el canon formativo y escolar en las aulas universitarias* [REDI-3CE5474]; and a university teaching network which must be refered as *La percepció de la identitat sexual de gènere i de raça en l'alumnat universitari a través de la lectura literària* [REDI-3CE5568].

REFERENCES

Adanti, D. (2017). *Disparen al humorista. Un ensayo gráfico sobre los límites del humor* [Shoot the comedian. A graphic essay on the limits of humor]. Astiberri.

Ahmed, M. (2016). *Openness of Comics: Generating Meaning within Flexible Structures.* University Press of Mississippi. doi:10.14325/mississippi/9781496805935.001.0001

Barthes, R. (1973). *Le plaisir du texte* [The pleasure of the text]. Editions du Seuil.

Bartual, R. (2014). *Narraciones gráficas. Del códice medieval al cómic* [Graphic narrations. From medieval codex to comics]. Self Published.

Berger, J. (2015). *Para entender la fotografía* [To understand photography]. Editorial GG.

Bordería Ortiz, E., Martínez Gallego, F. A., & Gómez Mompart, J. L. (Eds.). (2015). *El humor frente al poder. Prensa humorística, cultura política y poderes fácticos en España (1927-1987).* [Humor versus power. Humorous press, political culture and factual powers in Spain (1927-1987)]. Editorial Biblioteca Nueva.

Bringel, B., & Pleyers, G. (Eds.). (2020). *Alerta global: políticas, movimientos sociales y futuros en disputa en tiempos de pandemia* [Global alert: policies, social movements and futures in dispute in times of pandemic]. Consejo Latinoamericano de Ciencias Sociales., doi:10.2307/j.ctv1gm027x

Bröckling, U. (2021). *Héroes postheoricos. Un diagnóstico de nuestro tiempo* [Post-Heoric heroes. A diagnosis of our time]. Alianza Editorial.

Brooks, S. K., Webster, R. K., Smith, L. E., Woodland, L., Wessely, S., Greenberg, N., & Rubin, G. J. (2020). The Psychological Impact of Quarantine and How to Reduce it: Rapid Review of the Evidence. *Lancet, 395*(10227), 912–920. doi:10.1016/S0140-6736(20)30460-8 PMID:32112714

Brottman, M. (2018). *Contra la lectura: un ensayo dedicado a los lectores que no creen que los libros sean intocables* [Against reading: an essay dedicated to readers who do not believe that books are untouchable]. Blackie Books.

Carrión, J., & Sagar. (2018). *Gótico* [Gothic]. Norma Editorial.

Christopher, J. C., Wendt, D. C., Marecek, J., & Goodman, D. M. (2014). Critical Cultural Awareness: Contributions to a Globalizing Psychology. *The American Psychologist*, *69*(7), 645–655. doi:10.1037/a0036851 PMID:24841336

Cohn, N. (2013). *The Visual Language of Comics*. Bloomsbury Academic.

Costa, J. (Ed.). (2018). *Una risa nueva. Posthumor, parodias y otras mutaciones de la comedia* [A new laugh. Post-humor, parodies and other comedy mutations]. Lengua de Trapo.

De Sousa Santos, B. (2020). *La cruel pedagogía del virus* [The cruel pedagogy of the virus]. Consejo Latinoamericano de Ciencias Sociales. doi:10.2307/j.ctv1gm01nn

Eco, U. (1962). *Opera aperta. Forma e indeterminazione nelle poetiche contemporanee* [Open work. Form and indetermination in contemporary poetics]. Bompiani.

Embid, J. (2018). *Con capa y antifaz: la ideología de los superhéroes*. Catarata.

Featherstone, M. (1992). The Heroic Life and Everyday Life. *Theory, Culture & Society*, *9*(1), 159–182. doi:10.1177/026327692009001009

Fontdevila, M. (2013). *No os indignéis tanto* [Don't be so unworthy of them]. Astiberri.

García, S. (2010). *La novela gráfica* [The graphic novel]. Astiberri.

Giordano, P. (2020). *En tiempos de contagio* [In times of contagion]. Penguin Random House Grupo Editorial.

González Cabeza, I. (2017). *Imágenes de la enfermedad en el cómic actual* [Images of the disease in the current comic]. Servicio de Publicaciones de la Universidad de León - Eolas Ediciones.

Gopegui, B. (2008). *Un pistolazo en medio de un concierto* [A gunshot in the middle of a concert]. Editorial Complutense.

Groensteen, T. (1999). *Système de la Bande Dessinée* [Comic Strip System]. Presses Universitaires de France.

Jenkins, H. (2003). *Transmedia Storytelling. Moving Characters from Books to Films to Video Games can Make them Stronger and more Compelling*. https://www.technologyreview.com/news/401760/transmedia-storytelling

Matly, M. (2020). *La función del cómic* [The function of the comic]. ACyT Ediciones (Asociación Cultural Tebeosfera).

Matos, D. (2017). *Periodismo cómic. Una historia del género desde los pioneros a Joe Sacco* [Comic journalism. A history of the genre from the pioneers to Joe Sacco]. Comunicación Social Ediciones y Publicaciones.

Mendoza Fillola, A. (2001). *El intertexto lector. El espacio de encuentro de las aportaciones del texto con las del lector* [The reading intertext. The meeting space of the contributions of the text with those of the reader]. Ediciones de la Universidad de Castilla-La Mancha.

Moix, T. (1968). *Los 'comics'. Arte para el consumo y formas pop* [The 'comics'. Art for consumption and pop forms]. Jarama.

Pizzino, C. (2016). *Arresting Development. Comics at the Boundaries of Literature*. University of Texas Press. doi:10.7560/309773

Porcel, P. (2002). *Clásicos en Jauja. La historia del tebeo valenciano* [The 'comics'. Art for consumption and pop forms]. Edicions de Ponent - Generalitat Valenciana.

Porcel, P., & Pons, A. (2007). *Viñetas a la luna de Valencia. La historia del tebeo valenciano (1965-2006)* [Vignettes to the moon of Valencia. The history of Valencian comics (1965-2006)]. Edicions de Ponent - Generalitat Valenciana.

Román Maestre, B. (2021). Les llibertats i els drets en temps de pandèmia: reflexions des de l'ètica [Freedoms and rights in times of pandemic: reflections from ethics]. *Qüestions de vida cristiana, 270*, 46-56.

Rovira-Collado, J. (2017). Canon artístico y criterios de selección de historietas: las propuestas de Unicómic [Artistic canon and comic selection criteria: the proposals of Unicómic]. *Umbral. Literatura para infancia, adolescencia y juventud, 12*(3), 3-19.

Saunders, B. (2011). Do the Gods Wear Capes? Spirituality, Fantasy, and Superheroes. *Continuum*.

Scolari, C. A. (2013). *Narrativas Transmedia. Cuando todos los medios cuentan* [Transmedia Narratives. When all media counts]. Deusto.

Sousanis, N. (2015). *Unflattening*. Harvard University Press.

Tebeosfera. (2020). Tebeos para una pandemia [Comics for a pandemic]. *Asociación Cultural Tebeosfera Blogspot*. https://asociacionculturaltebeosfera.blogspot.com/2020/03/tebeos-para-una-pandemia.html

WHO. Regional Office for Europe. (2020). *Mental Health and Psychological Resilience During the COVID-19 Pandemic*. http://www.euro.who.int/en/health-topics/health-emergencies/coronavirus-covid-19/news/news/2020/3/mental-health-and-psychological-resilience-during-the-covid-19-pandemic

Yrigoyen, E. (2020). Con la fuerza de lo real. Pandemia, relato y ficción en época de coronavirus [With the strength of the real. Pandemic, story and fiction in times of coronavirus]. In N. Escutia, B. Fleitas, & T. Oñate y Zubía (Eds.), Pandemia, globalización, ecología. ¿Qué piensa la hermenéutica crítica? 34 filósofas y filósofos responden a estas cuestiones (pp. 149-158). Universidad Nacional de Educación a Distancia (UNED).

Yus Ramos, F. (1997). *La interpretación y la imagen de masas* [The interpretation and the image of masses]. Institut de Cultura «Juan Gil-Albert» - Conselleria de Cultura, Educació i Ciència de la Generalitat Valenciana.

Žižek, S. (2020). *Pandemia. La COVID-19 estremece al mundo* [Pandemic. COVID-19 is shaking the world]. Anagrama.

Zurita, C. (2020). La realidad, la ficción. Apuntes sobre pestes y plagas en la literatura [Reality, fiction. Notes on pests and plagues in literature]. *Trabajo y sociedad: indagaciones sobre el empleo, la cultura y las prácticas políticas en sociedades segmentadas, 35*, 203-208.

ADDITIONAL READING

Bringel, B. (2020). Geopolítica de la pandemia, escalas de la crisis y escenarios en disputa [Geopolitics of the pandemic, scales of the crisis and scenarios in dispute]. *Geopolítica, 11*(Especial), 173–187. doi:10.5209/geop.69310

Davies, D., & Rifkin, C. (Eds.). (2009). *Documenting Trauma in Comics. Traumatic Pasts, Embodied Histories, and Graphic Reportage*. Palgrave Macmillan.

Groensteen, T. (2006). *Un objet culturel non identifié* [An unidentified cultural object]. Editions de l'An 2.

Jonas, H. (1995). *El principio de responsabilidad* [The principle of responsibility]. Herder.

Mayor Serrano, M. B. (Ed.). (2018). Medicina y cómic [Medicine and comics]. *Tebeosfera, 9*(3). https://www.tebeosfera.com/numeros/tebeosfera_2016_acyt_-3_epoca-_9.html

Wang, C., Pan, R., Wan, X., Tan, Y., Xu, L., Ho, C. S., & Ho, R. C. (2020). Immediate Psychological Responses and Associated Factors During the Initial Stage of the 2019 Coronavirus Disease (COVID-19) Epidemic Among the General Population in China. *International Journal of Environmental Research and Public Health, 17*(5), 1729. doi:10.3390/ijerph17051729 PMID:32155789

Zeno, F., & Zimbardo, P. (2006). The Banality of Heroism. *Greater Good, 53*(2), 30–35.

Ziolkowski, T. (2004). *Hesitant Heroes. Private Inhibition, Personal Crisis*. Cornell University Press. doi:10.7591/9781501711275

KEY TERMS AND DEFINITIONS

Bruguera School: Based on both the graphic and storytelling style developed by comics artists who worked from the 1940s onwards for Editorial Bruguera, the most popular publishing house during classic Spanish comics period, critic Terenci Moix coined this term in 1968 to refer to its general traits. The usual tone was halfway between children's entertainment and satirical rendering, accompanied by sociopolitical and socioeconomic comments as a hidden reading. Likewise, its starring characters usually got frustrated by their lack of success when they tried to escape poverty, which served as a mirror for the desires of the unlucky contemporary Spanish society. Graphics were simple though meaningful, tending towards a certain geometric abstraction and possessing a high metaphorical value, and the backgrounds were minimalist. This publishing house closed in 1986 but its influence is still evident throughout new generations of creators.

COVID-19 Pandemic: A global pandemic caused by severe acute respiratory syndrome coronavirus 2 (SARS-CoV-2). Also known as the coronavirus pandemic, it began between late 2019 and early 2020, and it caused the authorities to take drastic measures to confine the population for prolonged periods of time in order to prevent an infections increase. It may not yet be fully eradicated, despite the fact that restrictive measures have almost disappeared in most countries.

Graphic Medicine: A movement which claims the use of comics to represent disease in images, especially based on a pedagogical will which may help patients heal or, at least, to help them understand the process they are going through. Additionally, it encourages empathy towards patients and their needs, with regard to both their families and society as a whole, especially concerning stigmatized illnesses such as mental issues.

Graphic Novel: An author-centered movement which claims, for the comics medium as an art, an absolute formal and thematic freedom, not dependent on business conditions. Likewise, it is conceived to appeal mainly to adult cross-sectional readers, who may be interested in reading a work not because a love for comics is prevalent to them but because of circumstantial motivations or because its specific topic converges with readers' interests in other artistic media. In contrast to conventional mainstream comics, they often reflect personal and intimate elements concerning its creators.

Iconic Solidarity: A term coined by theoretician Thierry Groensteen in 1999 to explain the stagement on a comics page as a unit of meaning, by which panels acquire coherence by coexisting across the same plane. It should be added that it refers to an intuitive and sensory reading conceptualization as opposed to the linearity developed throughout artistic media which are essentially word-based.

New Valencian School: A term which refers to a group of comics artists who, in the late 1970s and the early 1980s, resignified the graphic and narrative legacy of *Valencian School* (check this key term as well), to adapt it to works aimed at an adult audience, although young fiction items were also produced. As far as page layout is concerned, they were much influenced by *Ligne Claire* trends (an extreme sense of geometrical balance which makes every element included in a page to be perfectly positioned) through *Tintin* and other Franco-Belgian series, which is the reason why this movement was also called *Valencian Ligne Claire*.

Opera Aperta: A term coined by semiotician Umberto Eco in 1962 by which it is suggested that there is not just one final meaning for a text at the expense of its creator, but it rather refers to a plurality of meanings, depending on various factors such as readers' background.

Reader Intertext: A term which, mainly developed by literary theoretician Antonio Mendoza Fillola, denotes, in relation with literary competence, that readers decode what a text means by integrating, selecting and, therefore, activating their previous knowledge, and also their strategies and linguistic-cultural resources.

Slice of Life: A term originating from *Bande Dessinée* tradition (*tranche de vie*), that is, from Franco-Belgian comics market, which describes works focused on everyday life filtered by a mundane perspective (complex job circumstances such as dismissal or bad relationships between co-workers; sentimental relationships in crisis, etc.). It is often linked to autobiographical comics and, therefore, it represents one of the most common subgenres within the *Graphic Novel* movement (check this key term as well).

Valencian School: A term which designates the graphic and storytelling style developed by comics artists who worked for various Valencian publishers, such as Editorial Valenciana or Maga, from the 1940s onwards. In contrast to *Bruguera School* (check this key term as well), sociopolitical burden used to be less frequently adressed as preferences were higher for a naive comedy kind of tale, supported also by a powerful *sense of wonder*. On the other hand, backgrounds were more detailed, and graphics were usually less abstract as smooth and rounded shapes were favoured.

Chapter 7
Pandemics, Illness and Impairment as Reflected in Borges' Literature and as Key Factor to Shape His Authorial Style:
Searching in Literature the Epic Fate Frailty Had Denied to Him

Belén Lozano Sañudo
Universidad de Valencia, Spain

ABSTRACT

The first part of this chapter, consisting of Sections 1 and 2, aims at explaining the apparent scarce presence of Spanish Flu in modernist literature in general and in Borges' literary work in particular. The reason seems to be threefold: the degrading demise associated with illness in comparison to the glorifying destiny attributed to casualties from war, the different metaphorization processes undergone by distinct pandemics and epidemics, and the fact that this 1918 pandemic coincided in time with World War I and artists were trying to avoid evocating more suffering. The second part of the chapter, Sections 3 and 4, focuses on how the threat of Black Death and later Spanish Flu, which confined Borges at home, together with his frail health condition, made him prone to immersing in literature and dreams to escape from reality and experience adventures as real for him as those in the outside world.

DOI: 10.4018/978-1-6684-4735-2.ch007

INTRODUCTION

Pandemic and war have been present all along history reminding us of the fragile and ephemeral nature of humankind. As a young adult, the renowned Argentinian author Borges, who was then 19 years old, lived in Switzerland at a time when World War I and Spanish Influenza were taking the lives of many of his contemporaries.

In this study, we have read and analyzed some of Borges' most significant literary works to trace the presence of war, pandemic, illness and impairment in them. Whereas multiple references to military men and battles are easily found, those to pandemic are rather scarce and covert. In addition to this, in those cases where epidemic is mentioned, it is yellow fever, which is often a metaphor of slavery and used by authors, among them Borges, to condemn the evil of colonialism.

By reading his autobiographical essay and some critical works to gain an insight on the historical-sociological framework within which Borges' work was conceived, we have tried to explain why there are no overt references to Spanish Influenza, which had such a great impact on his education and creation of this own authorial style since, in the confinement it forced on him, he devoted many hours to translating, reading and rewriting some of the most significant works of literature of all times.

Borges idea of lives lived by reading literature and in dreams being as significant as those to which others refer as "real lives" is also exemplified in this chapter, since the oneiric and literary worlds are the only ones left to us in times of confinement. In these other ways of living Borges is given the opportunity of escaping from his fragile, impaired body and searching for a glorifying destiny met by his military ancestors and denied to him due to his weak physical condition.

To close the chapter the idea of his visual impairment and how, far from posing an obstacle to his artistic development, it was crucial in the shaping of his unmistakable style has been briefly addressed.

PRESENCE OF PANDEMICS AND SPANISH FLU IN LITERATURE

According to its autobiography Borges family arrived to Europe 1914, just four years before the worldwide H1N1 pandemic, best known as Spanish flu, struck the world. This febrile disease that began mildly in the summer 1918, swept around the world in just a few weeks. It broke out near the end of World War I and had an unusually high mortality for young adults. It devastated whole communities being one of the deadliest pandemics in human history and killing over 50 million people around the globe.

Opposite to what has been the case with other plagues the world has been in the grips of a long history, and as stated by Vazquez-Espinosa et al. (2020, p. 3), literature about the Spanish flu is rather scarce: "Instead the literature of the plague (Bocaccio´s Decamerone, Camus´s The plague), or tuberculosis (such as Thomas Mann´s The Magic Mountain), the 1918-1919 pandemic has hardly been the subject of novel or realistic descriptions by writers."

Virginia Woolf, one of the authors whose works Borges was well-acquainted with, admired and a couple of which he even translated, contracted influenza herself and was confined to bed, among other occasions in the early months of 1918 and at the end of 1919. These experiences with illness led her to write her essay *On Being Ill*, in which she, Woolf (1926) points out that in times in which our body is affected by pain, ailments and suffering there are two things we are left to turn to: our inner life and poetry.

In this essay, she also wonders how it can be that in times of the Spanish flu, the consequences of which were shaking the grounds of human existence, writers seemed to turn their back to illness, refusing it the place it should have as main theme of literature. Woolf (1926, p. 32) wrote:

CONSIDERING how common illness is, how tremendous the spiritual change that it brings, how astonishing, when the lights of health go down, the undiscovered countries that are then disclosed, what wastes and deserts of the soul a slight attack of influenza brings to light [...] with the greeting of the Deity stooping from the floor of Heaven to welcome us—when we think of this and infinitely more, as we are so frequently forced to think of it, it becomes strange indeed that illness has not taken its place with love, battle, and jealousy among the prime themes of literature.

In her book *Viral Modernism. The Influenza Pandemic and Interwar Literature* Outka (2020, p. 1) refers to this oblivion as a "modern mystery, and describes as "astonishing" the fact that, in spite of the flu having such a lethal impact on population and causing such deep effects on writers and artists, "it is rarely considered in modernist scholarship."

The author of the aforementioned book ibidem (2020, p. 2) agrees with that sustained in the previously cited article, Vazquez-Espinosa et al. (2020, p. 3), which attributes this forgetfulness to the fact that the 1918 pandemic coincided in time with World War I. Nevertheless, whereas Vazquez-Espinosa (2020, p. 3) seeks the explanation in the fact that writers and poets were trying to avoid evocating more suffering, Outka (2020, p. 2) rather points out that for some "The millions of flu deaths didn't (and don't) count as history in the ways the war casualties did." This is attributed to the fact that demises due to illness have been traditionally considered less dignified, worthy of admiration and more feminine ways of passing away.

In line with this idea of causing a casualty in war being a much more glorifying fate than dying of an illness, Borges in his autobiographical essay explains how he felt ashamed and even unworthy of love or attention because, contrary to many of his ancestors, he was denied taking part in valiant adventures and was not meant to be remembered by any military heroic deeds. In his own words, Borges (1971, p. 140):

So, on both sides of my family, I have military forebears; this may account for my yearning after that epic destiny which my gods denied me, no doubt wisely [...]I was always very nearsighted and wore glasses, and I was rather frail. As most of my people had been soldiers—even my father's brother had been a naval officer—and I knew I would never be, I felt ashamed, quite early, to be a bookish kind of person and not a man of action.

One other reason for this scarce presence of Spanish flu in literary texts in comparison with other plagues, pandemics and epidemics is the metaphorization and mystification processes plagues and other epidemics such as tuberculosis have undergone. Just to mention a couple of examples, whereas plagues have been traditionally related to divine punishment for corrupt societies, phthisis, in the 19th century was seen as associated to extraordinary characters with profound spiritual lives and sensitivities. As stated by Pôrto (2007, p. 1):

In the middle of the 19th century, those who suffered from tuberculosis had an aura of exceptionality that put them in a position of certain refinement in the eyes of their contemporaries. The concept of tuberculosis pertained to a markedly romantic sensibility, which was spreading about, especially among intellectuals and artists.

Great heroines of the most celebrated novels of the first half of the 19th century were victims of the white plague. Margarita Gautier, main character of Alexandre Duma's *The Lady with the Camellias*, is consumed by this illness that symbolizes the purification of her soul through sacrifice and abnegation. A character that appears at first sight as superficial, materialistic, and vain redeems herself from the dissolute life she had been leading by renouncing the love of Armando, putting his career and wellbeing before her own happiness. Sontag (1978, p. 16) writes about this imagery of purification of the soul and mystical metaphors associated to tuberculosis:

For over a hundred years TB remained the preferred way of giving death a meaning—an edifying, refined disease. Nineteenth century literature is stocked with descriptions of almost symptomless, unfrighten, beatific deaths from TB, particularly of young people, such as Little Eva in Uncle Tom's Cabin. [...] The dying tubercular is pictured as made more beautiful and more soulful.

Sontag (1978, p. 17) explains how myths associated to an illness greatly influence our perception of it. In this sense she points out how, in spite of the fact that the tubercle bacillus can also affect other parts of the body, such as the brain, the kidneys or the spine, it has been traditionally associated to lungs (breath, life), which are part "of the upper, spiritualized body". In her own words Sontag (1978, p. 18): "A disease of the lungs is, metaphorically a disease of the soul."

Contrary to what is the case with these other epidemics, as we have previously pointed out silent seems to surround the Spanish flu pandemic in literature and arts. Nevertheless, this apparent omission is not such if we learn to identify its subtle presence. Outka (2020, p. 2) invites us to search for the traces of the pandemic in the works of modernist writers for, contrary to what appears at first sight, and as she states:

If we know what to look for, the literature of the era emerges as particularly adept at representing the pandemic's particular qualities and its vast yet hidden presence. [...] When we recognize the terror and subsequent evasion that such a threat produced, modernism's indirect qualities emerge as subterranean echoes of the pandemic's horrors and the very ways these horrors go underground.

By thoroughly analyzing some of the most emblematic writings of modernism, such as *Mrs. Daloway, The Waste Land* and "The Second Coming", by Virginia Woolf, T.S. Eliot and W.B. Yeats respectively, the author reaches the conclusion that the presence of what she refers to as "viral tragedy" in them, although subtle, is very significant. In fact, she concludes Outka (2020, p. 4): "These texts showcase how central elements of modernist style— from elongated sentences to plotless structures to amorphous characters— provided the ideal form to represent the pandemic's presence."

PANDEMICS AS REFLECTED IN BORGES' LITERARY WORK

Although Borges lived at the time when the world was in the grips of Spanish Influenza, we don't find overt references to it, neither in his works, nor in his autobiographical essay (1971). In his Conversations with Osvaldo Ferrari (2014) when talking about his affinity with the Argentinian intellectual and writer Domingo Faustino Sarmiento, who according to Borges had brought sparrows and eucalyptus from Australia to Argentina, he cursorily refers to it:

I have a memory about a eucalyptus. When an epidemic of Spanish Flu broke out after the First World War, eucalyptus leaves were burnt in great pots. I guess they were supposed to be curative. That was in Geneva; I smelt the eucalyptus which I hadn't smelt for ages, and thought: Goodness, I am in the Hotel Las Delicias in Adrogué or in our quinta or country house La Rosalinda. I felt I was back in Adrogué thanks to the smell of those supposedly curative eucalyptus leaves in 1918 in Geneva.

Although he doesn't seem to be very convinced of its medicinal effects, its smell helps Borges travel in his mind to a safer moment in his life escaping the reality of World War I and Spanish Flu severely striking the world, for although Switzerland maintained armed neutrality, the 1918 pandemic was as harsh in this country as in the rest of the planet and war created great tension between Germaphone Swiss and their French- and Italian-speaking country men.

It is curious that, in spite of the Spanish Flu being one of the most devastating events in Swiss history (25.000 people died and half of the population was infected) and bearing in mind that the deadliest wave struck in October 1918, while Borges family was still living in Geneva, it is not present in Borges literature. Furthermore, the virus claimed more men than women and out of the deaths, 60% were victims aged 20 to 40 years old and at that time Jorge Luis Borges was 19.

Infected people could die within hours of falling seek, they often suddenly bled from the mouth or nose and the dead had to be buried immediately to prevent contagion. Switzerland was completely closed down, company and entertainment were nowhere to be found, concerts and theater performances were cancelled, and churches and schools were shut down or turned into emergency hospitals.

In spite of this apparent lack of attention to Spanish flu, we find references to other epidemics both in his stories and in his poems. For instance, his story *The Dread Redeemer Lazarus Morrell* (1975, 21), published as part of his work *Universal History of Infamy* reads: "Up-stream, between the Arkansas and the Ohio, is another stretch of lowlands. Living there is a sallow race of squalid men, prone to fever, who avidly gape at stone and iron, for in their environs there is little but sand, timber, and muddy water."

As we have mentioned in the previous section when explaining the metaphorization process undergone by pandemics, epidemics and plagues, there are different imageries associated to them, which are reflected in arts. Yellow fever often symbolizes the negative effects of colonialism and slavery trade. As explained by Lee (1998, p. 676):

[…] it was the geographical movement of this disease that determined its interpretative implications. Because these early medical studies nearly always referred to yellow fever as a Caribbean disease, and since the Caribbean was synonymous with the slave trade and colonial slavery, yellow fever itself became intimately tied to the physical and philosophical effects of slavery.

Studying Coloridge's poem *The Rime of the Ancient*, Lee (1998, p. 677) highlights the fact that a number of readers and critics have seen the poem as "an indictment of British maritime expansion" and a protest against the enslavement of native people. Lee (1998, p. 678) refers to yellow fever as the disease of "tyranny and subjection".

If we compare the imagery of tuberculosis to that of yellow fever, we can observe that whereas the former enthrones the individual bringing out his/her extraordinary spiritual value, creativity and sensitivity, in short is singularity, the second tends to rather characterize a civilization, a group. The illness and its effects are reflected in the collectivity on which a divine punishment is inflicted. As Sontag (1978, p. 37) explains:

Cholera is the kind of fatality that, in retrospect, has simplified a complex self, reducing it to sick environment […] In contrast to the great epidemic diseases of the past (bubonic plague, typhus, cholera), which strike each person as a member of an afflicted community, TB was understood as a disease that isolates one from the community.

Borges addresses the topic of imperialism and colonialism picturing a terrible, merciless world dominated by politic and economic interests in several of his short stories. We find an example in his short story *The Man on the Threshold* published as part of *The Aleph and Other Stories*. In this story British imperialist government sends a new governor to Colonial India to restore order. It reads Borges (1971, p. 88):

God, in his wrath, had allowed people to fall into corruption; the mouths of men were full of blasphemy and of deceit and of fraud. Yet not all were evil, and when it was known that the queen was about to send a man who would carry out in this land the law of England, those who were less evil were cheered, for they felt that law is better than disorder. The Christian came to us, but it was not long before he too was deceiving and oppressing us, concealing abominable crimes, and selling decisions. We did not blame him in the beginning; the English justice he administered was not familiar to anyone, and the apparent excesses of the new judge may have obeyed certain valid arcane reasoning.

At the beginning England, the metropolis is identified with law, justice and order, whereas the colony represents chaos and disorder. As we continue reading Glencairn, who stands for the colonizers, is described as descending from an "illustrious clan of warriors" and bearing "in his blood a tradition of violence". On the one hand "illustrious" as an adjective used to portray the character embodying civilization has in principle positive connotations ("illustrious" is someone honorable deserving respect). "Tradition" in turn conveys the meaning of something that is well established and consolidated. Nevertheless "violence" is already anticipating the oppression he soon started to exert on the colonized natives.

As we continue reading the story, the colonizing Christian is depicted as "deceiving" and "oppressing", concealing "abominable crimes", corrupt, since he is said to be "selling decisions", and in short, he is said to be a "wicked man". In the passage the words quoted above "corruption", "fraud", "deceit" (of the same word family as "deceiving", which is subsequently used to describe Glencairn) and evil are attributed to the natives.

Borges's notion of recurrent universal patterns is present in this story through the reference in the first line to Bartolomé de las Casas as archetype of cruel redeemers. As noted by Lawrence (2011, 167) in reference to Las Casas, he had "[…] a long-standing tradition among *americanistas*, stretching back to Bolívar and beyond, of viewing [him] as a savior among the slaughters of the Conquest […] yet seems anything but a philanthropist on the subject of black slaves."

Other references to yellow fever are to be found in his poem Deaths of Buenos Aires, *Chacarita* published in San Martin Copybook in 1929, Borges (1972, p. 73):

Porque la entraña del cementerio sur

fue saciada por la fiebre amarilla hasta decir basta;

porque los conventillos hondos del Sur

mandaron muerte sobre la cara de Buenos Aires

y porque Buenos Aires no pudo mirar esa muerte,

a paladas te abrieron en la punta perdida del oeste,

detrás de las tormentas de la tierra

y del barrial pesado y primitivo que hizo a los cuarteadores

[…]

Trapacerías de la muerte—sucia como el nacimiento del

hombre—

siguen multiplicando tu subsuelo y así reclutas

tu conventillo de ánimas, tu montonera clandestina de huesos

que caen al fondo de tu noche enterrada lo mismo que a la hondura de un mar,

hacia una muerte sin inmortalidad y sin honra.

[When the Southside's graveyards,

crammed full of yellow fever, cried out of their depths: Enough,

when the Southside's clustering tenements

spread death on the face of the city

until Buenos Aires could look at the carnage no longer,

shovel by shovel, they opened you up on the city's verge where the west drops away—

behind dust storms

and a weight of primordial muck left behind for the teamsters

[…]

The frauds of mortality—stained as in childbirth—

still fatten your subsoil; so you muster up souls

for your compounds, for your hidden contingent of bones

dropped into holes or buried away in your night

as if drowned in the depths of a sea,

preparing a death without hope of eternity, without honor.]

[Translation by Ben Bellit]

In this poem, and more specifically in the line that closes this stanza "preparing a death without hope of eternity, without honor" we find a good example that takes up what we have previously mentioned quoting Outka (2020, p. 2), who explained the lack of interest of modernist literature in reflecting Spanish influenza by pointing as main reason the fact that demises caused by illness were not considered as worthy of admiration, honorable or glorifying as casualties from war.

This idea of achieving a destiny of glory by taking part on military actions is not only reflected in his considerations about his personal life, as we have previously seen by quoting his autobiographical essay, but it is also very recurrent in his literary work. Just to mention a couple of examples, in his poem *Allusion to the Death of Colonel Francisco Borges (1833-74)*, published in his poem book *The Self and the Other* (1964), Borges (1972, p. 149) describes how his parental grandfather met his death in what Borges describes as an "epic world". Colonel Francisco Borges is depicted as a hero.

The poem *Sepulchral Inscription,* part of *Fervor of Buenos Aires* (1923), is dedicated to his great-grandfather Colonel Isidoro Suárez, who, as Borges writes in his autobiographical essay (1971, p. 139), in 1824, at the age of twenty-four "led a famous charge of Peruvian and Colombian cavalry, which turned the tide of the battle of Junín, in Peru. This was the next to last battle of the South American War of Independence." Borges (1972, p. 9) reads:

Dilató su valor sobre los Andes.

Contrastó montañas y ejércitos.

La audacia fue costumbre de su espada.

Impuso en Junín término venturoso a la lucha

y a las lanzas del Perú dio sangre española.

Escribió su censo de hazañas

en prosa rígida como los clarines belísonos.

Murió cercado de un destierro implacable.

Hoy es un poco de ceniza y de gloria.

[His valor passed beyond the Andes.

He fought against mountains and armies.

Audacity was a habit with his sword.

At Junín he put a lucky end to the fight

and gave Spanish blood to Peruvian lances.

He wrote his roll of deeds

in prose inflexible as battlesinging trumpets.

He died walled in by implacable exile.

Now he is a handful of dust and glory.]

[Translation by Robert Fitzerald]

Colonel Isidoro Suarez is embellished with attributes such as "valor", "audacity" and "glory". It is also worth highlighting how Borges uses the metaphor "he wrote his roll of deeds in prose inflexible as battlesinging trumpets", where "to write" is put on a level with "to live". This idea of literature and dreams being as significant in life as what others would call real experiences is also repetitive in Borges.

This is surely influenced by the fact that confinements forced on population due to pandemics were not new to him, since as we have previously mentioned, his family was still living in Geneva in 1918, when the deadliest wave of pandemic flu struck Switzerland, the country was shut down and its people forced to stay at home and lead a passive life.

In an interview with Burgin (2013) when Borges is asked about his writing always having its source in other books, he answers that for him what he experiences when reading a book "is no less an experience than travelling or falling in love." He makes no distinction between what other people would refer to as real life "toothache, headache, travelling and so on" and imaginary life and phantasy that "means the arts."

It is worth noticing that two out of three examples he gives of real life are related to corporal pain, no wonder that he, having suffered from such a frail health condition since his childhood years, seeks refuge in this imaginary life represented by the arts. In the aforementioned book by Burgin (2013) when asked about his story *The Circular Ruins* he explains how at the time when he was writing that story, which lasted one week, he felt that the regular life he was leading, working at a library and meeting friends for dinner every now and then, was unreal. He felt closer to the story he was writing.

BORGES' FRAIL HEALTH, CHILDHOOD CONFINED AT HOME AND AUTODIDACTIC LITERARY EDUCATION

Jorge Luis Borges did not attend school but rather received education at home until the age of 9. In its autobiographical essay (1971, p. 143) he attributes this to the distrust of his father of enterprises run by the State due to his condition of anarchist, but surely the fact that during his early years the world was under the threat of Black Death and his fragility he refers ibidem (1971, p. 140) also contributed to his parents making this decision.

Be that as it may, the point is that the boy was confined to his home, deprived of the chance to play with other children except for his sister and this fostered his imagination to the point that they invented nonexistent characters. In his own words ibidem (1971, p. 140): "[…] I spent a great deal of my boyhood indoors. Having no childhood friends, my sister and I invented two imaginary companions, named, for some reason or other, Quilos and The Windmill. (When they finally bored us, we told our mother that they had died.)"

He spent far more time among the books of his well-nourished father's library, which in his autobiographical essay Borges (1971, p. 140) refers to as "the chief event in his life", than among other children. He lived through literature and approached it from all its angles from a very early age: reading, writing, rewriting using texts he read as pretext for the creation of his own, literary critic, translation. As he explains in the foreword of his work *Evaristo Carriego*, Borges (1984, p. 33):

For years I believed I had grown up in a suburb of Buenos Aires, a suburb of dangerous streets and showy sunsets. The truth is that I grew up in a garden, behind a fence of iron palings, and in a library of endless English books. The Palermo of the knife and guitar throve (I am told) just around the corner, but those who populated my days and gave a pleasant shiver to my nights were Stevenson's blind buccaneer, dying under the horses' hooves, and the traitor who left his friend behind on the moon […]

According to his autobiographical essay (1971, p. 142) he starts writing at the age of six-seven years. At an age in which most children are learning to read in the sense of understanding how letters combine with one another to form words and start decoding short, simple sentences, autodidactic Borges imitates Spanish classics, such as Miguel de Cervantes, to develop his own authorial style.

And he not only succeeds in developing his style in just one language, but in two, for Borges (1971, p. 142) states: "I had set down in quite bad English a kind of handbook on Greek mythology, no doubt cribbed from Lempière." This bilingualism of his childhood, which turned into multilingualism later on in his life, opened the door to him to other literatures.

It was this mastery of several languages which enabled him to exercise translation, which he considered to be a paradigm of reading, writing and critical interpretation. In Borges we can observe two of the main functions of translation: finding, creating and refining one's style while importing themes, genres, models and values from other literary traditions.

At the tender age of nine he published his translation of Oscar Wilde's *The Happy Prince* in *El País*, one of the Buenos Aires dailies. In this translation as Lozano (2011, p. 43) points out and exemplifies, the creative infidelity Borges displays in his works as a translator can already be observed, since he seeks to reproduce the aesthetical emotion, rather than opting for a translation closer adhering to the wording of the original.

As we have seen, autodidactic learning plaid a central role in Borges education, in fact in his autobiographical essay he mentions how his father, despite being himself an English and Psychology teacher, Borges (1971, p. 42): «[...] never interfered. He wanted me to commit all my own mistakes, and once said, "Children educate their parents, not the other way around."

Nevertheless, it is his father, Jorge Guillermo Borges, Borges (1971, p. 138), who was a lawyer, writer, philosopher and translator himself, who taught Jorge Luis Borges his first lessons of philosophy and brought poetry close to him. "It was he who revealed the power of poetry to me- the fact that words are not only a means of communication but also magic symbols and music."

Borges' literature develops in parallel to that of Argentina, they are both the result of combining vernacular elements with foreign ones. After the migration wave of the beginning of the 19th century, in the streets of Buenos Aires Italian, German and English were spoken and the influence of all these languages and cultures got mixed with Creole traditions. Borges, for his part, exposed since his birth to English language and culture, attended from the age of fifteen a school in Geneva, where classes were given in French and he started learning German in an autodidactic way reading with the help of a German-English dictionary the first poems of Heine.

The level of mastery he reached of the German language was such that he was able to translate some of the great German expressionists as Klemm and Heynicke and even Schopenhauer, father of metaphysical pessimism, who saw in the aesthetics of art a way of escaping suffering and considered intellectual work the zenith of a happy life.

INFLUENCE OF ILLNESS, CORPORAL PAIN AND IMPAIRMENT ON HIS LITERARY WORK

Almost as fundamental for his literary and philosophical development as his father's library, which, as we have previously mentioned he, in his autobiographical essay, referred to Borges (1971, p. 140) as "the chief event in his life", is a near death experience he had. At Christmas Eve 1938 Borges had an accident while he ran up a staircase and hit his head on an open window casement that had just been painted, apparently because he had not seen it, due to his visual impairment, inherited from his father and which started already in his childhood, being already at a very advance stage.

Glass became embedded in his forehead and the injury was not properly cleaned what caused a septicemia leading to very high fever, hallucinations, and loss of the capacity to speak. For a month he, Borges (1971, p. 170), "hovered, all unknowingly, between life and death". He was terrified that on recovering he would not be able to write, read or think imaginatively anymore. In order to prove himself that he was still capable of writing he set himself the challenge of writing something he had never written before a story. The result was *Pierre Menard, Author of Don Quixote.*

This experience is reflected in his story in *The South*, first published in Spanish in *La Nación* in 1953, in which Juan Dahlman, who has many things in common with Borges: he is of German descent and has criollo military ancestors in his maternal part of the family he is very proud of (just like Borges himself, except that Borges' paternal family is of British rather than German descent).

Dahlman, just like Borges has an accident like the one Borges suffered, and after lying in bed at home with great pain and high fever causing hallucinations is taken to the hospital. Semi-delirious and confined in an anonymous room, he feels humiliation and self-hatred, as though he were in hell.

While struggling between life and death, he dreams that he has recovered and in his dream he is attacked by three farm hands and he gets involved in a knife fight. Although he has never wielded a knife and he is sure to die in the encounter, he feels that this, contrary to being defeated by illness, would be an honorable death. As explained by Gyurko (1988, p. 216) when exemplifying the influence of this story on Cortazar's *La noche boca arriba*:

[…] the sedentary but dream-prone protagonist Juan Dahlmann in reality dies ignominiously in a sanitarium, the victim of septicemia, but in his private, romantic, oneiric world is about to die heroically in a knife fight on la pampa. In both "El Sur" and "La noche boca arriba", fantasy seems to offer an escape from a mundane, threatening, dehumanizing reality

. […] In Borges, fantasy serves as a liberating force; within Dahlmann's hallucinatory world, his stature is increased […]. In the sanatorium, Dahlmann has come to loathe his weak, passive self, but his fantasy gives him the opportunity to prove his valor and feels a sense of exhilaration and joy as he confronts his opponent.

Once more, we find one of the recurrent themes of Borges: the confusion between reality, dream, and oneiric illusions as an escape from a humiliating, degrading reality. This, together with the ideas of time and infinity, memory and oblivion, self and double, free will and fate, cyclic time and space and the Eternal Return - and the symbols of these metaphysical preoccupations: the mirror, the labyrinth, the tiger, the knife are to be found over and over again both in his literary work and in that of the authors Gyurko (1988, p. 215) refers to as his literary "descendants".

Besides this accident, which as we have observed was crucial in his literary evolution, other impairments, mainly his declining vision, have also greatly contributed to shaping his style and literary evolution. Wilson (2006) attributes to his blindness the fact that Borges is not a descriptive writer, and he recurrently plays with memory.

Wilson (2006, p. 133) gives us some very illustrative examples on how this condition influenced Borges literary work: "At first, Borges 1955 blindness forced him to write poems. He had to abandon free verse as he needed mnemonic devices like meter, rhyme, and assonance to remember what he was dictating or composing in his mind."

In Borges it can be observed how on some occasion's disability is not to be considered as an obstacle, impeding artistic creation. As Snyder (as cited in Krentz, 2016, p. 37) argues, impairments are often an integral part of artistic achievement. Some artists succeed as a result of their impairments rather than in spite of them. By pointing to great Anglo-American literary figures such as Pope, Lord Byron and Henry James Snyder makes the point that, as stated by Krentz (2016, p. 37), "corporeal difference has sometimes contributed to celebrated works of Western literature". This has been, no doubt, the case with Borges, whose blindness has contributed to shape his unmistakable style.

CONCLUSION

This paper is divided in two parts. The first one, consisting in sections one and two, deals with the way Spanish flu and other pandemics were reflected both in Western literature and most particularly in Borges Work. The second one focuses on how Borges frail physical condition forced him to spend most of his childhood confined at home and how this fact, together with the accident he suffered at New Year's Eve in 1938 and his visual impairment greatly determined his style and themes.

Although Borges was a young man at the time when Spanish flu struck the world and he was surely confronted with the devastating reality caused by the pandemic all around the globe and, most specifically, in Switzerland, where Borges family was living at the time, he does not refer to it in his literary work. This is in line with what seemed to be the case with modernist literature in general.

The reasons put forward by academics and scholars to justify this apparent oblivion are threefold. On the one hand, the fate of people losing their lives to an illness was considered degrading and humiliating in comparison to those meeting a glorifying destiny causing casualty in war.

On the other hand, Spanish flu made its appearance during the years of World War I and some experts consider authors were trying to avoid reflecting more pain and suffering in their works.

The third explanation offered is the metaphors associated with the different illnesses, epidemics, and pandemics. Whereas tuberculosis has traditionally been associated with extraordinary characters, worthy of admiration and undergoing a beatifying death, other epidemics, or illnesses such as cholera or yellow fever have been used in arts as symbols of the oppression of colonizing powers and simplify the individual dissolving him/her in a community.

In this paper, examples have been provided of how Borges, most surely because of his ascendants being "men of action", indeed was ashamed and suffered from low self-esteem due to the fact that his physical condition had doomed him to be rather a "bookish" person. Epic stories about brave militaries meeting their destiny in the battlefield is an obsession in his work.

It has also been illustrated how yellow fever is present in his work as a symbol of dominating powers and their atrocious impact on natives and their lives, since it was Europeans who brought African slaves to the Caribbean and by doing so, they imported the illness.

In the second part of the paper, we have pictured Borges as a frail, overprotected boy and young adult who experimented the world through literature, confined at home and isolated from other children, instead of getting involved in the action of the streets of his native Buenos Aires.

Several examples are given of how for him what he experimented in dreams and by reading and writing was no less of an experience as that others call real life. He uses literature to escape from a reality at times too harsh to be faced.

Due to the fact that he spent so many hours among books, thanks to his infinite curiosity and his eagerness for constant learning, he came to master German, Latin and French, in addition to the two languages used in his family, Spanish and English. This gave him access to different literary traditions and through translation, while developing his own style, he helped import into Argentinean literature new genres, themes and styles.

His ailments, frailty, and visual impairment instead of representing an obstacle for his great artistic achievement, rather contributed to enthrone him as one of the key figures of universal literature. A clear parallelism can be stablished with the Vice-Admiral Nelson he describes in his writing signed with a pseudonym, who in spite of his fragile physical condition manages to defeat all fever attacks to encounter his glorifying destiny in Trafalgar battle, being enthroned as one of the most renowned English heroes of all times, Borges (1995, p. 105).

REFERENCES

Borges, J. L. (1971). *The Aleph and Other Stories 1933-1969*. Bantam.

Borges, J. L. (1972). *Selected Poems 1923-1967*. Allen Lane The Penguin Press.

Borges, J. L. (1975). *A Universal History of Infamy*. Penguin Modern Classics.

Borges, J.L. (1984). *Evaristo Carriego*. E.P. Dutton, Inc.

Borges, J.L. (1995). *Premio Cervantes 1979* [Cervantes Prize 1979.] Universidad de Alcalá.

Borges, J. L., & Ferrari, O. (2014). *Conversations* (Vol. 1). Seagull Books.

Burgin, R. (2013). *Jorge Luis Borges. The Last Interview and other Conversations*. Melville House.

Gyurko, L. A. (1988). The Metaphysical World of Borges and its Impact on the Novelists of the Boom Generation. *Ibero-amerikanisches Archiv. Neue Folge, 14*(2), 215–161.

Krentz, C. (2016). Borges in the Mind's Eye. *Journal of Literary & Cultural Disability Studies, 10*, 1.

Lawrence, J. (2011). *An American History of Infamy. Variaciones Borges, 31*, 161–179.

Lee, D. (1998). Yellow Fever and the Slave Trade: Coleridge's "The Rime of the Ancient Mariner." *ELH, 65*(3), 675-700. https://www.jstor.org/stable/300301

Lozano Sañudo, B. (2011). Borges y la traducción. Análisis de su primera incursión práctica: El príncipe feliz de Oscar Wilde [Borges and translation. Analysis of his first practical foray: Oscar Wilde's The Happy Prince]. *Mutatis Mutandis, 4*(1), 38–47.

Outka, E. (2019). *Viral Modernism. The Influenza Pandemic and Interwar Literature*. Columbia University Press. doi:10.7312/outk18574

Porto, Â. (2007). Social Representations of Tuberculosis: Stigma and Prejudice. *Revista de Saude Publica, 41*(Supl.1), 1–7. PMID:18038090

Sontag, S. (1978). *Illness as Metaphor*. Farrar, Straus and Giroux.

Vázquez-Espinosa, E., Laganà, C., & Vazquez, F. (2020). The Spanish Flu and the Fiction Literature. *Revista Espanola de Quimioterapia, 33*(5), 296–312. doi:10.37201/req/049.2020 PMID:32633114

Wilson, J. (2006). *Jorge Luis Borges*. Critical Lives. Reaktion Books.

Woolf, V. (1926). On Being Ill. *The New Criterion, 4*(1), 32–45.

Chapter 8
The Contribution of Children's Literature to the Development of the Child:
Book Therapy and Narrative Therapy

Marinos Bouchtsis
https://orcid.org/0000-0003-0170-1522
Universidad de Alicante, Spain

ABSTRACT

The influence of children's literature on the general development of the child is important. The initiation of the child in the book contributes to the spiritual, cognitive, and linguistic development to the mental and emotional maturation, to the aesthetic cultivation, the wealth of ideas, and offers entertainment, improves expressive ability, and contributes to the formation of the reader's character. "Pandemic" may have been the word of the year 2020, but perhaps, it should have been "coped." Many families have had to adapt to home education, financial hardship, and losses as well as their daily stressors, and this has had an emotional impact on the children. It turns out that books can be powerful coping tools. Books can help children cope with conversations when difficult things happen. Books can also provide parents, guardians, or teachers around them with the best tools to help children during this pandemic time.

INTRODUCTION

The influence of Children's Literature on the general development of the child is important. The initiation of the child in the book contributes to the spiritual, cognitive and linguistic development, to the mental and emotional maturation, to the aesthetic cultivation. Reading books brings the child in contact with intellectual creations, increases the wealth of ideas, offers entertainment, improves expressive ability, contributes to the formation of the reader's character (Anagnostopoulos & Delonis, 1988).

After all, the progress of man, and especially of the child, is interwoven with the spiritual and moral development, with the responsibility towards the society and himself. Literature and reading books play

DOI: 10.4018/978-1-6684-4735-2.ch008

a key role in achieving this progress (Theodoulou, 1988). Preparing children, therefore, for success in life presupposes a balanced education that ensures them both the acquisition of academic knowledge and the readiness to develop into responsible citizens, which is why the school, but also the family, must apply scientifically substantiated approaches that promote the social, emotional and cognitive development of children (Kourmousi & Salagianni, 1988).

Literature offers the child opportunities to discover and recognize his feelings, but also to find solutions to problems, through his identification with the heroes of the story. The benefits of reading books to the child have been utilized by book therapy, whether it is a case of cure or prevention. The method of using books to find solutions to readers' problems was called book therapy by Ireland in 1930 (Patera & Tsilimeni, 2012).

THE CONTRIBUTION OF CHILDREN'S LITERATURE TO THE DEVELOPMENT OF THE CHILD

Cognitive Development

Cognitive development is intertwined with the maturity of the child and is influenced by the experiences offered by his social environment. Children's books can help the child to understand basic concepts and develop his thinking. Children's Literature, moreover, is effective in shaping important functions related to thought, such as observation, comparison, categorization, hypothesis, organization, summary, application, and critique (Norton, 2007).

Children's books, with rich and colorful illustrations, are ideal for the exercise of observation, in young and old children. Literary books can be used to develop the ability of comparison. The comparison can be focused between two or more books, which present the same subject, in order to motivate the child to compare the external appearance of the book, the way each author presents the story, the illustration, the style, the language. and other elements. The comparison may also involve the approach of a story from different translations or adaptations, but also from variations of the story itself, encouraging the child to identify similarities and differences between them.

Books that refer to concepts are a stimulus for practicing classification and categorization. Some books help the younger child to understand the relationship between objects and concepts, such as color, shape, size. The classification can also refer to the characteristics of a story, about the main characters, the scenes, the elements of the narrative and the plot. Older children can classify books, either according to a given classification system, under the guidance of an adult, or by creating their own system, with criteria and categories, based on the content of the material they want to classify (Karpozilou, 1994).

Reading and listening to a literary work can develop and improve a child's organizational skills. His ability to place events in a logical order of causation but also in chronological order is cultivated by reading books, and especially traditional stories, which have a coherent plot and are based on repetition and description. After all, reading extends the reader's experience in space and time and helps him to gain a sense of time periods and evolution (Spink, 1990).

Social Development

Children's first relationships develop in the immediate family environment and then extend to the wider social environment (school, friends, peers). Literature can be a useful aid for the development of children's relationships, encouraging them to become aware of the feelings of others (Norton, 2007) and to discover the thoughts and actions of other people, but also new human relationships (Theodoulou, 1988). Books often describe problems faced by family members, but also the possibilities that exist to overcome these difficulties. A common theme, also in children's books, is brotherly relationships and feelings of friendship.

Children's books provide opportunities to cultivate children's social skills (Glazer, 1986). Books offer children the experience of drawing conclusions about the feelings and intentions of others. As the stories unfold, the characters constantly reveal more and more of their emotions, but also the reasons why they act that way each time. Children can make assumptions and find out, as the story progresses, whether their guesses were correct. Even from the pictures in the books, children can interpret the body language of the heroes and the expressions on their faces, as captured by the illustrator.

By following similar practices, when reading children's books, children will be able to show greater sensitivity to the feelings of others. When they are in such a position, they may be asked to empathize with a hero and think about how they would feel if they experienced a similar situation with him, or even talk about their relevant personal experiences. Identification, after all, with the characters of a story, allows children to understand the feelings of others and to observe behaviors that are similar to their own (Karpozilou, 1994).

Emotional Development

The term emotional development refers, on the one hand, to the emotions themselves, as experienced by the person and on the other hand to the regulation of emotions, i.e. the ability of the person to control his emotions depending on the situation in which he is (Hatzichristou, 2011). Emotional, social, and cognitive development are closely linked.

Children, in order to shape their personality traits, go through various stages of personal development. Progress through the stages of a child's personality development means the development of his / her maturity, and children's books can play a decisive role in this process (Norton, 2007). Reading literary works can help the child to understand but also to accept his feelings, to adopt new perceptions and to form his personal identity. Most books help to understand the feelings of others and at the same time the reader, thus helping the child to come to terms with his own feelings and behavior (Spink, 1991).

Literature can play a complementary role, as children's books contribute to emotional development in various ways (Karpozilou, 1994). Initially, they enable the child to realize that negative emotions (aggression, impulsive actions, jealousy, etc.) are familiar to his peers, since they are experienced by them, so they are normal. At the same time, through a story, the child can watch an event from the different perspectives of the heroes, but also accept that a person may have different contradictory emotions. It is also important that children's books offer alternative solutions to problems that may concern the child. Literary characters, through their actions, create patterns of behavior, which help the child to face similar difficulties and problems, such as parental divorce, loss of a loved one, moving, attending a new school. Books on family and interpersonal relationships can contribute to the formation of the child's self-esteem (Androtsopoulou, 1997).

Many children's books help, either directly or indirectly, to manage the various emotional states they experience, such as feelings of jealousy, fear, or anger (Norton, 2007). The problems that the characters face, especially the feeling of fear, can help in the development of the children's personality, since the characters overcome similar fears and feelings, with those that a child feels. Continuing, it is pointed out that Literature can play a catalytic role in the development of positive emotions in relation to themselves.

BOOK THERAPY

Book therapy, as an aid through books for children, was used in 1946, including the benefits that arise from the discussion between children and the teacher, which presupposes their involvement with a literary book (Papadopoulou, 2008). As the first educational approach of the term, book therapy is the use of books to help young people solve their problems (Papadopoulou, 2004). It is important, when using pediatric book therapy, to match the appropriate book with the problems they are experiencing (Pardeck & Markward, 1995) and with their level of reading, and also to present the problem in a realistic way, but in accordance with the emotional and developmental needs of children (Pardeck, 1995).

The method of book therapy has several benefits (Prater et al, 2006). Initially, it encourages children to express their problems and concerns, as some refuse to deal with traumatic events. Books can bring problems to the forefront and thus reduce the repression that children feel about them. In addition, book therapy can be a tool that provides information to help them solve their problems. Utilizing the messages associated with the picture and text of the book, children are introduced to ways in which others have tried, or succeeded, in solving their problems (Burnett, 1997).

In addition, book therapy contributes to the emotional relaxation and linguistic discharge of the child's emotions, which can result in both his mental rehabilitation and his linguistic maturation, through the dialogue that will follow the reading of a book (Papadopoulou -Mantadaki, 2003). Book therapy can also be a means by which teachers can teach appropriate social, emotional, and developmental skills (Sullivan & Strang, 2002). Also, book therapy can help students deal with real life situations, thus enhancing their chances of success both academically and socially.

NARRATIVE THERAPY

The narrative approach is based on the assumption that narratives are not representations or reflections of identities, but that narratives are identities. Narrative identity is the internalized and evolving story of a person's life, which incorporates the reconstructed past and the imaginary future to give life a degree of unity and purpose. The importance of identity and the recognition of transition support the idea that narrative approaches to therapy could be useful. Because narrative therapy considers identity to be the story of one's life, people are encouraged to look at and possibly rewrite their life story, past, present, and future (Leonard et al., 2017).

Narrative therapy argues that the interpretation of an event or experience by the individual is influenced by culture, context, and language. Interpretations of an experience, which are sometimes experienced as negative and problematic, influence his thoughts and actions. In therapeutic practice, one of the goals is to redefine how the individual sees the problem, shifting it from part of his or her identity to an external challenge that is not a fundamental aspect of identity (Leonard et al., 2017).

The application of narrative therapy is observed mainly in a variety of people, including those experiencing substance abuse, young people with autism spectrum disorders, refugees with post-traumatic stress disorder, students with learning disabilities and attention deficit hyperactivity disorder and hyperactivity and hyperactivity. Treatment can take place individually or in groups. (Panina-Beard & Vadeboncoeur, 2019)

USE OF LITERATURE TO COPE CHILDREN'S LONELINESS DURING THE PANDEMIC

Drawing from biological research, humans appear to be fundamentally a social species that needs to recognize and form relationships with others in order to survive (Bowles & Gintis, 2013; Tomasello & Vaish, 2013). A large body of research has shed light on how social relationships positively impact mental well-being in humans during different stages of life (Cacioppo & Cacioppo, 2014; Haslam, Jetten & Alexander, 2012; Holt-Lunstad & Smith, 2012; Huxhold, Fiori & Windsor, 2013; Seppala, Rossomando & Doty, 2013), with other studies showing the negative outcomes of lack or absence of social relationships (Santini et al., 2015).

Although social isolation can be considered a socially constructed concept, it can actually be quantifiable and observable (Holt-Lunstad, Smith & Baker, 2015). Loneliness, on the other hand, is defined as the perception of social isolation. That is to say, the individual's subjective experience of perceiving himself alone (Holt-Lunstad, Smith & Baker, 2015). However, it is important to emphasize the main role that an individual's cognitions play as a mediator in which one individual may prefer to be alone and still feel happy and connected, while another individual may be surrounded by family and friends and still feel alone. Consequently, there is evidence to suggest that these two concepts are not significantly related and may act as independent variables (Coyle & Dugan, 2012; Perissinotto & Covinsky, 2014). However, there is no agreement between disciplines on how best to define and measure these concepts (Courtin & Knapp, 2017). Other scholars define social isolation as "disengagement from social ties, institutional connections or community participation" (Pantell et al., 2013. p. 2056), which appears to be very much in line with the idea currently used by governments around the world during COVID-19.

"Pandemic" may have been the Word of the year 2020, but perhaps it should have "coped". Many families have had to adapt to home education, financial hardship, and losses as well as their daily stressors, and this has had an emotional impact on the children.

It turns out that books can be powerful coping tools. "Counselors have been using books to help children cope with adversity or difficult times for decades," says Michele Borba (2021), author of *Thrivers: Surprising Reasons Why Some Kids Struggle and Others Shine*. Associating a book with a problem, whether it be grief, loneliness, or anxiety, can help children process their emotions through the story's narratives and characters.

For example, a book with brave and independent protagonists, whether it's a classic like Louisa May Alcott's *Little Women* or a graphic novel like Gene Yang's *American Born Chinese*, can promote self-sufficiency in children. A grieving child can benefit from Susan Varley's Badger's *Parting Gifts*, which is about a group of woodland animals processing the loss of their friend.

And after a year of physical isolation from friends and family, literature can also help children cope with feelings of loneliness and learn to enjoy their own company. A missing friend may find solace in Tim J. Myers and Priscilla Myers' *Full of Empty,* a story about a lonely princess. For a child who is afraid of breaking out of the bubble, Frances Hodgson Burnett's *The Secret Garden* is a story of optimism and courage.

In addition to helping children cope with complex feelings, parents can also appeal to books as an entry point for difficult discussions on all sorts of issues. ("Remember how [character name] had a problem with [blank]?")

Books can help children cope with conversations when difficult things happen. For example, in Mildred Taylor's *Song of the Trees,* someone can talk about racism through the eyes of one of the characters.

Similarly, in Beverly Cleary's *Ramona Forever*, eight-year-old Ramona Quimby's father works double shifts while looking for a better job. When parents were unhappy, the whole world seemed to go wrong. This level of realism is what allows children to think about real-life issues that may be relevant during the pandemic and beyond.

When children see themselves on the pages, the experience can be encouraging. Books give children a sense of power. They have the power to mention the things that annoy them. This type of empowerment can be good for mental health - they don't seem to be powerless and can't do anything.

A recent moderate-quality systematic review identified 51 articles examining the benefits of recreational reading (for fun or learning) across different populations, including children (The Reading Agency, 2015).

Studies clearly show that reading promotes pleasure, relaxation, a better understanding of oneself and one's social identities. As a form of entertainment, it can also help people to "escape" from difficult times, but also to open up to other cultures and points of view. Reading also promotes empathy, social inclusion, self-esteem and community cohesion. Finally, some studies show that reading books can also improve memory and attention.

CONCLUSION

In recent years, psychology has been using more and more alternative methods of psychotherapy. Book therapy and therapeutic writing play a leading role in psychoanalysis and help individuals overcome their phobias or traumas. When people read a book or write a poem, for example, they organize the information in specific ways so that a meaning can be achieved, even if only aesthetically.

Researchers found that even six minutes of reading can reduce a person's stress levels by two-thirds. They believe this is because the distraction of entering a new world allows people to get away from their worries and this releases tension in both their minds and their bodies. In fact, they found that reading works faster than any other way to relieve stress, such as listening to music while walking or even enjoying a hot drink.

Reading books can help children cope with worries, feel better and cope with difficult times, with a list of books chosen and recommended by leading health professionals and co-produced with children and families. Opening conversations with children about anxiety and worry through reading can be really important in helping children identify and cope with how they are feeling. Books can also provide parents, guardians, or teachers around them with the best tools to help children during this pandemic time.

REFERENCES

Anagnostopoulos, B. D., & Delonis, A. (1988). Children's Literature and school. Pataki.

Androtsopoulou, A. (1997). The choice of modern stories for children as a means of book therapy: Rationale and applications. *Routes*, (49), 12–17.

Bowles, S., & Gintis, H. (2013). *A cooperative species: Human reciprocity and its evolution*. Princeton University Press.

Burnett, J. (1997). *Opening the World to Children: Using Books to Develop Problem-Solving Strategies*. Academic Press.

Cacioppo, J. T., & Cacioppo, S. (2014). Social relationships and health: The toxic effects of perceived social isolation. *Social and Personality Psychology Compass*, *8*(2), 58–72. doi:10.1111pc3.12087 PMID:24839458

Courtin, E., & Knapp, M. (2017). Social isolation, loneliness and health in old age: A scoping review. *Health & Social Care in the Community*, *25*(3), 799–812. doi:10.1111/hsc.12311 PMID:26712585

Coyle, C. E., & Dugan, E. (2012). Social isolation, loneliness and health among older adults. *Journal of Aging and Health*, *24*(8), 1346–1363. doi:10.1177/0898264312460275 PMID:23006425

Glazer, J. (1986). Literature for Young Children. Merrill.

Haslam, C., Jetten, J., & Alexander, S. H. (2012). *The social cure: Identity, health and well-being*. Psychology Press.

Hatzichristou, C. (2011). Social and Emotional Education at school (vol. 3). Typothito.

Holt-Lunstad, J., Smith, T. B., Baker, M., Harris, T., & Stephenson, D. (2015). Loneliness and social isolation as risk factors for mortality: A meta-analytic review. *Perspectives on Psychological Science*, *10*(2), 227–237. doi:10.1177/1745691614568352 PMID:25910392

Huxhold, O., Fiori, K. L., & Windsor, T. D. (2013). The dynamic interplay of social network characteristics, subjective well-being, and health: The costs and benefits of socio-emotional selectivity. *Psychology and Aging*, *28*(1), 3–16. doi:10.1037/a0030170 PMID:23066804

Karpozilou, M. (1994). The child in the land of books. Kastanioti.

Kourmousi, N., & Salagianni, M. (2016). Social and Emotional Learning. In Social and Emotional Learning through Children's Literature and the "Steps for Life" Program. Hellenic Committee of the World Preschool Organization.

Leonard, R., Horsfall, D., Noonan, K., & Rosenberg, J. P. (2017). *Identity and the End-of-Life Story: A Role for Psychologists: Identity and EOL*. Academic Press.

Norton, D. (2007). Through the eyes of a child. In Introduction to Children's Literature. Epikentro.

Panina-Beard, N., & Vadeboncoeur, J. A. (2019). *Narrative therapy*. Salem Press Encyclopedia.

Pantell, M., Rehkopf, D., Jutte, D., Syme, S. L., Balmes, J., & Adler, N. (2013). Social isolation: A predictor of mortality comparable to traditional clinical risk factors. *American Journal of Public Health*, *103*(11), 2056–2062. doi:10.2105/AJPH.2013.301261 PMID:24028260

Papadopoulou, S. (2004). The Emotional Language. Typothito-George Dardanos.

Papadopoulou, S. (2008). Book Therapy as a Teaching Approach through Linguistic Art and as a Body of Culture. In Education Sciences: Former "School and Life" (pp. 113-118). Academic Press.

Papadopoulou-Mantadaki, S. (2003). The socio-emotional teaching of language through the children's realistic novel. Metaichmio.

Pardeck, J. (1995). Bibliotherapy: An Innovative Approach for Helping Children. *Early Child Development and Care, 101*(1), 83-88. doi:10.1080/0300443951100106

Pardeck, J. & Markward, M. (1995). Bibliotherapy: Using books to help children deal with problems. *Early Child Development and Care, 106*(1), 75-90. doi:10.1080/0300443951060108

Patera, A. & Tsilimeni, T., (2012). *Literacy and socio-emotional development of the child. Theoretical approaches, activities and games*. Epikentro.

Perissinotto, C. M., & Covinsky, K. E. (2014). Living alone, socially isolated or lonely—What are we measuring? *Journal of General Internal Medicine, 11*(11), 1429–1431. doi:10.100711606-014-2977-8 PMID:25092012

Prater, M., Johnstun, M., Dyches, T.T., & Johnstun, M. (2006). Using Children's Books as Bibliotherapy for At-Risk Students: A Guide for Teachers. *Preventing School Failure, 50*(4), 5-13.

Santini, Z. I., Koyanagi, A., Tyrovolas, S., Mason, C., & Haro, J. M. (2015). The association between social relationships and depression: A systematic review. *Journal of Affective Disorders, 175*, 53–65. doi:10.1016/j.jad.2014.12.049 PMID:25594512

Seppala, E., Rossomando, T., & Doty, J. R. (2013). Social connection and compassion: Important predictors of health and well-being. *Social Research, 80*(2), 411–430. doi:10.1353or.2013.0027

Spink, J. (1990). Children as innovators. Kastanioti.

Sullivan, A. & Strang, H. (2002). Bibliotherapy in the classroom: using literature to promote the development of emotional intelligence. *Childhood Education, 79*(2), 74-80.

The Reading Agency. (2015). *Literature review: The impact of reading for pleasure and empowerment*. BOP Consulting.

Theodoulou, D. (1988). Children's Literature and the Toddler. In *Children's Literature and the Toddler*. Kastaniotis.

Tomasello, M., & Vaish, A. (2013). Origins of human cooperation and morality. *Annual Review of Psychology, 64*(1), 231–255. doi:10.1146/annurev-psych-113011-143812 PMID:22804772

Chapter 9
Algerian Literature as Socio-Educational Therapy During the 2020-2021 Pandemic

Mourad Kacimi
Universitat de València, Spain

ABSTRACT

This chapter focuses on the therapeutic function of Algerian literary production during the pandemic between 2020 and 2021. It describes the socio-educational environment of the Algerian population before the lockdown and highlights the effect of the pandemic on the cultural life of Algerian intellectuals and citizens. Also it reveals the importance of new technological media such as television, the internet, social networks, and digital books for transmitting literary works as well and then reflects on the contribution of Algerian writers and artists in this exceptional period. Likewise, the use of digital media as an option to replace traditional media in the literary environment is valued.

INTRODUCTION

The current study focuses on the socioeducational role of literary production during the COVID-19 pandemic on Algerian society, and the role of writers and mass media as intermediaries on the transmission of this literary contribution to society. This community was deeply affected by the pandemic: on one hand, the impact of the disease on their health; on the other, the impact on social life as a result of health measures.

This article highlights the characteristics of human relations in Arab societies, such as home visits, greetings, social spaces such as cafeterias, mosques, libraries, souks, etc. This social life had to adapt to the new situation, and in turn this happened thanks to artists and writers who have always had a crucial role in entertaining and guiding the population with their work. Algerian society´s interest in art and literature has served as a relief during this period.

Literature has been able to describe with precision the characteristics of the pandemic and individual suffering, and contemporary novel has much to say about mankind and nature. The exceptional circum-

DOI: 10.4018/978-1-6684-4735-2.ch009

stances we live can be an exceptional framework for writers. Literature has always dealt with pandemics and throughout history, all situations that provoked an upheaval of regular life was a source of inspiration for literary creativity. Likewise, this current pandemic has also been a catalyst for the creation of excellent literary works. Because the pandemic is like war, it makes us think again on humankind, on the basic elements of our lifestyle, on ways of escaping the shadow of death, a death that has come to dwell among us involuntarily.

When faced with this critical situation, the reaction of many writers was geared towards on two essential functions: first, making the population aware with informational works that reflected the gravity of the situation and the obligation to follow the norms created by health authorities. To do so, studies were published on how to deal with the pandemic that narrated similar historical events, and other works abounded on the consequences of this type of disease. The second function of the work of writers and artists was to offer consolation to people in order to relieve the lack they experienced in their social life as motivated by the current circumstances.

The sanitary measures adopted by health authorities severely limited social activities. After closing cultural, educational, and religious centers, mobile phones, television, radio, social media and mass media have been responsible for keeping readers up to date about literary novelties. Relevant artists and writers have taken advantage of digital tools such as electronic journals and books to keep their production abreast. Numerous artists used their YouTube and Facebook, etc. accounts to communicate with their followers. This situation has moved population at large to use digital tools to follow literary novelties. Nonetheless, we must mention some disadvantages of this technology and its effect on the literary production and social life in general in the world and Algerian society in particular.

ALGERIAN LITERARY PRODUCTION BEFORE THE PANDEMIC

Because of historical factors and the geographical location of Algeria in the Mediterranean, a large part of Algerian population –in addition to their mother languages, Arabic and Amaziġ– reads and uses French. As for the languages of other neighboring countries, Spanish and Italian are present among a reduced élite who has received their education in these countries; we can also say the same about English and German. These characteristics allow Algerian authors to publish in Arabic and French, and even in other languages.

Before the pandemic, most works by Algerian writers and artists revolved around topics related to customs, cultural traditions, social problems, etc. These contents were dealt with in genres such as classical and dialectal poetry, letters, messages, essays, discourses, short stories, novels, and theater.

Among them, we could underscore the Algerian novel which had reached an international stature due to important authors. In another study we already classified Algerian authors into two generations. The first one is represented by authors like Mohammed Dib, Mouloud Feroune, Abdelhamid Benhadouga, Assia Djebar, etc., and we said that they are characterized by writing in French in order to take advantage of it as a platform to project the Algerian cultural identity to the world and to defend the cause of Algerian society under French colonial rule (Kacimi, p. 420). The second generation includes authors like Ahlam Mostaghanemi, Yasmina Khadra, Rachid Boudjadra, Malika Mokaddem, and Amara Lakhous. They are interested in different topics and are far from a colonial life they did not live personally (Kacimi, pp. 422-424).

Among the first-generation Algerian authors who achieved recognition inside and outside Algeria, we must highlight Mohammed Dib. Some of his works have been translated into other languages, including Spanish. Among his novels we can mention *L'incendie* [*The fire]* (1954) and *Un été africain* [*An African summer*] (1959), translated into Spanish as *El incendio* (1979) and *Un verano en África* (1976). His novel *Incendie* and *La Grande Maison* [*The Big House*] were adapted as soup operas for Algerian TV under the direction of Mostapha Badi (1974).

Similarly, Mouloud Feraoun has been selected by the quality of his novels, such as *Le fils du pauvre* (1950), also translated into Spanish (2001). Novelist Abdelhamid Benhadouga wrote in Arabic and French. Among his works we can mention *Rīḥ al-ğanūb* [*The South Wind*] (1971), translated into French as *Le Vent du Sud* (1978) by Marcel Bois. Marcelino Villegas, his Spanish translator with the title *Viento del sur* (1981), called it a masterpiece. This novel was made into a film by the Argelian director M. Salim Riad (1975).

In this phase, female authors were represented above all by Assia Djebar. She has dealt with the role of women in Algerian society in his collection of short stories *Femmes d'Alger dans leur appartement* [*Women of Algiers in their apartment*] (1980). Among her best works we could mention *Les Nuits de Strasbourg* [*The Nights of Strasbourg*] (1997), translated into Catalan as *Les nits a Estrasburg* (2002), and into Spanish as *Las noches de Estrasburgo* (2015).

Currently, there are numerous important authors in Algeria. Most are known at a national level, but some have been recognized internationally. Among them, we could mention female author Ahlam Mostaghanemi, who has gained recognition by important literary figures such as Nizar Qabbani; his appreciation of Ahlam´s novel *Dākirat al-ğasad* (1993) is included by Sihām Al-Samarrā'ī in his *al-'Atabāt al-naṣṣiyya fī riwāyat al-ağyāl al-'arabiya* (2016, p. 43). The novel had 19 editions until 2004, and by then it had sold more than 3 million copies. It was translated into English by Baria Ahmar Sreih with the title *Memory in the flesh* (2000) and by Mohamed Mokeddem into French as *Mémoires de la chair* (2002).

Yasmina Khadra is the *nom de plume* of another Algerian international figure who has written novels on diverse topics. His real name is Mohammed Moulessehoul. He has written his latest novels in French, later translated into other languages. For instance, *Les Sirènes de Bagdad* (2006) was translated by Wenceslao-Carlos Lozano González into Spanish (2015) and by Caroline Miller into English as *The Sirens of Baghdad* (2008). His novel *Ce que le jour doit à la nuit* (2008) was also translated into Spanish by Wenceslao-Carlos Lozano González as *Lo que el día debe a la noche* (2009).

Algerian playwright, poet and novelist Rachid Boudjedra is known in Algeria and worldwide. Many of his works were translated into other languages. For instance, *La Répudiation* (1981) was translated by Roxana Páez as *El repudio* (2002) and his poetry in *Pour ne plus rêver* (1965) and *Cinq Fragments du désert* (2001) was selected and translated by Leonor Merino in a book entitled *Para no soñar más y cinco fragmentos del desierto* (2005).

Algerian-Italian Amara Lakhous is a prolific novelist who writes about contemporary topics and is read throughout the world. His work *Scontro di civiltà per un ascensore a Piazza Vittorio* (2006) was translated into English by Ann Goldstein as *Clash of Civilizations Over an Elevator in Piazza Vittorio* (2008), and *La zingarata della verginella di Via Ormea* (2014) was translated into English by Antony Shugaar as *The Prank of the Good Little Virgin of Via Ormea* (2016).

At a national level, there are many writers who write in Arabic. Among them, we should mention Azzedine Djelaoudji who is the author of more than 40 titles including novels, literaty criticism, plays, short stories and children´s literature. In 2001, he founded the Authors League and in 2003 he was chosen to be a member of the Union of Algerian Writers. Among his works as a literary critic we could mention *al-Masraḥiyya al-ši'riyya fī-l-adab al-magāribī al-mu'āṣir* (2012).

SOCIAL AND CULTURAL ATMOSPHERE IN ALGERIA

Algeria is a North African country which belongs to the islamic world. Its official language is Arabic, although a large part of the population speaks Amaziġ, which includes dialectal varieties such as Kabil, Chawí, Terguí, and Mizabi. Nonetheless, most of these ethnic groups are united by their islamic character. It is obvious that this double identity results in a cultural diversity in traditional dress, music, arts and crafts, etc. Regarding religious identity, we also find another type of cultural diversity regarding schools of law. Maliki sunnis are the majority, but sufi orders and confraternities as a manifestation of popular islam are also present in Algeria, particularly in the desert. The *ibāḍī* school centers around Ghardaya, and there is a Christian minority in the kabil region, as reflected by Yasmina Saduki (2018, pp. 184-185).

Social relations in Algeria are displayed in a variety of ways. Family relationships are reflected in the obligation to visit family for any social occasion, either to congratulate, offer support, or just visit. These visits have a religious basis, for islamic religion recommends strengthening family ties. 'Abdelsalam Aichouni explains the role of these social values and their religious background (2021, pp. 147-150). This is also explained by Souhila Laghresse when dealing with celebrations and festivities of a religious character in Algerian society (2021, p. 297).

Another aspect of Algerian public life consists of going to public places and institutions such as souks, mosques, libraries and cultural and sports centers. In addition, cafeterias are considered places of social interaction, as well as literary gatherings for intellectuals.

The mosque is a religious institution that plays a crucial role in muslim life. Islamism requires muslims to pray five times per day, at the mosque rather than at home. Al-Buḫārī includes several of Muhammad´s hadiths that place public above home prayers (2002, p. 131). In addition, going to the mosque to listen to Friday´s sermon and praying in group are muslim obligations, such as explained by imam Malik Ibn Anas (1994, p. 233). To these religious collective activities, we must add the attendance to funerals and weddings.

Another common custom in the Mediterranean, including Algeria, consists of greetings, that include close contact among people. A large part of Algerian population kisses and hugs when greeting family and friends. Handshakes are utilized for unknown people.

SOME EFFECTS OF THE PANDEMIC IN ALGERIA

A week after the declaration of March 16th about the COVID-19 pandemic by WHO (OMS), in which a worldwide health and social emergency was declared that required and effective and immediate governmental intervention and the collaboration of people and companies, the Algerian government decreed a partial lockdown in the capital city and the city of Blida due to the large number of cases in this region (2020, p. 9).

Later on, Algerian authorities decreed other health measures to halt the pressure on public health (2020, p. 15). These measures had a notable impact on the economy and social life, as well as negative effects on the psychology of a part of the population.

Part of the population was not infected but suffered mentally the effects of an unexpected crisis in their lives. This pandemic has significantly complicated the live of citizens, both the infirmed and the health workers, or people who have suffered other type of indirect consequences such as unemployment because of the closing down of many companies and services. Due to this, the psychological impact has been evident.

Stress and anxiety have increased because of the menace represented by the pandemic, and the measures adopted by many governments such as lockdowns, quarantines, closing of public, cultural, and educational institutions have augmented the psychological pressure. According to Victoria de la Caridad Ribot Reyes et al.,

we should urge the boosting of resilience, personal growth, interfamily relations and personal attention to vulnerable groups so that we can minimize the psycho-social impact of the epidemic on the population (Reyes et al., 2020, para. 5).

In addition to the effects of COVID-19 on the health and the social life of people, state institutions have also suffered a management crisis, such as the legal system that has been affected by the accumulation of urgent cases, which had to be delayed. With regard to this, Mohamed Zidane describes this situation and explains how Algerian legislation has adapted to this circumstance (2020, p. 627).

Soufiane Kheloufi deals in his study with the impact of the COVID-19 pandemic on the world economy in general and the Algerian economy more in particular. He indicates its effect on international commerce and the price of energy. The pandemic has caused serious effects to the Algerian economy, which is mostly based on the exportation of gas and oil. This obliged Algeria to change its strategy regarding expenditures and the management of resources (2021, pp. 1666-1668).

In view of the situation, it is recommended that people adopt activities and hobbies previously abandoned because of lack of time such as reading, learning languages, playing and listening to music or computers, among others. At home, it was recommended to keep in touch with loved ones through phone and social media, as well as to learn relaxation techniques. TV and other media such as radio, broadcasted guidelines from experts and mental health professionals on how to take advantage of the social isolation to develop experiences at a personal and familial level.

In order to reduce the psychological effect of social isolation created by the lockdown or quarantine conditions, mental health is promoted starting with environments that allow adopting and keeping healthy ways of life. The work of health professional, culture, mass media, as well as family and the community in general has been presented as fundamental to guarantee mental health.

To all these elements we must add the contribution of artists and writers, who through their works provide guidelines to society and offer with proposals or reflections on social behaviors and traditions. In addition, it serves to describe and document what is currently happening to future generations.

THE SOCIAL ASPECT OF LITERATURE DURING THE PANDEMIC

The traditions and customs we mentioned in the previous section are part of daily life in Algeria. Any curtailment of this way of life will find it difficult to be socially accepted. Due to this, the application of the restrictions under the exceptional circumstances of the pandemic made it necessary to count with the collaboration of all intellectuals in order to make people conscious of it.

The COVID-19 health crisis has been a real challenge for humankind. All countries organized themselves to overcome it in every health, social and economic level. These circumstances required an important contribution by writers all over the world.

In reality, pandemics have been a literary topic throughout the history of literature. In fact, several novelists and poets have dealt with human stories related to the pandemic such as conciliation, separation, the feelings of those who lost loved ones because of the pandemic, as well as the loneliness of those who had to be quarantined, or fear of contagion and death.

In this regard, any literary creation, be it a poem, a short story, a narrative text or any other fictional work can offer historical data about a given period. Literature in turn can offer a contribution, and each literary genre has its place in the reader´s imaginary regardless of whether the work was written before or after the pandemic. In fact, when we read famous works that deal with pandemics, such as Albert Camus´s *La peste* or G. García Márquez´s *El amor en los tiempos del cólera* we discover more data about the pandemic period and we remember the difficult conditions endured by humankind, as is the case with the current pandemic of coronavirus. Because of this, we would like to highlight another of literature´s functions, that of providing representative scenarios of particular moments in history.

Literary creativity is not a mechanical job but requires inspiration, dedication, confidence, creativity and even discipline. It is obvious that artists are influenced by their environment, and their experiences and daily circumstances are the source of inspiration for their literary work. The pandemic has also influenced Algerian Arabic writers, and they have left their imprint during this period.

In this critical period, we observe that Algerian literary production in Arabic played two essential roles. First, to make population aware about the severity of the virus and the obligation to follow the directives and recommendations issued by authorities. To do so, several works have been published on how to deal with the pandemic and how to behave during it.

The second function has been, on one hand, to entertain and distract people in their social isolation through a varied and attractive production. On the other hand, it has consisted in offering consolation to the population for their losses, alleviating the feeling of loneliness created by the forced absence of social relations. This has made some poets to perform supportive actions in favor of the affected population.

In the Arab world, the literary contribution can be seen in literary studies and criticism on the pandemic, either books, articles, or blogs. Poetry and novel have also been very present when dealing with this phenomenon.

LITERARY STUDIES AND CRITICISM

We must highlight in this field the studies by the Kuwait writer and journalist Taleb Alrefai. In his book *Lawn al-ġad: ru'yat al-muṯaqqaf al- 'arabī li-mā ba'da Corona* (The color of tomorrow: the vision of the Arab intellect about the post COVID-19), he gathers and analyzes the opinions of 88 intellectuals from 19 countries. He affirms that the massive use of technology was one of the main causes of the terror felt during the pandemic and that people were as many victims from the social media as from the virus. He states that technology has made any national individual into an international person who can disseminate and receive information at home (2020, p. 18).

Likewise, Moroccan Ahmad Sharrak wrote a book entitled *Corana wa-l-ḫiṭāb: muqaddimāt wa-yawmiyāt* on the effects of the pandemic at the social and educational levels.

Some literary studies have focused on the narrative of the historical events, pointing at the consequences of these types of diseases. In this regard, the Algerian literary critic Saïd Boutadjin (2020) published on a webpage from the Ministère de la Culture et des Arts an article entitled *Marāyā ʻākisa, al-adab wa-l-awbiʻa* (Reflected Mirrors: Literature and Pandemics). In it, he analyzes writers´ treatment of pandemic throughout history. Likewise, Lybian historian and writer Ali Al-Salābī (2020), who is very famous in the Arab world, published in his blog of the Al-Jazeera webpage an article describing how Muslims have lived epidemics throughout history.

As for young people, and representing something exceptional, the Arab Youth Center published a work in which more than one hundred youths participated from all over the Arab world. It deals with their experiences during the social lockdown.

From a scientific point of view, the Egyptian doctor Hussein al-Churà (2020) provides the reader in his book *Asrār corona: Kaifa taḥmī nafsak wa-usratak* (The Secrets of COVID-19: How to Protect Yourself and Your Family) with instructions on how to protect themselves from the pandemic.

Researcher Hassiba Mahieddine dealt with the pandemic from a legal aspect and focused on the legal punishments for not complying with the health measures and contributing to the dissemination of the virus. His goal was to make citizens conscious and make them take responsibility for their actions (2021, p. 1057).

From a sociological point of view, Naoual Belghelifi deals with the population´s perception of the idea of a pandemic; for her, understanding the social mentality of the population is crucial for the adoption of adequate measures against the dissemination of the virus (2021, p. 100). With a similar approach, Djilali El Mestari deals with the role of social and educational institutions in the management of the pandemic (2020, pp. 2-10). As for Nourdine Bessadi, she underscores in her article the positive side of the pandemic as reflected in the solidarity displayed by the Algerian population (2020, paragr. 4-7).

Literary production with a religious content has also had a role in this period. For instance, researcher Salima Abdelsalam studied how religious rites adapted to the health crisis. In her work, and taking as a point of departure the basic rules of Islamic law, she explains how the obligation to perform a collective prayer at the mosque was substituted by individual prayers at home. Likewise, she deals with other questions such as the obligations of health workers, which patients have priority in case the system is overburdened, etc. (2021, pp. 209-214).

Literary criticism has appeared more in articles than in books. Among the latter, Azzedine Djelaoudji (2020) wrote on theater in Algerian literature. As for articles, we underscore the work of Raḥma al-Qurašī (2020) on the poets´ view of the COVID-19 virus; and the article by ʻAbdu Wāzan (2020) where he gathers the testimony of 17 Arab writers on the lockdown. Along similar lines, Annahar (2020) deals with the writers´ obsession with the topic of the pandemic, highlighting that the virus has been a catalyst for the production of literary works.

Salih Shuaib et al. (2020) published a study of the effect of epidemics on Arab poetry, including an analysis of Hashem al-Bashir´s poem on the current pandemic.

POETRY OF THE PANDEMIC

Because Arab poetry is a reflection on society and the expression of everything that takes place in it, be it happy or sad occasions in every aspect of life, there has been in Arabic literature a clear interaction between poets and pandemics, which have provoked fear and threatened humankind since past times. The current coronavirus pandemic has had the most impact across the world. Because of it, contemporary poets have analyzed it from a variety of perspectives: religious, philosophical, psychological, and social, because of its great impact on societies.

In the current situation, many writers refer to past poets who lived similar situations. Among them, we could mention the poet Ibn al-Wardī who composed in 749 H/1348 AD a poem of the plague that says:

I do not fear the plague like others do,

It is only two good things,

If I die, I rid myself of my enemies,

If I survive, my eyes and ears will be healed (1986, p. 94).

Poet ʻAlī al-Ǧārim also dealt with this topic when the cholera hit his region in 1985. He composed a poem entitled *al-wabā'* that reflects human pain and sadness because of a disease that provoked thousands of deads. The poem reads:

O microbe slowly please,

You have caused terror along the way,

You are not shaped like a j, but like a sickle,

You reap many souls, how vicious! (2012, p. 591).

Iraki female poet Nazik al-Malā'ika, who revolutionized modern poetry, wrote in 1947 a poem entitled *The cholera* in which she describes the disease as a cruel tool used by Death to take revenge on humankind regardless of gender and age. It killed many people, provoked ruin, caused pain and sadness to many people (986, p. 138).

Regarding the contemporary pandemic, among the poems that circulate in the Arab world we can highlight that by Syrian Nizār 'Ābidīn (2020) entitled *al-Ḥub fī zaman Corona* (Love in Times of COVID-19). It replicates the meter and rhyme of Ibn Zaydūn in his famous poem dedicated to his lover Wallāda (the famous quasida "*nūniyya*") and describes the changes that the pandemic brought to the story of two lovers.

Saudi Arabian poet, Masra'ī Ġarīd Ǧāzān (2020), from a religious perspective, has composed a poem that expresses his sadness for the closing of the Mecca mosque due to COVID-19.

Similarly, his compatriot Saad 'Aṭiyya Alghamdi (2020) beseeches God to make the disease disappear. On another occasion, the newspaper *Akhbar24* (2021) includes an exchange of verses between him and his friends after falling sick with the disease. He announced he fell ill despite being vaccinated and having followed the restrictions of social isolation. Faced with the news, his friends sent him consolatory verses.

Al-'Ašmāwī (2020) describes the virus as something invisible that came to remind humankind how powerless they are in front of God. 'Abd Allāh al-'Awāḍī (2020) published a poem entitled *Layālī Corona* (The nights of COVID-19) in *Šabakat al-Alūka*, where he describes fear and its effect on social life during the lockdown. Six months later, 'Abd al-Laṭīf Išūlā (2020) published his poem *Virus Corona* on the same webpage and describes in it the danger of the virus through its symptoms and explains personal and collective measures to be adopted in order to be safe.

On the other hand, poems by Fawwāz al-La'būn (2020) attempt to transmit hope and calmness to readers. Al-Qurašī also quotes some of his verses:

We shall soon see happiness blossom

Disillusioned sadness will disappear

Black anguish will quickly fade away

There is a solution for every problem. No doubt (2020, paragr. 9).

Conversely, Ḥāšim al-Bašīr (2020) in his poem *Ğā'iḥat Corona* (COVID-19) talks about his sadness, pain, and anguish, and describes the effects of the pandemic on every aspect of life.

In Algeria, the health crisis captured the interest of Algerian poets, who did not refrain from expressing their feeling about it. Salima Melizi (2020), in an exercise of solidarity, dedicates his poem to the inhabitants of Blida, a city affected by COVID-19, thus expressing his support and desire to see the end of the pandemic. we quote some verses of his poem:

I sing the most beautiful song

To Blída the city of roses

Andalusian essence and Amaziġ roots

From grandfather Ṣāliḥ and the Banī Masrā

From the language of Banī Ya'rub spreads

A fragrance equivalent to that of Paris

Form each letter of poem

Emerged between the times and the fields

His presence is kept in the heart

It's my gift to the city of roses. (Salima Melizi, 2020)

Researcher Mohamed Bakadi includes two poems by Mobarak Goumni on the pandemic, the first in classical Arabic entitled *Qalbun munīb*, the second in Algerian dialect entitled *Yā laṭīf* (2021, pp. 224-225).

THE NOVEL

Novel is clearly the most prominent literary genre in our time. The pandemic has also been an inspirational motif for many novelists. In fact, very early on, Egyptian'Abd-al-Ḥalīm Qandīl published *Corona wa-sinīnu-hā: taḥawwulāt al-'ālam wa-qtiṣādi-hī wa-ṯawarāti-hī ba'da al-ğā'iḥa* (Coronavirus and Its Time: World Changes and Revolution after the Pandemic) in which he underscores the effects of the pandemic in Arabic and African countries at a social, economic, political, and mental health levels (2020, p. 3).

Syrian poet and novelist Jan Dost (2020) in his novel *Fī qabḍat al-kābūs: Ṯalāṯuna yawman mina ḥiṣār Corona* (Nightmare´s Grasp: Thirty Days Besieged by COVID-19) describes life in his city during the lockdown and its consequences on families. Qatari writer Jassim Salman (2020) wrote *Corona al-ḥubbu wa-l-ḥarb: malḥama kutibat aṯnā' al-ḥağr* (Coronavirus between Love and War: a Battle Written during the Lockdown) in which he describes the difficulties and the positive side of the lockdown during the pandemic.

Likewise, Lybian female writer Stefani Awini (2020) in her novel *Ḥub fī zaman Corona* (Love in the Time of COVID-19) invites the reader to live the exciting protagonists´ life events.

Aicha Bassry (2020) was inspired by events that developed with the first news on the coronavirus and immersed herself in the feelings lived by people at the beginning of the pandemic in her *Ka-ğutta fī riwāya būlisiyya* (Like a Corpse ion the Detective Novel).

The pandemic has also been the topic of the novel by Mohamed Ould Mohamed Salem (2020) entitled *Alā'īb Ḫālid ma'a Corona* (The Tricks of Ḫālid with the Pandemic). In it, he uses the diaries of a Mauritanian boy who likes to play outside his house. His family emigrates to the United Arab Emirates where he makes new friends, but all of a sudden, the pandemic arrives and the authorities issue lockdown orders. The boy does not understand it (nor accepts it) and he constantly makes something up to break the restrictions and go out to play.

Jordanian author Mustafa al-Qarna (2020) wrote the novel *al-Hurūb min corona* (The escape of COVID-19) in which the protagonist is the virus, an invisible being that travels throughout the world causing terror.

Algerian writer Wacini Laredj (2020) also published a novel entitled *Layliāt Ramada* in which he deals with a love story during the pandemic full of sadness. In it, he portrays the resilience of human beings when facing both pandemics as well as corrupted systems.

The literary production generated during the pandemic that does not deal with the health crisis nor its effect in a direct way is also the object of our work. We consider it a creative work that alleviates loneliness for individuals, entertains them and distracts them so that they do not feel in an enclosed space and with limited freedom. This type of production makes them feel that they are communicating with the outside world from their homes. In this regard, the novel *Mā yušbih al-qatl* (What Seems an Assassination) by Aḥmad al-Malwānī (2020), narrates a magic journey of four people in search of the tree of wisdom which in reality is a search for themselves trying to find answers about freedom, destiny and other contradictions of the human soul. The novel by Kamal Raḥīm (2020) entitled *Qahwat Ḥabaši* also deals with topics unrelated to the pandemic. It shows readers the ways of life of a marginalized community in a small village, and describes the traditions and the social problems that the population is immersed in. Likewise, Raġad al-Nābulsī (2021) in his novel *Imra'a min ṣūf* (A Woolen Woman) invites readers to reflect on the life of a woman in her 50s who has spent her life sewing wool and then wonders about the possibility of changing the past.

International literary production also reached Arab readers through translations. For instance, *Diez mujeres* by Marcela Serrano was translated into Arabic in 2015, and most of Dostoyevski´s works which were translated into Arabic by the Syrian ambassador Sami Droubi (d. 1976) were reedited between 2010 and 2020 such as his novel *The Insulted and Humiliated*, republished in (1861/2020).

OTHER MEANS OF LITERARY DISSEMINATION

Nowadays, we live in the digital era and the measures adopted as a result of the current health crisis have given an advantage to digital tools as the best way to disseminate information in these new times. This has made us study and analyze the work done by different media in their function as bridges between the Algerian population and their artists and writers. During the lockdown, after educational, cultural and religious places were closed down, mobile phones, TV, radio, social media and other mass media have been fundamental in keeping citizens informed about news. Prominent artists and writers have used these digital tools to continue their activity. Numerous artists used YouTube channels, Facebook accounts, etc. to communicate with their followers.

TV and Radio

TV and radio have been a great communication tool for the public. They are also communication channels among artists, writers and their followers. In fact, we find numerous TV cultural programs where important literary figures are invited to enrich the program´s content. For instance, in Algerian national TV2, the program *Jarka* edited by Director Samir Ayat al-Amara, invited Abdelkader Chercham together with the literary critic Mohamed Serir. In Algeria, the population is very attracted to cultural programs and thanks to technology they can access a great number of TV stations. In fact, Sa'īd Khatibi (paragr. 1) affirms that the TV program *La grande librairie* by the French TV5 has a large Algerian audience.

Radio also broadcasts literary programs, as evinced by *Misāḥa li-l-adab* (A Space for Literature). Miftāḥ Bakhouche, the presenter of the program, always invites writers to discuss literary topics. For instance, on September 23, 2021 he invited doctor Mohamed Serir to explain the literary value of popular poetry.

Internet

During this period, through internet, several platforms have been very active in disseminating content on several disciplines. On YouTube we can find several channels interested in literature. For instance, al-Nahar´s channel includes the program *Ṣā'at Amal* (The Hour of Hope). During the pandemic, the program invited poet Muḥammad Zawād, who, in a supportive act, dedicated a marvellous poem to the city of Blida after it suffered many losses. Al-Jazeera Documentary also broadcasts frequently documentaries on literature and writers. Two years ago, there was an interesting documentary on female poet Nazik al-Malā'ika (2019) and ten of her poems were read out loud, including comments by great literary critics.

Through their platforms, many cultural centers have also participated with numerous works during the pandemic. Among them, we can highlight the Goethe Institute and its channel (2021), which has published videos of artists and writers in a series entitled *Ibdā': al-fan fī zaman corona* (Creativity. Art in the Times of COVID-19). These Arab protagonists from different countries reflect on the situation and their activity as artists. This same center offered the population 19 links to free courses as well as numerous pages of cultural content (2020).

Currently, internet is also utilized for disseminating the activities of many academic, cultural or political institutions. At present in Algeria all journals, newspapers, etc. have electronic editions.

Social Media

Social media have become a way of dissemination and communication among writers and their followers. In fact, among Algerian authors novelist Ahlam Mosteghanemi (2022) is very active on social media and frequently uploads her literary texts on her Facbook account. This is also the means used by other writers such as Azzedine Djlaodji (2020b) to inform her followers about her new works, and by Mustapha Benfodil to comment and interact, depending on the circumstances.

On the other hand, researchers Omar Benaichouhe and Hacene Boussersoub underscore the contribution of social media to make people aware about the situation and for the dissemination of health information through internet (2020, pp. 306-307).

Electronic Libraries

Equally important has been the role of digital or electronic books. Digital libraries solve the problem of access to physical libraries. With a tablet or a computer, or even a mobile phone, connected to internet, the reader can access digital libraries that include books on many topics. Thus, we can find open-access libraries with thousands of books such as the Maktabah al-Waqfeya, and other pay-per-view libraries that offer new works, such as eKtab.

During the pandemic, the different platforms have offered Arab readers thousands of electronic books to read or download for free. For instance, the webpage of al-Maktabah includes many novels. The same applies to the electronic library Noor that allows to read and download thousands of scanned Arab books.

CONCLUSION

In sum, it was obvious that Algerian writers would be affected by the pandemic, both in a negative and positive manner. They have attempted to adapt themselves to this new circumstance both personally and professionally. As we have seen, many of the texts that received inspiration from this pandemic belong to a group of literary genres the most relevant among which are literary studies and criticism, poetry, novel, and the many articles that have flooded journals and social media.

This reaction on the part of writers has been positive for society, because through these publications they have contributed to making people aware of the situation and to alleviating their pain, making them forget their loneliness and the restrictions imposed on them with their works.

Finally, after knowing the role of electronic resources, we have confirmed their help to readers, becoming an alternative to the function played by other cultural spaces such as libraries and theater. Even so, we should mention the possible disadvantages of this technology. If the social isolation continues, this will also have negative effects on the writers´ production, for, in the end, writers are just sensitive people and need motivation, travel, etc. These resources reduce social life and create an imaginary world away from reality. In fact, researchers Ibtissam Ghanam and Karima Bensghir have stressed that the use of digital screens has had a negative effect in the educational values of children (2021, pp. 448-449). On the other hand, the massive use of these screen causes fatigue to our eyesight and, from the point of view of mental health, they can become addictive, which would then be a new problem to be solved.

REFERENCES

Abdelsalam, S. (2021). Understanding balances and its impact on the new events of the Corona pandemic (selected issues). *Mağallat al-Šihāb*, *1*(7), 195-222.

'Ābidīn, N. (2020, May 12). Al-Ḥub fī zaman Corona [Al-Hub is better tan Corona]. *Al-Watan*. https://www.al-watan.com/news-details/id/231225/

Aichouni, 'A., & Adjal, A. (2021). The impact of value communication on family bonding in Algerian society during the Covid 19 crisis. *Mağallat al-riwaq li-l-dirāsāt al-iğtima'iyya wa-l-insāniyya*, *2*(7), 141-168.

Al-'Ašmāwī, 'A. (2020, April 7). Yā ḫāliqa al-kawni luṭfan anta munqiduna [Oh cosmic affair of Louvain, you are our bound]. *Ğarīdat al-Umma*. https://al-omah.com/

Al-'Awāḍī, 'A. A. (2020, March 31). Layālī Corona [Corona nights]. *Šabakat Al-Alūka*. https://www.alukah.net/literature_language/0/139424/

Al-Bašīr, Ḥ. (2020, May 6). Ğā'iḥat Corona [Corona Cases]. *Alrakoba*. https://www.alrakoba.net/31394213/

Al-Buḫārī. (2002). *Ṣaḥīḥ al-Buḫārī* [Sahih Bukari] (M. Z. Ben Nāṣir, Ed.). Dār Ṭūq al-Nağāt.

Al-Churà, H. (2020). *Asrār corona: kaifa taḥmī nafsak wa-usratak* [Corona's secrets: How to feed yourself and your family]. Kitāb al-Yawm.

Al-Ğārim, 'A. (2012). *Dīwān 'Alī al-Ğārim*. Mu'asasat Hindāwī.

Al-La'būn, F. [@fawaz_dr]. (2020, March 10). *Ṭāla al-zaman wa-Corona tuṭāridunā* [Time and Corona hit us] [Tweet]. Twiter. https://twitter.com/fawaz_dr/status/1237407639245594628?lang=es

Al-Maktaba. (2021). *Plataforma de libros electrónicos* [E-book platform]. https://books-library.net/free-835057225-download

Al-Malā'ika, N. (1986). Dīwān Nāzik al-Malā'ika vol. 2 [Diwan Nazik Angels Vol. 2]. Dar al-'Ūda.

Al-Malā'ika, N. (2019). 'Ašr qasā'id. *Al-Jazeera Documentary*. https://www.youtube.com/watch?v=Ub9CZ_c5fTE&t=268s

Al-Malwānī, A. (2020). *Mā yušbih al-qatl* [What a killer]. Al-Dār al-Miṣriyya al-Lubnāniyya.

Al-Nābulsī, R. (2021). *Imra'a min ṣūf*. Dār al-Warda.

Al-Qarna, M. (2020). *Al-Hurūb min min corona* [The war from Corona]. Dār al-Riwaya al-'Arabiyya.

Al-Qurašī, R. (2020, April 27). Corona fī 'uyūn al-šu'arā' [Corona in the eyes of poets]. *Al-Jazirah*. https://www.al-jazirah.com/2020/20200417/cm4.htm

Al-Salābī, A. (2020, March 19). Kayfa ta'āmala al-muslimūn ma'a al-awbi'a wa- ātāruhā fī-marāhil tārīḫihim [How do Muslims work with epidemics and Ataroh in the pits of Tarhim]. *Aljazeera*. https://www.aljazeera.net/blogs/2020/3/19/

Al-Samarrā'ī, S. (2016). *Al-'Atabāt al-naṣṣiyya fī riwāyat al-ağyāl al-'arabiya*. Al Manhal.

al-Wardī, I. (1986). *Dīwān Ibn al-Wardī*. Dār al-Qalam.

Alghamdi, S. A. [@Saad_Alghamdi] (2020, March 5). *Poetic Verses* [Tweet]. Twitter. https://twitter.com/Saad_Alghamdi/status/1505981971595468809?cxt=HHwWkoC58finqeYpAAAA

Alghamdi, S. A. (2021, February 10). Acadīmī uṣība bi-Corona. *Akhbar24*. https://akhbaar24.argaam.com/article/detail/531646

Alrefai, T. (2020). *Lawn al-ġad: ru'yat al-muṯaqqaf al-'arabī li-mā ba'da Corona* [The color of the return: a vision of Arab attitudes after Corona]. Almutawassit.

Annahar (Ed.). (2020, November 7). Corona hāğis al-kuttāb [Corona book pilgrims]. *Al-Ğarīda*. https://www.annahar.com/arabic/culture/

Arab Youth Center. (Ed.). (2021). *Al-Šabāb al-'arabi wa-l-COVID-19: Ḫawāṭir ibdā'iyya arabiyya fī zaman al-wabā* [Al-Habbab Al-Arabi and Covid-19: Arab Creative Paths in the Time of Al-Waba`ah]. Qindeel.

Awini, S. (2020). *Ḥub fī zaman Corona* [Hub in the time of Corona]. Dar Abaad.

Badi, M. (Director). (1974). *Al-Ḥarīq* [The Hammer] [TV Series]. Télévision Algérienne.

Bakadi, M. (2021). Corona pandemic manifests in the poetry of the poets of the Tamanraset region goumni mobarek in his poems; ya latif, and kalb mounib, as a model. *Mağallat al-Kalim*, *1*(6), 216-234.

Bakhouche, M. (2021). *Misāḥa li-l-adab* [Maya Literature] [Radio Series]. Al-Iḏā'a al-Ṯaqāfiyya. https://radioalgerie.dz/culture/ar/

Bassry, A. (2020). *Kağutta fī riwāya būlisiyya* [Kaguta is better than the police]. Al-Dār al-Miṣriyya al-Lubnāniyya.

Belghelifi, N. (2021). Mass memory and the epidemic's representations in the Machira area: Corona is a model. *Mağallat Wiḥdat al-baḥṯ fī tanmiyat al-mawārid al-bašariyya. CRASC*, *3*(16), 98–121.

Benaichouhe, O., & Boussersoub, H. (2020). The role of Facebook in promoting health awareness about Corona Covid 19 A field study of a sample of Facebook users, Corona virus news page, and health education as an example. *Mağallat al-Tamkīn al-Iğtimā'ī*, *2*(2), 288-309.

Benfodil, M. [@Mustapha Benfodil] (2022, February 23). *Mes pièces "End/Igné"* [My "End/Igneous" pieces] [Status update]. Facebook. https://www.facebook.com/benfodilmustapha

Benhadouga, A. (1971). *Rīḥ al-ğanūb* [Alien head]. Sned editions.

Benhadouga, A. (1976). *Le Vent du Sud* [The South Wind] (M. Bois, Trans.). Sned editions. (Original work published 1971)

Benhadouga, A. (1981). *El Viento del sur* [The South Wind] (M. Villegas, Trans.). Instituto Hispano-Árabe de Cultura. (Original work published 1971)

Bessadi, N. (2020). Al-Muǧtama'al-ǧazā'irī yašhad izdihāran aṯnā' al-ǧā'iḥa. *Ru'ya*. https://www.goethe.de/prj/ruy/ar/covid/21853154.html

Boudjedra, R. (1965). *Pour ne plus rêver* [To stop dreaming]. ÉNA.

Boudjedra, R. (1981). *La Répudiation* [The Repudiation]. Gallimard Folio.

Boudjedra, R. (2001). *Cinq Fragments du désert* [Five Fragments of the Desert]. Barzakh.

Boudjedra, R. (2002). *El Repudio* [The Repudiation] (R. Páez, Trans.). Emecé editores. (Original work published in 1981)

Boudjedra, R. (2005). *Para no soñar más, y cinco fragmentos del desierto* [Not to dream anymore, and five fragments of the desert]. (L. Merino, Trans.). Huerga y Fierro Editores. (Original work published 1965)

Boutadjin, S. (2020). *Marāyā ʿākisa, al-adab wa-l-awbiʿa* [Reflective Mirrors - Literature and Epidemics]. Ministère de la Culture et des Arts. https://www.m-culture.gov.dz/index.php/ar/2-non-categorise/3063-

Camus, A. (2002). *La peste* [Plague]. EDHASA.

Dib, M. (1952). *La Grande Maison* [The Big House]. Le Seuil.

Dib, M. (1954). *l'Incendie* [The fire]. Le Seuil.

Dib, M. (1959). *Un été africain* [An African summer]. Points.

Dib, M. (1976). *Un verano en África* [A summer in Africa]. (O. C. Alegre, Trans.). Arte y Literatura. (Original work published 1959)

Dib, M. (1979). *El Incendio* [The fire]. Arte y literatura. (Original work published 1954).

Djebar, A. (1980). *Femmes d'Alger dans leur appartement* [Women of Algiers in their apartment]. Éditions des Femmes.

Djebar, A. (1997). *Les Nuits de Strasbourg* [The Nights of Strasbourg]. Actes Sud.

Djebar, A. (2002). *Les nits a Estrasburg* [Nights in Strasbourg] (A. Casassas, Trans.). Edicions 62. (Original work published in 1997)

Djebar, A. (2015). *Las noches de Estrasburgo* [The nights of Strasbourg]. (M. S. Crespo, Trans.). Alfaguara. (Original work published 1997)

Djelaoudji, A. (2012). *Al-Masraḥiyya al-šiʿriyya fī-l-adab al-maġāribī al-muʿāṣir* [Standard play in warrior literature]. Dār al-Tanwīr.

Djelaoudji, A. (2020). *Al-Naṣ al-masraḥī fī-l-adab al-ǧazā'irī* [The Egyptian Naas in Azeri literature]. Dār al-Muntahà.

Djlaodji, A. (2020, June 15). *Ġilaf riwāyatī al-ǧadīda* [Elaf new novels]. Facebook. https://www.facebook.com/265532643874402/posts/908025542958439/

Dost, J. (2020). *Fī qabḍat al-kābūs: ṯalāṯuna yawman mina ḥiṣār Corona*. Dār Ḫuṭūṭ.

Dostoyevski F. (2020). *Mudhillūn muhānūn* [Humiliated and Insulted] (S. Droubi Trans.). Dār al-Tanwīr lil-Ṭibā'ah wa-al-Nashr. (Original work published in 1861)

El Mestari, D. (2020). *Covid-19 en Algérie: enseignements et regards croisés (premiers éléments de réflexion)* [Covid-19 in Algeria: lessons and crossed views (first elements of reflection)]. Centre de Recherche en Anthropologie Sociale et Culturelle CRASC.

Feraoun, M. (1950). *Le fils du pauvre* [The poor man's son]. Cahiers du Nouvel Humanisme.

Feraoun, M. (2001). *El hijo del pobre* [The por man's son] (G. F. Parrilla & M. E. López, Trans.). Ediciones del Oriente y Mediterráneo. (Original work published 1950)

García Márquez, G. (2021). *El amor en los tiempos del cólera* [Love in the time of cholera]. Debolsillo.

Ghanam, I., & Bensghir, K. (2021). Children's use of electronic screens in light of the Corona epidemic, and its effects on educational values from the points of view of children's parents and teachers. *Mağallat wiḥdat al-Baḥṯ fī Tanmiya al-Mawārid al-Bašariyya, 3*(16), 427-451.

Goethe Institut (Ed.). (2020). Tis'ata 'ašara rābiṭ li-dawarāt tadrībiyya maǧǧāniyyawa-'urūḍ ṯaqāfiyya. *Ru'ya*. https://www.goethe.de/prj/ruy/ar/covid/rethink.html

Goethe Institut (Ed.). (2021). Ibdā': al-fan fī zaman corona. *Ru'ya*. https://www.goethe.de/prj/ruy/ar/covid/rethink.html

Ibn Anas, M. (1994). *Al-Mudawwana* [Blog]. Dār al-Kutub al-'Ilmiyya.

Išūlā, 'A. (2020, October 5). Virus Corona. *ŠabakatAl-Alūka*. https://www.alukah.net/spotlight/0/142334/

Kacimi, M. (2017). Wāqi' al-riwāya al-ǧazā'irriyya fī-l-kitābāt al-ağnabiyya, al-luġa al-isbāniyya namūdağan [The Protector of the Aghazirian Novel in Foreign Writings, the Spanish Brigade of the Namdani]. In Al-Riwāya wa-l-funūn bayna al-tağrīb wa-l-naqd (pp. 420-428). Mu'assat Tšīcū li-l-Ṭibā'a wa-l-Našr.

Khadra, Y. (2006). *Les Sirènes de Bagdad* [The Sirens of Baghdad]. Julliard.

Khadra, Y. (2008). *Ce que le jour doit à la nuit* [What day owes to night]. Julliard.

Khadra, Y. (2009). *Lo que el día debe a la noche* [Whatday owes to night] (W.-C. L. González, Trans.). Ediciones Destino. (Original work published 2008)

Khatibi, S. (2021, August 20). Barāmiğ al-ṯaqāfa fī al-tilivision [Attached software in the phone area]. *Al-Quds Al Arabi*. https://www.alquds.co.uk/

Kheloufi, S. (2021). The impact of the Coronavirus Covid-19 pandemic on global economic indicators during the first quarter of 2020. With reference to the state of the Algerian economy. *OEB Univ. Publish. Co, 3*(8), 1650–1677.

Laghresse, S. (2021). Habits and traditions the celebration of the Laylat al-Qadr in Algerian society (Socio anthropological study in the city of Oran). *Mağallat Atropoloğia al-adyān, 2*(17), 296-312.

Lakhous, A. (2006). *Scontro di civiltà per un ascensore a Piazza Vittorio* [Clash of civilizations for an elevator in Piazza Vittorio]. Edizioni e/o.

Lakhous, A. (2008). *Clash of Civilizations Over an Elevator in Piazza Vittorio* (A. Goldstein, Trans.). Europa Editions. (Original work published 2006)

Lakhous, A. (2014). *La zingarata della verginella di Via Ormea* [The Prank of the Good Little Virgin of Via Ormea]. Edizioni e/o.

Lakhous, A. (2016). *The Prank of the Good Little Virgin of Via Ormea* (A. Shugaar, Trans.). Europa Editions. (Original work published 2014)

Laredj, W. (2020). *Layliāt Ramada* [Ramada Nights]. Dār al-Ādāb.

Mahieddine, H. (2021). Criminal liability for coronavirus (covid-19) transmission in Algerian legislation. *Mağallat al-dirāsāt al-qānūniyya al-muqārana, 2*(7), 1056-1074.

Maktabat, N. (2021). *Plataforma de libros electrónicos* [E-book platform]. https://www.noor-book.com/

Masra'ī, Ġ. Ğ. [@ryany_2015]. (2020, March 5). *Badā muhībān ğalīlan* [Two loved ones started] [Tweet]. Twiter. https://twitter.com/ryany_2015/status/1235595864036511746?lang=es

Melizi, S. (2020, March 28). Al-Bulaida madīna al-ward [Blida, the city of roses]. *Diwān al-'Arab.* https://diwanalarab.com/

Mostaghanemi, A. (1993). *Dākirat al-ğasad* [Memory in the flesh]. Dār al-Ādāb.

Mostaghanemi, A. (2000). *Memory in the flesh* (B. A. Sreih, Trans.). American University in Cairo Press. (Original work published 1993)

Mostaghanemi, A. (2002). *Mémoires de la chair* [Memory in the flesh] (M. Mokeddem, Trans.). Albin Michel. (Original work published 1993)

Mosteghanemi, A. [@ahlammostaghaanmy]. (2022, February 28). *Mimma qara'tu* [Status update]. Facebook. https://www.facebook.com/search/posts/?q=ahlem%20mosteghanemi

People's Democratic Republic of Algeria. (2020). *Fixant des mesures complémentaires de prévention et de lutte contre la propagation du Coronavirus (COVID-19)* [Laying down additional measures to prevent and combat the spread of Coronavirus (COVID-19)] (Décret exécutif n° 20-70). Journal officiel Algerie. https://www.joradp.dz/FTP/jo-francais/2020/F2020016.pdf

People's Democratic Republic of Algeria. (2020). *Portant mesures supplémentaires au titre du dispositif de prévention et de lutte contre la propagation du Coronavirus (COVID-19)* [Introducing additional measures under the system to prevent and combat the spread of Coronavirus (COVID-19)] (Décret exécutif n° 20-446). Journal officiel Algerie. https://www.joradp.dz/FTP/jo-francais/2021/F2021001.pdf

Qandīl, A. (2020). *Corona wa-sinīnu-hā: taḥawwulāt al-'ālam wa-iqtiṣādi-hī wa-ṯawarāti-hī ba'da al-ğā'iḥa.* Dār al-Taqāfa al-Ğadīda.

Raḥīm, K. (2020). *Qahwat Ḥabaši* [Abyssinian Coffee]. Dār al-'Ayn.

Reyes, V. C. R., Paredes, N. C., & Castillo, A. L. G. (2020). Efectos de la COVID-19 en la salud mental de la población [Effects of COVID-19 on the mental health of the population]. *Rev. Haban. Cienc. Méd.*, *1*(19). http://scielo.sld.cu/scielo.php?script=sci_arttext&pid=S1729-519X2020000400008

Riad, M. S. (Director). (1975). *Film Rīḥ al-ǧanūb* [Ronin] [Film]. Television Algerienne.

Saduki, Y. (2018). Maḍāhir wa-natā'iǧ al-tanawwu' al-ṯaqāfī fī-l-Ǧazā'ir [Maher and the scope of Al-Haqafi diversity on the surface]. *Maǧalat dā'irat al-buḥūṯ wa-l-dirāsāt al-qānūniyya wa-siyyāsiyya*, *2*(4), 180-193.

Salem, M.O.M. (2020). *Alā'īb ḫālid ma'a Corona*. Al-Mu'asasa al-'Arabiyya li-l-Dirāsāt wa-l-Našr.

Salih, S. S., & Ismail, M. A. (2021). *Corona's Reflections on Contemporary Arabic Poetry (Corona Pandemic Poem by Hashem Al-Bashir As a model)*. Academic Press.

Salman, J. (2020). *Corona al-ḥubbu wa-l-ḥarb: malḥama kutibat aṯnā' al-ḥaǧr*. Al-Dār al-'Arabiyya li-l-'Ulūm.

Samir, A. (Director). (2022, January 5). *Jarka. Ma'a Lila Borsali* [Episodio de serie de televisión]. Televisión Nacional Algerienne 2. https://www.youtube.com/watch?v=YtZ08gDsSYA&t=2181s

Serrano, M. (2015). Ašr nisā (Ṣ. 'Ilmānī, Trans.). Qatar Foundation Publishing. (Original work published in 2011)

Sharrak, A. (2020). *Corana wa-l-ḫiṭāb: muqaddimāt wa-yawmiyāt*. Mu'assasat Muqārabāt.

Wāzan, 'A. (2020). Sab'ata 'ašara kātiban 'arabiyyan yašhadūn alà laḥẓat al-'uzla al-tārīḫiyya fī 'ālam corona. *Independent Arabia*. https://www.independentarabia.com/node/105711/

World Health Organization WHO. (2020, March 3). *Joint ICC-WHO statement: An unprecedented call to action for the private sector to tackle COVID-19*. https://www.who.int/es/news/item/16-03-2020-icc-who-joint-statement-an-unprecedented-private-sector-call-to-action-to-tackle-covid-19

Zawād, M. (2020, May 13). *Al-Kātib al-ǧazā'irī Moḥammad Zawād yuhdī al-Bulaida qaṣīda ši'riyya* [Video Archive]. YouTube. https://www.youtube.com/watch?v=ZH3vHuc6KpI

Zidane, M. (2020). Effects of the corona virus pandemic COVID19 on a legal's limits times in algérian law. *Annales de l'Université d'Alger*, (34), 625-642.

Chapter 10
Coronavirus Pandemic and the Isolation of Deaf and Hard-of-Hearing Children in Greece

Evangelia Gkigkelou
University of the Basque Country, Spain

ABSTRACT

On March 11, 2020, the World Health Organization (WHO) declared the outbreak of COVID-19 as a worldwide pandemic affecting all people around the world. In order to control pandemic spread, governments, including Greece, took some public measures concerning health and social distancing. This has affected nearly every sector of the economy and education as well. Governments were forced to suspend students' attendance at schools and start distance education. As schools have been shuttered and the lives of students have been changed, it is crucial to consider the extreme isolation suddenly facing a special group of pupils: deaf and hard-of-hearing children who rely on sign language, lip reading, and facial expressions. That type of education and the obligatory use of facemasks acted as obstacles in their participation in school procedures and communication with their teachers and peers. However, those two years were transitional and have changed a lot of things regarding the data of these areas. There has been significant growth with innovations that should have been made long ago.

INTRODUCTION

The pandemic had started in the first months of 2020 and many people have faced the experience of exclusion from their ordinary life, being cut off their, until then, reality and experiencing the feeling of daily isolation, according to the World Economic Forum (WEF) as many measures must be taken in order to reduce the transmission of the virus. The remaining closure of schools for a quiet long time led to distance education. Such huge change affected the inclusive education regarding the students with special education needs/ disabilities. For those children, who are more likely to be isolated or victimized, and especially for the deaf and hard-of-hearing children, in this case, the feeling of isolation and everyday experience of exclusion in the COVID-19 period was enlarged.

DOI: 10.4018/978-1-6684-4735-2.ch010

Despite the fact that social isolation is not automatically relative with loneliness, early intimations in the pandemic situation show that more than 30% of kids and adolescents report high levels of seclusion and anxiety. Moreover, the extensive and intensive use of protective face masks or/and coverings, in order to prevent disease transmission, led to various communication problems and acted as barrier for deaf and hard-of-hearing people, especially pupils, as they made them feel that they kept out of the rest world.

Aim

The present paper will explore the impacts of the coronavirus pandemic crisis on the hearing impairment community in Greece, especially on children and adolescences and the isolation they have encountered during the pandemic and somehow continue to face. Recent research has shown that minorities, such as deaf and hard-of-hearing pupils, are suffering directly from the pandemic effects as they do not have access to services and welfare and in an extent viewpoint, to education. This study's primary goal is to point out the isolation that deaf and children with hearing impairments face during COVID-19, in Greece, the first difficulties in distance learning, the lack of communication through the obligatory mouth and nose covering and the, after two years, improvement in these factors the subsequent period.

METHODOLOGY

This paper was carried out after an intensive and systematic literature review, utilizing government and journalistic sources, as well as detailed and useful articles, in order to provide an appropriate and comprehensive synthesis of evidence and to inform about the imperative educational policy decision-making regarding the first distance education, the systematic use of face masks in schools and the isolation which is faced by deaf and hard of hearing children through the COVID-19 period. This review observes to the basic principles of systematic bibliographic reviews, including the inflexibility of the scientist, clarity, and reproducibility. It uses brief systematic review procedure, including limiting search criteria and quick data eradication.

Distance Learning

During the coronavirus pandemic emergency which started in the first days of March of 2020 and lasted almost until the end of the school year, which means the last days of May/ beginning of June, schools in Greece were closed. After this decision and during the months of the prohibition, as it is called lockdown, there was a short period that the government was searching the best solutions in order pupils continue their academic reality. The central planning, which was set as primary from the Greek Ministry of Education, regarding primary and secondary education, designed in strengthening technological infrastructure at national level while, simultaneously, ensured free access from mobile phones and computers on services and applications, concerning the platforms e-me and e-class, of the PanHellenic School Network. So, after some ambiguous and difficult moments and with the data that existed until then, schools began to organize their "distance learning" mainly through asynchronous teaching.

Based on the official data published on the Greek Ministry of Education website (2020), during this unique and bizarre situation, there was a deep and large response to manufacturing online education. Analyzing the data it can be said that the response of teachers and students exceeded all expectations

(PanHellenic School Network, 2020), as until the end of autumn 2020: 85% of the total number of teachers have been registered and approximately 1,022,864 students in a total of 1,448,916 (70.5% of the total). As it concerned the synchronous platform it is used the Webex platform but the first time of the pandemic crisis there were few teachers that they were using it. Additionally, in a very short time the educational television, through the channel ERT, took over support of distance education, mainly, with creation of videotaped lessons especially for primary school students, while at the same time ensuring the free access to all available digital services and their integration into Internet learning environments (Papadimitriou, 2020).

However, there were obvious and objective difficulties which acted as a deterrent to the design and implementation of a coherent framework of actions for distance education at a central level and this attempt made all the students face new challenges and many difficulties, specifically the deaf and the hearing impaired ones. While school community used video conferencing in real-time lessons many technical issues may had been raised. Most importantly, there had been that there was no plan for real-time transcription and subtitling of what the teacher were saying on camera. This, obviously, for deaf, hard-of-hearing and with severe hearing impairment children, who have to rely on lip reading and/or sign language or both, was a huge obstacle. Moreover, there was no targeted feedback when those children needed it. The material provided at the beginning was mostly standardized and did not arouse their curiosity and interest, preventing them from engaging effectively. In fact, the interventions that were carried out were not structured in such a way as to be able to give the desired results and operated procedurally. Their effect was only superficial (Mantzikos & Lappa, 2020). Furthermore, there was a lack of collaboration between teachers and students, teachers (the general and special education ones) among themselves and as well as between teachers and parents, which if it was achieved, it could deliver multiple benefits, social and cognitive, for deaf and hard of hearing children. As something like this never happened the first period, the feelings of loneliness, depression and isolation had increased even further (Khalil & Ebner, 2014). Also, there had been no useful adjustments and adaptations to the teaching material that was presented by the educators and as a matter of fact differentiated instruction was not applied either.

All of the above, also, applies to courses that conducted via educational television. It is important to be mentioned that, in the first period of the pandemic, on this specific educational television programs, it seemed that lessons were not took place using pedagogical and practical approaches that would benefit both disabled and non-disabled pupils. Moreover, it also seemed that teachers who were conducting the lessons were not aware of the pupils' profiles and their abilities. For instance, they were not aware of whether the pupils had any disability, of their level of understanding the Greek language (pupils from other countries), learning level, etc.

Despite the fact that those lessons, provided through this educational TV, were accessible to students with hearing problems with interpretation at Greek Sign Language, in essence they were more standardized. The lack of meaningful feedback was also important. Educational television was just aimed to cover the curriculum of the basic lessons and follow the same attitudes as follow the schools before the COVID-19 pandemic. In other words, educational television did not promote a severe and meaningful, actually, learning. In addition, by teaching the same content in the exact same way on educational television, marginalization and exclusion of certain pupils was enlarged as it is not considered the elements of heterogeneity that are essential in the learner population (Mantzikos & Lappa, 2020).

Moreover, mentioning the distance education in general, the resume is that there was not a single lesson designed for deaf and hard-of-hearing pupils who attend either mainstream or special education schools and was mostly intended for non-disabled pupils. Despite their inalienable right to have access to information and educational material, they were left out of distance learning on the assumption that they constitute a difficult to manage population that requires more specialized educational approaches (Liasidou & Symeou, 2016). As it was implemented, it was no surprise that distance learning followed a separated education path, and that, during this cruel period, the learning level, that these children had managed to reach before the COVID-19 crisis, dropped substantially, and learning gaps gradually arose (e.g., Levinson, Cevik, Lipsitch, 2020). The Greek Ministry of Education seemed to had taken into consideration only what is implemented at homogeneous schools, mainstream schools, that are only in theory inclusive and not in reality.

As for teachers, the fact that they acted as individuals rather than a part of a team led to lack of communication and cooperation with each other, with their students and the students' parents as well. As a result, disabled pupils are further marginalized and, probably, stigmatized, and many aspects of their development are negatively affected (Mantzikos & Lappa, 2020). Many parents had increased their anxiety levels because they were not ready for this difficult situation. Their anxiety was not unjustified. They had to address the needs of their child to a much larger extent than previously and face the feelings of anxiety, isolation and loneliness in every sector of education, and not only, that their children had to deal with. In literature is mentioned that students with disabilities are "among the most vulnerable individuals" in crisis that may affect them and their families' emotional and mental health on the long run (Alshawabkeh et al, 2021).

In order for parents to be able to help their children, as much as they can, during distance learning, they had to work more closely with the classroom and special education teachers but this collaboration between the two sides became more complicated and it led to an ineffective communication. It was based on the exchange of standard material via e-mail or sometimes the two sides communicated through phone calls or video calls only for a few minutes and as it comes to mind that was not enough. Through various researches it appeared that a number of parents indicated they were not very satisfied with their collaboration with the special education teacher (Mantzikos & Lappa, 2020). As a result, this affected the learning, social and emotional development of their hearing impaired child (Apple, 2016). In general, research shows high prevalence of anxiety and depressive symptoms in children and adolescents, due to COVID-19 crisis, distance education, social isolation and parents' stress.

Use of Face Masks

In response to the increasing number of coronavirus, when schools open on June, deaf and hard of hearing children faced two important barriers: the one was the use of face masks and coverings which became mandatory and, the other, was the 1 and a half meter social distancing rule. During face-to-face mode, mask-wearing impoverishes communication and interaction between educators and children. Such constraints are particularly pertinent for teachers and students with special needs, such as deaf and hearing impaired young children who going to school for the first time, and foreign language learners. (Kefalaki, 2021)

Speaking specifically for the deaf and, generally, for the hearing impaired pupils who rely on sign language it is obligatory to be said that facial expressions is a need in order to understand completely of what is being communicated, and those with hearing aids or cochlear implants during rehabilitation rely on lip reading in order to understand better what is being said and heard (Homans & Vroegop, 2021). As a matter of fact, anyone with hearing impairment will have difficulty with muffled speech that most people have due to the obligatory use of facemask. Thus, covering of face by mask can cut down on the ability to connect, and the about two meters recommendation for physical distancing during the pandemic posed, and still poses, a problem for the hard-to-hear population due to inaudible voice, resulting in social isolation and mental health implications. With the return of children to schools, it is outstanding to refer to these communication issues. As teachers and other students at schools wear masks, many parents have expressed worries and concerns that their deaf and hard-of hearing children will experience greater difficulties in speech understanding, as the visible cues from the mouth and lips had been removed.

As teachers in mainstream and special education schools are afraid about the transmission of COVID-19 within schools, they did not want to put themselves and the health of all children in danger and fully implemented the instructions for the mandatory use of the mask. However, mask-wearing, as it mentioned above, may delay or block lip reading and make teachers' voices not very clear. This with the 1 and a half meter social distancing rule that has to be abided by all people within the classroom makes the whole project even more difficult, aggravating the anxiety of the children. Also, it is important to mention that Greek public schools have experienced spending cuts on teaching materials and that reducing of money spending on education leads disabled students to feel a sense of isolation and this has huge consequences for their mental health (Oliver, 2009).

The Improvement of Distance Learning

Although online education has been carried out, advanced, and promoted at higher education before early 2020, it was not widespread for primary and secondary schools. The classic and usual form was in-class education, where all students were physically present. However, when COVID-19 declared as a pandemic by World Health Organization (WHO), measures such as lockdown and social distancing were introduced in many countries all around the world (Marinoni, 2020). According to UNESCO (2020), school closures in more than 180 countries as the date of March 27 caused by the COVID-19 pandemic have affected over 1.5 billion students and families, and 63 million of educators.

As a result, education could no longer be provided in its current form and was therefore provided online. Consequently, students were forced to follow another way, the education from home way, in order to continue their education. Due to the immediate changes in society, the teaching practices had to be adapted rapidly to new situations. The Coronavirus pandemic has shifted the academic community into new landscapes that require educators and students to adjust and manage their expectations and has presented various challenges for teaching students with disabilities in an online didactic and pedagogical environment. Also, it gave opportunities for collaboration, training, and communication between general and special educators with their students and became an chance to meet their needs, in this case meet the needs of the deaf and hard-of-hearing ones.

Many "how can" questions are being presented, as such as:

- how can a whole system change to an online just in few days, especially when it is based mainly on classroom teaching;
- how can teachers deal with students without the financial resources to access the required technology and the internet;
- how can children be excluded from the teaching procedure;
- how can be supported educators with no training or experience in online education;

- how can teachers and the whole system determine the 'value' of students; and
- how can be preserved quality and excellence in the delivery of education in this new and difficult paradigm [International Association of Universities (IAU), 2020].

The new conditions in the life of people during the pandemic have identified a number of new opportunities for the individual – the development of individual strategies of self-development and self-education, for the business - the creation of new educational resources and improve their quality, for the society - the formation of a new quality of human capital, which has such competence as creativity, critical thinking, cooperation and communication (Maqableh & Alia, 2021). There are plenty of online tools available which is important for an effective and efficient learning environment. Digital Literacy that is created, is the alertness, perspective and the ability of individuals to use, appropriately, digital tools and facilities to classify, approach, manage, assimilate, appraise, analyze and synthesize digital resources, erect new knowledge, create media expressions, and communicate with others, in the context of specific life situations, in order to enable effective social action (Martin, 2008, p. 167). So, under these circumstances, people evolved in terms of technology and made their life easier.

During the 2nd period of the pandemic (October-November 2020), talking about a central level design, was upgraded: a) the role of educational television with the addition of new ones objects, which should be further enriched and mainly to be interconnected with the school every day (to be used as asynchronous supplementary educational material by teachers), b) the level of technological capabilities of the PanHellenic Network and specifically the access to asynchronous learning environments of e-class and e-me and c) was secured the technological access to the environment of modern distance education in all teachers and students despite their dysfunctions first days managed to respond to an unprecedented for the data technological venture (Anastasiadis, 2020).

The deaf and hard-of-hearing students noticed that online learning was a difficult and challenging experience. But at the same time, those students said that it intensified their skills in technology and their competences in adapting to a new environment (Alshawabkeh et al, 2021). Also, this whole new world, led them to gain direct contact with technology and find new ways of communicating with their peers that were not so widespread. A huge benefit is that the educational materials, in the e-learning platforms, e-me and e-class, are available to the students at any time they want, 24 hours a day. Also this material can be enriched with audio and visual files (multimedia) using subtitles, which can facilitate the understanding of complex concepts, especially for students with hearing impairments. In addition, since realism can be incorporated into an e-learning curriculum, it is possible to increase the motivation of learners through the use of interactive activities (electronic game, virtual world) or sensory simulation tools (Ally & Prieto-Blázquez, 2014).

Hopefully, this health, and not only, crisis could also yield social and educational benefits from a reassessment of ambition, aims and goals that could constantly change the nature of education and literacy as we know it. One of these benefits could be imagining ways of conceiving of the relationships between society, literacy, and schooling anew, so as to be able to posture significant problems for literacy and learning in while and post-pandemic times and come to terms with the risks and uncertainties that have assailed us all (Martin, 2008). Hence, education through the development of technological tools and their use can help people, and especially children, the disabled and no-disabled ones, not only to cope with the educational process but to be able to find different ways of communication that bring them closer to each other and help them to avoid their feeling of isolation and the sense that they are alone.

Face Masks with Clear Windows

Face masks not only disrupt access to the acoustic and visual aspects of speech, but they also break apart the social aspects of face-to-face communication (smiles, frowns, smirks, etc.) that serve as subtle nonverbal cues, context for verbal content, and emotion. Individuals use a variety of cues in their face and body in order to communicate on the one hand and perceive emotion on the other hand (Bänziger et al., 2009). The face, however, provides particularly prominent cues that "photograph" the emotional situation of the communication partner. Despite the fact that the eyes and mouth are both able to communicate aspects of emotion, both static and dynamic mouth positions tend to do a better job (Blais et al., 2012). However, emotion perception may be altered when social interaction involves the obligatory use of face masks (Grieco-Calub, 2021).

Face masks with clear windows could be a solution as they allow access to facial expressions and lip movements. Thus, deaf people and people with hearing problems have the opportunity to communicate to a greater extent with their interlocutor without fear of spreading the disease of coronavirus. Nevertheless there are few manufacturers who produce these types of transparent masks and as a result the supplies are low those masks gave a solution to many people. Moreover, administrative barriers to the use of clear masks remain in medical settings and are not widely used. Clearing these barriers is an essential priority, especially for those people who have not another choice. All around the world, deaf and hard-of-hearing people are fashioning their own clear masks in order not to be excluded and be part of the community. This will be an area for product innovation and activism in the future (Grieco-Calub, 2021).

Focusing on this idea, recent studies confirm that listeners' speech recognition improves through a transparent mask if there is access to the talker's mouth (i.e., access to visual speech) (Thibodeau et al., 2021). It is important to note, however, that the materials used to make transparent masks and face shields have variable acoustic filtering properties and variable transparency due to reflections or fogging. Thus, the benefits observed with transparent equipment—and thus access to visual speech—may be limited if the material itself causes too much degradation to the speech signal (Grieco-Calub, 2021).

Another solution and strategy that is effective at improving speech recognition in the presence of acoustic signal degradation, despite the clear masks, is the use of FM systems or remote microphones (e.g., Roger microphone from Phonak). These systems are designed to advance the intensity of the talker's voice related to other sounds present in the environment. FM systems are frequently utilized in classrooms in order to provide in deaf and/or hard of hearing children better access to their teacher's and classmate's voices. If masks and social distancing continue to be mandatory within schools, FM systems and remote microphones may be crucial to provide that children are able to hear talkers in schools and, especially, in the classroom (Grieco-Calub, 2021).

If listeners are better able to recognize speech because they have access to visual speech or because they have access to an improved signal-to-noise ratio, then the onus on the talker to overcome the acoustic filtering of face masks and social distancing is less. Consistent with this idea, the benefit of hearing amplification to both the adult users with hearing loss and their communication partners has been showed (Beechey et al., 2020). As a result, finding ways to improve the fidelity of the speech signal may be critical to ensuring communication efficiency for people who use face masks and execute social distancing, especially for deaf and hard-of-hearing.

CONCLUSION

The coronavirus pandemic has created the largest disruption of education systems in human history, affecting nearly 1.5 billion learners in more than 200 countries. Closures of schools, institutions and other learning spaces have impacted more than 94% of the world's student population and have changed the world in many aspects. Most of the countries all around the world suspended schools and provided alternative educational methods, synchronously and asynchronously. Deaf and students with hearing impairments in Greece were excluded from alternative education methods during this situation, especially from the synchronous method and many problems arose mainly the first period of the pandemic crisis, especially the feeling of isolation and the sense of loneliness. Additionally, there were no adequate reactions from their teachers to resist this exclusion or to offset the absence of educational provisions for these students (Madhesh, 2021).

Many schools across the word, including those which serve individuals who are deaf or hard-of-hearing, are now open in various capacities for face-to-face lessons. For all children, especially those who are deaf and hearing impaired, or utilize cochlear implants and/or hearing aids to communicate, access to quality auditory information is critical for speech perception and learning. However, the consistent use of masks in the classroom and out of it created and still creates, to a degree, other difficulties to these people and as a result did not and do not help the education and communication procedure.

However, face masks and the 1 and a half meter social distancing have been proven to be successful measures at mitigating the spread of COVID-19. Despite this success, they may create challenges to effective communication, which can have negative downstream effects on speech production, speech recognition, language processing, and cognition. As time passes, more and more solutions and choices come to light (Grieco-Calub, 2021). The last two years have been made many efforts in distance learning and there is a general improvement in digital literacy and the use of technology in order people come closer to each other and none student be excluded from the educational procedure. Also, there is a severe trial to give several solutions regarding the materials used in the masks in order none of the people be excluded. The times we live in require radical changes and genuine interest for these changes to be effective. To make this possible, strategies and methods should be adopted, which will be based on an inclusive educational model focusing on pupils, adolescents and university students (Apple, 2016).

REFERENCES

Ally, M., & Prieto-Blázquez, J. (2014). What is the future of mobile learning in education? *RUSC Universities and Knowledge Society Journal*, *11*(1), 142–151. doi:10.7238/rusc.v11i1.2033

Alshawabkeh, A. A., Madhesh, A., Woolsey, M. L., & Kharbat, F. F. (2021). Using online information technology for deaf students during COVID- 19: A closer look from experience. *Heliyon*, *7*(5), e06915. Advance online publication. doi:10.1016/j.heliyon.2021.e06915 PMID:34013080

Anastasiadis P. (2020). Η Σχολική Εξ Αποστάσεως Εκπαίδευση στην εποχή του Κορωνοϊού COVID-19: το παράδειγμα της Ελλάδας και η πρόκληση της μετάβασης στο «Ανοιχτό Σχολείο της Διερευνητικής Μάθησης, της Συνεργατικής Δημιουργικότητας και της Κοινωνικής Αλληλεγγύης» [Distance learning in the era of COVID-19, focusing on the Greek Educational System]. *Open Education - The Journal for Open and Distance Education and Educational Technology*, *16*(2).

Apple, M. W. (2016). *Εκπαίδευση και εξουσία* [Education and Power]. Epikentro Publishers.

Bänziger, T., Grandjean, D., & Scherer, K. R. (2009). Emotion recognition from expressions in face, voice, and body: The Multimodal Emotion Recognition Test (MERT). *Emotion (Washington, D.C.)*, *9*(5), 691–704. doi:10.1037/a0017088 PMID:19803591

Beechey T., M. Buchholz M. J., & Keidser G. (2020). *Hearing aid amplification reduces communication effort of people with hearing impairment and their conversation partners*. doi:10.1044/2020_JSLHR-19-00350

Blais, C., Roy, C., Fiset, D., Arguin, M., & Gosselin, F. (2012). *The eyes are not the window to basic emotions*. doi:10.1016/j.neuropsychologia.2012.08.010

Greek Ministry of Education. (2020). https://mathainoumestospiti.gov.gr/

Grieco-Calub, M. T. (2021). COVID-19, Face Masks, and Social Interaction: How a Global Pandemic Is Shining a Light on the Importance of Face-to-Face Communication. *Perspectives of the ASHA Special Interest Groups*, *6*(5), 1097–1105. Advance online publication. doi:10.1044/2021_PERSP-21-00037

Homans, N. C., & Vroegop, J. L. (2021). Impact of Face Masks in Public Spaces during COVID-19 Pandemic on Daily Life Communication of Cochlear Implant Users. *Laryngoscope Investigative Otolaryngology*, *6*(3), 531–539. doi:10.1002/lio2.578 PMID:34195375

Kefalaki, M., Rudolph, J., Tan, S., & Diamantidaki, F. (2021). Face masks in education: The cases of Greece and Singapore. *Thesis*, *10*(1), 3-42.

Khalil, H., & Ebner, M. (2014). MOOCs completion rates and possible methods to improve retention - a literature review. In J. Viteli & M. Leikomaa (Eds.), *Proceedings of Ed Media 2014—World Conference on Educational Media and Technology* (pp. 1305-1313). Association for the Advancement of Computing in Education (AACE). https://cutt.ly/8omp9lH

Levinson, M., Cevik, M., & Lipsitch, M. (2020). Reopening Primary Schools during the Pandemic. *New England Journal of Medicine*. https://www.nejm.org/doi/full/10.1056/NEJMms2024920

Liasidou, A., & Symeou, L. (2016). Neoliberal versus social justice reforms in education policy and practice: Discourses, politics and disability rights in education. *Critical Studies in Education*, *59*(2), 149–166. doi:10.1080/17508487.2016.1186102

Madhesh, A. (2021). Full exclusion during COVID-19: Saudi Deaf education is an example. *Heliyon*, *7*(3), e06536. Advance online publication. doi:10.1016/j.heliyon.2021.e06536 PMID:33842703

Mantzikos, N. C., & Lappa, S. C. (2020). Difficulties and barriers in the education of deaf and hard of hearing individuals in the era of COVID-19: The case of Greece- A viewpoint article. *European Journal of Special Education Research*, *6*(3). DOI:57 doi:10.46827/ejse.v6i3.33

Maqableh, M., & Alia, M. (2021). Evaluation online learning of undergraduate students under lockdown amidst COVID-19 Pandemic: The online learning experience and students' satisfaction. Elsevier. *Children and Youth Services Review*, *128*, 106160. doi:10.1016/j.childyouth.2021.106160

Marinoni, G., Land, H., & Jensen, T. (2020). The impact of COVID-19 on higher education around the world. IAU Global Survey Report. International Association of Universities.

Martin, A. (2008). Digital Literacy and the "Digital Society. In C. Lankshear & M. Knobel (Eds.), *Digital Literacies: Concepts, Policies and Practices* (pp. 151–176). Peter Lang Publishing.

Oliver, M. (2009). *Αναπηρία και Πολιτική* [The Politics of Disablement]. Epikentro Publishers.

Papadimitriou S. (2021). Η συμβολή της Εκπαιδευτικής Τηλεόρασης στην εξ Αποστάσεως Σχολική Εκπαίδευση [The contribution of Educational Television to Distance School Education]. *Proceedings of the Conference: Εξ Αποστάσεως Εκπαίδευση και Σχολική Πραγματικότητα*. doi:10.12681/online-edu.3226

Thibodeau M. L., Thibodeau-Nielsen B. R., Quynh Tran C.M. & Tangerino de Souza Jacob R. (2021). *Communicating During COVID-19: The Effect of Transparent Masks for Speech Recognition in Noise.* doi:10.1097/AUD.0000000000001065

Chapter 11
E-Inclusion and the COVID-19 Pandemic:
Inclusive Digital Classrooms and Collaboration Between General and Special Education Teachers

Maria Mouchritsa
https://orcid.org/0000-0002-2021-7173
University of the Basque Country, Spain

Urtza Garay Ruiz
https://orcid.org/0000-0001-7298-9274
University of the Basque Country, Spain

Ainara Romero-Andonegui
University of the Basque Country, Spain

Spyridon Kazanopoulos
https://orcid.org/0000-0001-8076-7057
University of the Basque Country, Spain

ABSTRACT

Extreme situations such as the COVID-19 pandemic have revealed important characteristics that can be used to improve inclusion in both face-to-face and distance modalities, such as strengthening connections between those involved and establishing activities in which technologies can be used to support inclusion effectively. This chapter aims to demonstrate that having a computer, tablet, or smartphone during a pandemic is not sufficient to ensure learning. To illustrate this point, several national online resources are inaccessible to students with disabilities, preventing them from participating in e-inclusion. Furthermore, because of a lack of collaboration and communication between classroom and special education teachers during COVID-19, teachers were unable to plan meaningful learning activities for their students. To achieve effective electronic inclusion, activities must be organized in such a way that they meet the needs of students with special needs, and modern, asynchronous tools must be available to assist in this process.

DOI: 10.4018/978-1-6684-4735-2.ch011

INTRODUCTION

Millions of schools around the world have been forced to close as a result of the COVID-19 pandemic. Consequently, teachers and educational leaders must devise novel approaches to delivering education to over one billion students worldwide. Even though the world is in a crisis, there is an opportunity to reconsider education. As a result, all should make the most of the new circumstances. While online education will not be able to replace all of the functions that schools perform in society, it will be able to do much more than simply serve as a less-effective version of traditional face-to-face education (Zhao, 2020).

Due to the coronavirus pandemic, schools around the world suspended personal teaching in the spring of 2020. Teachers all over the world were forced to convert their classrooms into distance classrooms for learning, often for a short period, a discouraging task for teachers who had planned their lessons for personal teaching (Petzold, 2020). Furthermore, important issues are raised, such as the need for the anthropocentric dimension of distance learning (Abidah et al., 2020), which focuses on issues of equal access (Reich et al., 2020). According to Camacho et al. (2020), a new role for teachers emerges, in which they must implement all necessary changes, media adaptations, techniques, and methods in terms of flexibility and accessibility for students to gain positive learning experiences in the context of distance learning. Teachers require time, resources, training, and material support to continue adapting their practices to the needs of distance learning (Zhao et al., 2020).

Furthermore, school closures affect all students, but the most vulnerable students suffer the most. People with disabilities, immigrants, refugees, ethnic minorities with differing gender identities and sexual orientations (OECD, 2020a), and those with special educational needs are denied opportunities for life, learning, social, and emotional development that schools provide (OECD, 2020b). When schools are closed, they are more likely to become isolated. If countries fail to promote educational justice and inclusion, this group of students will be more likely to suffer negative educational outcomes and receive inadequate school support (OECD, 2020c). The "digital divide" continues to impede a future inclusive education model, and it has been identified as a major inhibitory factor in several studies (Scully et al., 2021).

Nevertheless, the importance of collaboration in inclusive education cannot be overstated. Education is expected to face any situation with collaborative practices among school professionals in inclusive education because it provides significant benefits to peers and all school professionals. Collaboration must be modified because the government decided that students should learn at home during COVID-19. Furthermore, collaboration in inclusive education entails the regular and special education teachers working together on activities with equal contribution status to discuss shared goals and problem-solving to improve student performance. Collaboration practices boost the success potential of inclusive education both before and during the pandemic by broadening opportunities for all school professionals based on their field backgrounds and expertise (Hardiani, 2021).

As a result, the main purpose of this chapter is to analyze key issues, such as inclusive education, ICT (Information and Communications Technologies) and special education, distance education, the collaboration between general and special educators, as well as e-inclusion, and then to raise concerns about the achievement of the goals of the inclusive e-classroom, as well as the cooperation of special and general education teachers to enhance e- inclusion during COVID-19.

BACKGROUND

Inclusive Education

The 1994 World Conference on Special Education in Salamanca, attended by 92 governments and 25 international organizations, was a watershed moment in international literature and the field of Special Education (Ainscow, 2005; Miles & Singal, 2008; Vislie, 2003). The conference laid the groundwork for inclusive education around the world. It has been argued that the most effective way to build an inclusive society is through inclusion. By improving the quality of the education system, this institution provided effective education for the majority of children (Ainscow, 2005). After many socio-political changes, the passage of time is now leading to a new system of education for children with disabilities, to a "School for All" based on a social model of disability (UNESCO, 1994).

Inclusive education allows both teachers and students to feel at ease with diversity, viewing it as a challenge and enrichment in the learning environment rather than a problem. Moreover, inclusive education concerns all students, with a particular emphasis on students with special needs and disabilities, as well as children from ethnolinguistic minority populations (UNESCO, 1994). Co-education of children with and without special educational needs creates frameworks and didactic practices that view individual differences as an opportunity to enrich the teaching and learning process (UNESCO, 1994). Furthermore, the curriculum, methods and techniques, and procedures are referred to flexibly and on a case-by-case basis to be adapted to the extent deemed necessary to meet the needs of all students. The term "inclusion" was proposed to describe the quality of education provided to children with disabilities in the context of the general school, with the collaboration of general and special education teachers (Sourtzi et al., 2013).

The term "co-education," according to Georgiadi et al. (2007), refers to the effort put forth to ensure the coexistence and co-teaching of the vast majority of students with special educational needs alongside their non-special classmates' educational needs in public schools at all levels of education, including elementary and secondary school classes. To accomplish this, qualified teachers or an interdisciplinary team must provide the necessary specialized pedagogical assistance and support. All over Europe, "co-education" has been one of the most important issues in planning for education for the last few decades (Georgiadi et al., 2007).

For the past two decades, Greece has been implementing the inclusion of students with and without special educational needs in general school classrooms. Co-education was implemented as (a) separate education for children with special educational needs; (b) partial integration of children in the classroom with simultaneous attendance of integration or supportive teaching; and (c) full integration into the classroom with two teachers in the same room (Polychronopoulou, 2003). Only in 2008, with the special education law (369/2-10-2008, Government Gazette 199), was the institution of parallel support established and implemented within the framework of inclusion, providing for the support of students with special educational needs in the general classroom.

The term "inclusion," and more specifically "inclusive education," refers to the process of transforming educational systems to respond to the diversity of their students (Ainscow, 2005; Meijer et al., 2003; UNESCO, 1994), and is related to the content of collaboration between general and special education teachers (Cook & Friend, 2004; Brownell et al., 2006).

Collaboration Between General and Special Education Teachers

Special education and general education teachers collaborate to design, create, and solve problems. Their collaboration is distinguished by the partners' mutual trust and co-responsibility in terms of the effects on the inclusion of all students in the educational process taking place in general education (Cook & Friend, 2004; Moreillon, 2007). The most important aspects of collaboration between general and special education teachers are individual work with students and solid assistance to teachers (Bouillet, 2013). According to Kirkpatrick et al. (2020), outside of the classroom, general and special teachers collaborate to plan lessons and assessments, obtain resources, and discuss the unique needs of their students. In the classroom, they employ similar instructional strategies.

Collaboration among teachers is based on the exchange of information and materials in lesson preparation, shared assignment planning, and working together to prepare, implement, and assess lessons and exercises in the context of co-construction (Jurkowski et al., 2020). Many studies have revealed that collaboration between special education and general education teachers is one of the most important factors related to the effectiveness of the education of students with special educational needs, as indicated in the relevant literature (Beaton, 2007; Tsakiridou & Polyzopoulou, 2014; Strogilos, et al., 2011).

As Wiggins and Damore (2006) point out, successful collaboration requires the following preconditions to be met: a) a positive attitude manifested through a shared philosophy toward the education of students with special educational needs and the recognition of the colleague's competencies; b) teamwork, in which members actively interact and communicate with one another; c) the development of one's professional skills and competences through participation in various in-service courses, seminars, lectures, and discussions; the sharing of best practices; and engaging in various modes of self-study; d) management and leadership, in which the leader demonstrates his or her firm position, can organize, and involves school personnel in joint activities by allowing every teacher to feel like a highly competent professional; e) resources, i.e., the ability to find and manage time and material resources to achieve quality education and f) operational effectiveness.

Apart from the importance of teacher collaboration, it is difficult to implement collaborative practices in and out of the classroom because general and special education teachers' collaboration forms are infrequent and insufficient in many cases. Despite similarities in the content of teachers' collaboration, such as co-planning and implementing students' educational programs, co-teaching, assessing, and discussing all students' issues, teachers emphasize poor collaborative behaviour among themselves (Mouchritsa et al., 2021).

ICT (Information and Communications Technologies) and Special Education

The term ICT (Information and Communications Technologies) refers to all available digital technologies (technological products as well as technological tools for design, production, and evaluation) based on the management of digital information (production, representation, processing, and storage) and its transmission through communication networks, especially the Internet. The systematic integration of digital technologies into the educational process to improve the quality of students' learning experiences and help them achieve higher levels of learning outcomes is referred to as "ICT in Education" (Dimitriadis, 2015).

In modern society, the main goal is to shift the educational philosophy toward individualized education and student-centeredness through curriculum adjustments, while the challenge is school reconstruction and the provision of equal educational opportunities for all students. The use of ITC in special education is a means of achieving the aforementioned goals. The ability of children with special educational needs to use and utilize new ICT contributes to the elimination of exclusion and the closing of the digital divide between students (Aggelopoulou, 2011).

Furthermore, modern pedagogical perspectives on the utility and effectiveness of integration, as well as continuous technological advancements, have sparked interest in utilizing the various applications of new ICT in individualized interventions as well as during the integration of students with special needs into general schools (Williams et al., 2006). For students who are unable to benefit from traditional educational programs, new technologies can play a critical role, particularly in Special Education, in improving teaching and learning effectiveness (Hadi et al., 2010; Hasselbring & Glaser, 2000).

The application of ICT in special education addresses the need to provide equal opportunities for all students. It specifically aids in the multisensory approach to teaching subjects, the acquisition of problem-solving skills, and the development of social skills (Aggelopoulou, 2011). Furthermore, the use of ICT benefits students with special educational needs because they can express their preferences and points of view through the computer and, at the same time, communicate in a variety of ways using the tools provided by the internet (Forzani & Leau, 2012; Williams, 2005). Underlined by Paraskevopoulos (2005), students can and do play a role in the main goal of their integration into the general classroom.

The use of a computer assists students with learning disabilities in maintaining their interest and motivation for learning as well as paying attention to the lesson areas in which they present significant challenges (Hennesy et al., 2005). Simultaneously, there are numerous benefits to using ICT for students with autism, who frequently show an interest in interacting with a computer because they operate according to predefined rules and the stimuli they receive are always predictable and controllable (Christinaki et al., 2013; Kalyva, 2005).

Concurrently, touch technologies (mobile phones and tablets) play an important role in the education of children with autism, mental retardation, and learning disabilities because their use improves their communication, social, and language skills (Campigotto et al., 2013; Fernadez-lopez et al., 2013). They also allow for freedom of movement within the school and the transfer of activities to the home (Fernadez-lopez et al., 2013). It also allows students with special needs to participate in teaching goals and activities that are matched to their level of ability (Aggelopoulou, 2011), which helps them learn.

The Internet, with its numerous applications and flexible, ready-made programs, is a valuable educational resource that can provide not only incentives but also didactic and learning benefits, provided that all of these services are aligned with the interests of students with special educational needs (Williams et al., 2006). Most of the time, it is possible for students with mild learning disabilities to participate in class activities with their peers if specific activities are planned for them and the right adaptive devices are used (Kourbetis et al., 2014; Koumaki & Haidi, 2015).

There have been various surveys (Gros, 2007; Habgood, 2007; Thomas, 2009; Whitton, 2010) indicating that the use of ICT is highly motivating for students and in the learning process integrates fundamental principles that promote learning, such as active involvement, social participation, constructive activities, the development of a strategy for understanding and problem solving, self-control, the reconstruction of pre-existing knowledge, and the organization of material around general principles and explanatory text.

According to UNESCO (2011), information and communication technology (ICT) is an invaluable tool in educating people with disabilities, and access to digital infrastructure must remain a timeless and strong goal. The development and cognitive improvement of several developmentally and cognitively delayed young children with disabilities can be attributed in large part to technological assistance

(Judge, 2000). As a result of the integration of information and communication technology (ICT) into the everyday teaching process, the levels of learning interest, hilariousness, enthusiasm, dedication, and motivation in many special schools and integration departments are extremely high today (Mastrogiannis & Anastopoulos, 2012).

Therefore, it is a pedagogical commitment to a modern school that gives equal opportunities to take initiatives to enhance, promote, and improve the learning of all students. The use of best on an individual basis with a focus on the student is defined as a priority (Kourbetis et al., 2014). Particularly, in Grece

Distance Learning

According to Sophos and Kron (2010), p. 134, the term "distance learning" is mentioned in educational data that we encounter in electronic form and which is used in both public and private schools to achieve learning and knowledge building, whether internet access is available or not. Furthermore, Keegan (2001) highlighted that distance learning has two dimensions: a) educational material created for the program's needs and b) the learning process in which the trainees' active participation is required.

Distance learning is classified into three types: asynchronous, synchronous, and mixed (Anastasiadis, 2014). According to Arkorful and Abaidoo (2014), synchronous distance learning includes simultaneous access for teachers and students, whereas asynchronous access allows participants to post announcements and download material whenever they want. Students in the modern form of distance learning communicate with teachers in real-time, using tools such as video conferencing and chat rooms, which provide direct feedback.

The term "school distance learning" refers to the organized distance education process that takes place in primary and secondary schools (Paleodimou, 2017). According to Holmberg (2003), school distance learning is an evolution that is addressed to students who are either forced to monitor learning programs remotely due to circumstances (e.g., school closure due to pandemic) or choose to attend courses that are not included in conventional training.

Due to complex social and economic factors, but also because of the rapid development of technological media, distance education methodology has become a primary major field of research interest in recent decades (Martin et al., 2020). According to research data (OECD, 2020d), the COVID-19 crisis has pushed the education system worldwide to look for alternative ways of education rather than lifelong teaching. As a result, teachers and students are using distance education on an unprecedented scale. Educational institutions were compelled to discontinue life courses, workshops, and other activities, transferring teaching from the traditional form to a physical presence in the distance via the internet and the services it provides. The new way of education is distinguished by a high degree of flexibility, is independent of place and time, and occurs at an unprecedented and shocking rate. However, the above procedure was stressful for teachers because the challenge of comparing distance learning with live teaching under current pandemic conditions is great and adds extra pressure (Zioga, 2021).

In the context of the COVID-19 pandemic, remote teaching was invited to assist in restoring communication and interaction between students and teachers following the suspension of school unit operations. This unexpected temporary transfer of the educational process from the conventional to the remote due to emergencies, as well as its idiosyncratic application without prior experience in such a universal application without preparation, training, and insufficient technological infrastructure, brought to the fore the new term "emergency remote teaching," which tries to describe and render this special treaty and the application of Distance Learning (Hodges et al., 2020).

The use of the platforms by the entire school unit, rather than individual teachers, over the last two years laid the groundwork for the integration of the traditional educational system with the open and distance education systems. The flipped classroom is an example of a relevant methodology that, according to the Flipped Learning Network, which includes teachers who use the inverted classroom (FLN, 2014), "transfers the delivery of the lesson (wherein the conventional class is usually a monologue) outside the physical space of the classroom (mainly through video), so that the teaching time in the classroom is dedicated to more interactive type activities where students are actively participating." As a result, this methodology shifts the passive (for the student) theoretical part of teaching at home, while the teacher has more time at school to apply student-centred and experiential teaching techniques (Makrodimos et al., 2017). In each case, the student and the teacher are separated by space but not necessarily by time (Valentine, 2002), given that Greenberg (1998) defined modern distance education as a planned teaching/learning experience that uses several different technologies to reach students digitally and is meant to promote learners' interaction and credentialing of learning, either synchronously or asynchronously.

Distance Learning first appeared in Greece in the field of school education in 2010, following a proposal from the Pedagogical Institute (PI), intending to create a Unified Digital Education Platform, with the main purpose of utilizing digital educational materials in the educational process and enhancing integration and inclusion of digital technologies by students (Pedagogical Institute, 2011).

Nevertheless, new data from the pandemic that erupted in the spring of 2020 all over the world compelled the Ministry of Education to take immediate action and make the provision for school distance learning mandatory for all students in the country, at least in terms of the asynchronous education provided. In the first phase, teachers registered on the Ministry of Education's existing asynchronous distance learning platforms (e-Class and e-me) and were then invited to create their virtual sections. The students' parents and guardians were then required to enrol their children in the Panhellenic School Network (Panhellenic School Network, 2022a, 2022b). Teachers were then tasked with developing content for their digital classrooms, utilizing the interactive textbooks as well as the various educational material repositories (e.g., Photodentro, Aesopos). Furthermore, the teachers who wanted to use the Cisco Webex digital platform to teach modern lessons were also given the chance (Panhellenic School Network, 2022c).

Furthermore, the Greek government adopted three key measures to ensure the inclusion of pupils with disabilities and the maintenance of their education. The circular letter 39317/GD4 "Distance learning for pupils with disabilities and/or special educational needs" was sent to all schools and stakeholders. A social measure was adopted with the distribution of 9,000 digital devices (at a cost of more than 1.48 million euros) to support distance learning during the lockdown. Other distance learning provisions have been made through the national television channel ERT2 TV, where students can follow some lessons with the contribution of Greek Sign Language interpreters (Drakopoulou, 2020).

MAIN FOCUS OF THE CHAPTER

E-Inclusion

E-inclusion was defined as follows by Bianchi et al. (2006), citing the final report of the European Commission's eEurope Advisory Group (working group 2 on e-inclusion): "E-inclusion" is defined as the extent to which information and communication technologies (ICTs) contribute to equalizing and encouraging participation in society at all levels' (eEurope Advisory Group, 2005). E-inclusion is defined as the use of information and communication technologies (ICTs) in compensatory uses to assist students in overcoming their limitations, as well as in participatory uses to enable students to participate actively and collaboratively in social learning contexts (Mitchell & Sutherland, 2020; Parmigiani et al.,2021; Rice & Dykman, 2018).

Distance education is viewed as a versatile and adequately inclusive method of providing inclusive education. Inclusion could be aided by technology. The advancement of technology and open distance learning could go a long way toward increasing access to education for the majority of children with disabilities, allowing the learning process to continue (Khokhar, 2007).

Distance education must be inclusive and adapted to the needs of students with special needs. Furthermore, distance education should broaden and improve access to training and education opportunities that are tailored to the student's specific needs (Masalela, 2008). Diverse learners should be able to recognize the importance of pedagogical approaches to recognition to enable them to recognize their own experiences and identities in the curriculum. Students should be valued as active meaning-makers with the ability to influence their own and others' educational experiences (Masalela, 2008).

Furthermore, students with learning disabilities benefit from the digital classroom because it increases personalization and compensatory processes in the classroom. Supportive technologies in a digital classroom, when combined with an inclusive didactic plan, can be considered scaffolding tools, which can be used to aid in the processes of learning acquisition as well as personal development (Gaggioli, 2018). More specifically, flipping the classroom assists teachers in differentiating instruction to meet the needs of students with learning disabilities. Self-paced, mastery learning gives students flexibility in how they learn content. The teacher's responsibility for learning is essentially transferred to the students. Collaboration and cooperative learning are encouraged in the flipped classroom. Students assist one another in learning rather than relying solely on the teacher to disseminate knowledge. Additionally, the flipped classroom allows for continuous and immediate formative feedback.

In Greece, for example, digital materials and software are available that promote differentiation of teaching for students with special educational needs while also being accessible to all students. The material is classified by disability type, but this classification is not legally binding. Students with visual and hearing impairments, motor impairments, moderate and mild intellectual disability, autism spectrum disorders, special learning difficulties, distraction and concentration issues are among those whose educational needs are met (*Universal Design and Development of Accessible Digital Educational Materials*, 2022).

E-Inclusion and Covid-19

When it comes to the developments that followed the COVID-19 pandemic, using technology in education provided a solution. It did so while also bringing to light barriers to the inclusion of students with special educational needs, as well as the fact that while online learning offers opportunities for some students, it is unlikely to work smoothly for large groups of students (Zhao, 2020).

Nevertheless, because of the nature of the Internet, the use of technology in education during the COVID-19 pandemic has also brought to light the difficulties that students with special education needs face, as online learning provides opportunities for some students while being unlikely to work smoothly for diverse groups of students (Zhao, 2020; Giannouli et al., 2021). Even before the pandemic, students with disabilities were at greater risk of being denied access to services, including appropriate education, when compared to their non-disabled peers (Bernard et al., 2020). This included appropriate education, even before the pandemic began (Gilmour et al., 2019). Most of the time, these students are at a disadvantage when there is a disaster or crisis, such as the pandemic of COVID-19 (Kuper et al., 2020).

In Germany, students, parents, and teachers took part in a national survey that revealed that, throughout the pandemic period, differentiated instruction was not used to include students with special education needs in online courses, according to the findings. Because of the uncertainty and difficulty of coping with the current situation, teachers have also reported increased levels of stress, nervousness, and anger (Letzel et al., 2020). When asked to identify barriers to the effectiveness of distance learning, special education teachers responded with a long list that included issues such as a lack of internet access, a lack of support staff for students with disabilities, and a lack of easily accessible digital materials, among other things. Some teachers claim that students with disabilities in their classrooms are not being adequately supported or trained, and this is a source of contention for some educators (McClain-Nhlapo et al., 2020; Giannouli et al.,2021).

According to Letzel et al. (2020), respondents' answers to questions about inclusive practices during homeschooling indicate that little differentiation was implemented to meet the needs of not only students with special educational needs but also all learners. This inherently leads to the conclusion, shared by both parents and teachers, that educational equality cannot be guaranteed in such a critical situation.

Modern research investigates the perceptions of students with and without special educational needs in a variety of educational contexts and levels, as it has been shown that their positive or negative attitudes have a significant impact on learning outcomes in a variety of educational settings. According to Stampoltzi et al. (2020), the perceptions and experiences of Greek students with learning difficulties or disabilities speak of a positive evaluation of distance learning, despite individual difficulties. Teachers can do a great deal to overcome barriers that may be caused by things such as perceptions, attitudes, experiences, knowledge, organizational issues, and so on, if they identify them early and link them to possible solutions and inclusive practices in the classroom or throughout the entire educational community for both students with and without disabilities, on this basis (Darrow, 2009).

Collaboration Between General and Special Education Teachers and E-Inclusion

Parmigiani et al. (2021) indicated that collaboration between regular and special education teachers regarding setting up inclusive online teaching/learning strategies and practices during the emergency due to COVID-19 was poor and limited, whereas high-level and effective collaboration enabled teachers to plan meaningful learning activities for their students.

As evidenced by the statements made by both classroom and special education teachers, the collaboration between the two groups was also critical for inclusion, particularly when the latter was teaching students with severe disabilities. As a result, collaborative efforts between regular and special education teachers have a significant impact on e-inclusion processes, particularly for students with severe disabilities. Researchers discovered that, in a completely online environment, a lack of relationships among teachers can result in the complete exclusion of students with special educational needs (Parmigiani et al., 2021).

One of the most difficult challenges for educators is the lack of physical coexistence of students and teachers in the same place, which reduces the quality of interaction and makes communication difficult (Orhan & Beyhan, 2020).

Even though the COVID-19 pandemic posed a threat to the Italian model of school inclusion, the consequences were not as severe as one might have anticipated. Human resources (a combination of classroom teachers and assistant educators), on which inclusion is based and in which it has been invested over the past decades, appear to have played an important role in ensuring students with disabilities right to an education and a fundamental connection to school (i.e., maintaining a daily relationship with assist educators) (Colombo & Santagati, 2021).

Parmigiani et al. (2021) demonstrate that teacher collaboration is particularly effective when teachers schedule recurrent online planning sessions to share the teaching strategies they intend to use and create individualized solutions for students. Weekly online meetings where teachers can share ideas and plan strategies with one another are essential if they are to improve their ability to work effectively together.

CONCLUSION AND FUTURE RESEARCH DIRECTIONS

A significant feature of e-inclusion in extreme situations such as the COVID-19 pandemic is the discovery of significant characteristics required to improve inclusion in both face-to-face as well as distance modalities, such as building stronger connections between those who are involved and establishing activities in which technologies can be used to support integration effectively (Parmigiani et al., 2021). Students' having computers, tablets, or mobile devices during the COVID-19 period does not ensure learning when learning materials are standardized for all, difficult to access, and fairly unappealing (Forteza-Forteza, et al., 2021). In addition to students with disabilities and language learners, state education agencies should continue to develop new guidance for a variety of vulnerable populations (Mississippi Department of Education, 2020).

Some national platforms' online materials and resources are inaccessible to students with disabilities or learning disabilities. For the most part, education providers have not received additional training to better serve students with disabilities. As a result, the vast majority of teachers are unqualified to provide inclusive education materials to distance learning students (Drakopoulou, 2020). In mainstream education, learners with disabilities are primarily supported through one-on-one parallel support with an instructor. Students enrolled in distance learning programs do not have access to this resource. Furthermore, students who need a lot of help may not be able to function independently enough to follow the teacher's instructions while participating in online learning activities. Finally, students with disabilities have experienced additional stress, anxiety about failing, and social isolation as a result of COVID-19, in addition to the disruption to their learning (Drakopoulou, 2020).

Parmigiani et al. (2021) stated that for functional electronic inclusion to occur, in addition to appropriate technological equipment, a satisfactory level of knowledge of computer handling, working with students' families and all teachers, and knowledge of online teaching strategies, the most important thing appeared to be the organization of activities that would focus on the special education needs of students with the contribution of modern and asynchronous tools.

Future research should focus on the application of new information and communication technologies to the educational environment and educational process in the modern rehabilitation process of inclusive education, which is critical. Another thing that needs to be studied is how teachers work together in digital classrooms so that all students can benefit from distance learning.

REFERENCES

Abidah, A., Hidaayatullaah, H. N., Simamora, R. M., Fehabutar, D., & Mutakinati, L. (2020). The Impact of Covid-19 on Indonesian Education and Its Relation to the Philosophy of "Merdeka Belajar". *Studies in Philosophy of Science and Education, 1*(1), 38–49. doi:10.46627ipose.v1i1.9

Aggelopoulou, D. (2011). Pedagogical utilization of new technologies and educational software for students with or without special educational needs. In E. Papanis, P. Giavrimis, & A. Vicky (Eds.), *Research and educational practice in special education* (pp. 187–214). Sideris.

Ainscow, M. (2005). Understanding the development of an inclusive education system. *Electronic Journal of Research in Educational Psychology, 3*(3), 5–20. https://www.redalyc.org/pdf/2931/293121928002.pdf

Altemueller, L, & Lindquist, C. (2017). Flipped classroom instruction for inclusive learning. *British Journal of Special Education, 44*(3), 341-358. doi:10.1111/1467-8578.12177

Anastasiadis, P. (2014). Research in e-learning in Greek Primary, Secondary and Higher Education: Review and perspectives. *Open Education - The Journal for Open and Distance Education and Educational Technology, 10*(1), 5-32. https://ejournals.epublishing.ekt.gr/index.php/openjournal/article/view/9809/9933

Arkorful, V., & Abaidoo, N. (2014). The Role of e-Learning, the Advantages and Disadvantages of Its Adoption in Higher Education. *International Journal of Education and Research, 2*(12), 397–410. https://www.ijern.com/journal/2014/December-2014/34.pdf

Beaton, L. J. (2007). *Stepping stones to success II. Collaboration: Working together for all students.* CTE Resource Center. Commonwealth of Virginia Department of Education.

Bernard, A., Weiss, S., Stein, J. D., Ulin, S. S., D'Souza, C., Salgat, A., Panzer, K., Riddering, A., Edwards, P., Meade, M., McKee, M. M., & Ehrlich, J. R. (2020). Assessing the impact of COVID-19 on persons with disabilities: Development of a novel survey. *International Journal of Public Health, 65*(6), 755–757. doi:10.100700038-020-01433-z PMID:32705300

Bianchi, A., Barrios, S., Cabrera, M., Cachia, R., Compañó, R., Malanowski, N., & Centeno, C. (2006). *Revisiting e-Inclusion: From vision to action.* Institute for Prospective Technological Studies, European Commission.

Bouillet, D. (2013). Some aspects of collaboration in inclusive education - Teachers' experiences. *CEPS Journal, 3*(2), 93–117. doi:10.26529/cepsj.241

Brownell, M. T., Adams, A., Sindelar, P., Waldron, N., & Vanhover, S. (2006). Learning from collaboration: The role of teacher qualities. *Exceptional Children, 72*(2), 169–185. doi:10.1177/001440290607200203

Camacho, A. C. L. F., Joaquim, F. L., de Menezes, H. F., & Sant'Anna, R. M. (2020). Tutoring in distance education in times of COVID-19: Relevant guidelines. *Research. Social Development, 9*(5), 1–12. doi:10.33448/rsd-v9i5.3151

Campigotto, R., McEwen, R., & Epp, C. D. (2013). Especially social: Exploring the use of an iOS application in special needs classrooms. *Computers & Education, 60*(1), 74–86. doi:10.1016/j.compedu.2012.08.002

Christinaki, E., Vidakis, N., & Triantafyllidis, G. (2013). Facial expression recognition teaching to preschoolers with autism: a natural user interface approach. In *BCI '13: Proceedings of the 6th Balkan Conference in Informatics* (pp. 141-148). Association for Computing Machinery. 10.1145/2490257.2490262

Colombo, M., & Santagati, M. (2021). The Inclusion of Students With Disabilities: Challenges for Italian Teachers During the Covid-19 Pandemic. *Social Inclusion (Lisboa), 10*(2). Advance online publication. doi:10.17645i.v10i2.5035

Cook, L., & Friend, M. (2004). *Co-Teaching: Principles, practices, and pragmatics.* New Mexico Public Education Department Quarterly Special Education Meeting.

Darrow, A.-A. (2009). Barriers to effective inclusion and strategies to overcome them. *General Music Today, 22*(3), 29–31. doi:10.1177/1048371309333145

Dimitriadis, S. N. (2015). *Learning Theories & Educational Software.* Kallipos.

Drakopoulou, E. (2020). *Inclusive Education and the Impact of COVID-19 on learners with disabilities.* Education Policy - European Disability Forum. https://www.edf-feph.org/content/uploads/2021/06/Inclusive-Education-and-COVID-19_Eleni-Drakopoulou.docx

eEurope Advisory Group. (2005). *eInclusion. New challenges and policy recommendations.* European Commission.

Fernández-López, Á., Rodríguez-Fórtiz, M. J., Rodríguez-Almendros, M. L., & Martínez-Segura, M. J. (2013). Mobile learning technology based on iOS devices to support students with special education needs. *Computers & Education, 61*(0), 77–90. https://dx.doi.org/10.1016/j.compedu.2012.09.014

Flipped Learning Network. (2014). *Definition of flipped learning.* https://flippedlearning.org/definitionof-flipped-learning

Forteza-Forteza, D., Rodríguez-Martín, A., Álvarez-Arregui, E., & Menéndez Álvarez-Hevia, D. (2021). Inclusion, Dyslexia, Emotional State and Learning: Perceptions of Ibero-American Children with Dyslexia and Their Parents during the COVID-19 Lockdown. *Sustainability, 13*(5), 2739. https://dx.doi.org/10.3390/su13052739

Forzani, E., & Leu, D. J. (2012). New Literacies for New Learners: The Need for Digital Technologies in Primary Classrooms. *The Educational Forum, 76*(4), 421–424. https://doi.org/10.1080/00131725.2012.708623

Gaggioli, C. (2018). Digital classroom and students with learning disorders: a study to improve learning processes and teaching practices. *Research on Education and Media, 10*(2) 26-35. doi:10.1515/rem-2018-0012

Georgiadi, M., Kourkoutas, E., & Kalyva, E. (2007). *Inclusion in Europe.* http://conf2007.edu.uoi.gr/Praktika/1236-1328.pdf

Giannouli, V., Sarris, D., & Papadopoulou, M. (2021). Distance education in the pandemic era: The views of Greek general and special education teachers of secondary education regarding readiness, challenges and the post-covid educational practices. *European Journal of Special Education Research, 7*(4). https://dx.doi.org/10.46827/ejse.v7i4.4050

Gilmour, A. F., Fuchs, D., & Wehby, J. H. (2019). Are Students With Disabilities Accessing the Curriculum? A Meta-Analysis of the Reading Achievement Gap Between Students With and Without Disabilities. *Exceptional Children, 85*. doi:10.1177/0014402918795830

Greenberg, G. (1998). Distance education technologies: Best practices for K-12 settings. *IEEE Technology and Society Magazine*, 3. *IEEE Technology and Society Magazine*, *17*(4), 36–40. https://doi.org/10.1109/44.7358626-40

Gros, B. (2007). Digital Games in Education: The Design of Games-Based Learning Environments. *Journal of Research on Technology in Education*, *40*(1), 23–38. https://files.eric.ed.gov/fulltext/EJ826060.pdf

Habgood, M. (2007). *The effective integration of digital games and learning content* (ID: 10385) [Doctoral dissertation, University of Nottingham]. Nottingham ePrints.

Hadi, M. Y. A., Mohamad, B., & Jaafar, M. S. A. (2010). Study of information and communication technology (ICT) usage in the technical and vocational special education programme. *Global Journal of Human Social Science Research, 10*(1), 35-43. https://globaljournals.org/GJHSS_Volume10/ghss_vol10_issue1_ver1_paper11.pdf

Hardiani, H. (2021). Collaboration practices between educators in inclusive education before and during Covid-19. In *Educational Innovation in Society 5.0 Era: Challenges and Opportunities.* doi:10.1201/9781003206019

Hasselbring, T. G., & Glaser, C. H. W. (2000). Use of computer technology to help students with special needs. The Future of Children. *Children and Computer Technology, 10*(2), 102–122. doi:10.2307/1602691

Henessy, S., Ruthven, K., & Brindley, S. (2005). Teacher perspectives on integrating ICT into subject teaching: Commitment, constraints, caution, and change. *Journal of Curriculum Studies*, *37*(2), 155–192. https://doi.org/10.1080/0022027032000276961

Hodges, C., Moore, S., Lockee, B., Trust, T., & Bond, A. (2020). *The Difference Between Emergency Remote Teaching and Online Learning.* https://er.educause.edu/articles/2020/3/the-difference-between-emergency-remote-teaching-andonline-learning

Holmberg, B. (2003). *Distance education in essence. An overview of theory and practice in the early twenty-first century*. BIS-Verlag, Carl von Ossietzky Universitat Oldenburg.

Judge, S. L. (2000). Computer applications in programs for young children with disabilities: Current status and future directions. *Journal of Special Education Technology*, *16*(1), 29–40. https://doi.org/10.1177/016264340101600103

Jurkowski, S., Ulrich, M., & Müller, B. (2020). Co-teaching as a resource for inclusive classes: teachers' perspectives on conditions for successful collaboration. *International Journal of Inclusive Education.* doi:10.1080/13603116.2020.1821449

Kalyva, E. (2005). *Autism: Educational and Therapeutic Approaches*. Publications Papazisi.

Keegan, D. (2001). *The basic principles of open and distance education.* Metaichmio.

Khokhar, B. (2007). Widening participation: How can new technologies best be used to enhance, learning and teaching and ensure educational inclusion and engagement for excluded groups? *Proceedings of the 12th forum on Open and Distance Learning*. http://www2.open.ac.uk/r06/conference/

Kirkpatrick, L., Searle, M., Smyth, R. E., & Specht, J. (2020). A coaching partnership: Resource teachers and classroom teachers teaching collaboratively in regular classrooms. *British Journal of Special Education*, *47*(1), 24–47. https://doi.org/10.1111/1467-8578.12296

Koumaki, E., & Haidi, E. (2015). Digital School: Digital learning for children with Special educational needs (EAA) of Special Primary School – Good Practices. *8th Panhellenic Conference of Teachers for ICT: Utilization of Information and Communication Technologies in Teaching Practice*, 1244-1258.

Kourbetis, B., Gelastopoulou, M., & Bombaridou, Ch. (2014). New perspectives in the field of special education: Design and development of accessible educational material for students with disabilities and/or special needs educational needs. In *4th Panhellenic Conference of Educational Sciences* (pp. 9-21). National Documentation Centre - ePublishing.

Kuper, H., Banks, L. M., Bright, T., Davey, C., & Shakespeare, T. (2020). Disability inclusive COVID-19 response: What it is, why it is important and what we can learn from the United Kingdom's response. *Wellcome Open Research*, *5*, 1–5. https://doi.org/10.12688/wellcomeopenres.15833.1

Law 3699. (2008). *Special Education and Training for People with Disabilities or Special Educational Needs*. Government Gazette 199.

Letzel, V., Pozas, M., & Schneider, C. (2020). Energetic Students, Stressed Parents, and Nervous Teachers: A Comprehensive Exploration of Inclusive Homeschooling During the COVID-19 Crisis. *Open Education Studies, 2*(1), 159–170. doi:10.1515/edu-2020-0122

Makrodimos, N., Papadakis, S., & Koutsoumba, M. (2017). Distance Education: a case study with the inverted class method for Mathematics of the 5th Primary school. *Open Education: the magazine for Open and Distance Education and Educational Technology, 13*(1), 26-37. doi:10.12681/jode.13975

Martin, F., Sun, T., & Westine, C. D. (2020). A systematic review of research on online teaching and learning from 2009 to 2018. *Computers & Education*, *159*, 104009. https://doi.org/10.1016/j.compedu.2020.104009

Masalela, R. K. (2008) *Inclusive education and the role of distance education*. http://www.ais.up.ac.za/digi/docs/masalela_paper.pdf

Mastrogiannis, A., & Anastopoulos, A. (2012). Dynamics, mathematics environments in Special Education. *6th Panhellenic Conference Hellenic Institute of Applied Pedagogy and Education with international participation and topic "Paideia kalliston Esti Ktima Vrotois: Humanitarian and Positive Sciences: Theory and Practice"*. http://www.elliepek.gr/documents/6o_synedrio_eisigiseis/57_mastrogiannis_anastopoulos.pdf

McClain-Nhlapo, C., Singh, R. K., Martin, A., Alasuutari, H., Baboo, N., Cameron, S., … Tucker, M. (2020). Pivoting to Inclusion: Leveraging Lessons from the COVID-19 Crisis for Learners with Disabilities. In Other Education Study. Washington, DC: World Bank Group.

Meijer, C., Soriano, V., & Watkins, A. (2003). *Special education in Europe*. European Special Education Agency. https://www.europeanagency.org/sites/default/files/special-needs-education-in europe_sne_europe_el.pdf

Miles, S., & Singal, N. (2009). The Education for All and Inclusive Education debate: Conflict, contradiction or opportunity? *International Journal of Inclusive Education*, *14*(1), 1–15. https://doi.org/10.1080/13603110802265125

Mississippi Department of Education. (2020). *Updates and Information in Response to COVID-19 (Coronavirus)*. https://www.mdek12.org/COVID19

Mitchell, D., & Sutherland, D. (2020). *What really works in special and inclusive education: Using evidence-based teaching strategies*. Routledge.

Moreillon, J. (2007). *Collaborative Strategies for Teaching Reading Comprehension: Maximizing Your Impact*. ALA Editions.

Mouchritsa, M., Kazanopoulos, S., Romero, A., & Garay, U. (2021). Collaboration between General and Special Education Teachers in Inclusive Classrooms: A Review of the Literature. *Journal of Education and Practice*, *12*(6). https://doi.org/10.7176/JEP/12-6-04

OECD. (2020a). *Supporting immigrant and refugee students amid the coronavirus pandemic*. https://oecdedutoday.com/immigrant-refugee-studentscoronavirus

OECD. (2020b). *How coronavirus is affecting students with special education needs*. https://oecdedutoday.com/coronavirus-students-special-education-needs/

OECD. (2020c). *Coronavirus school closures: What do they mean for student equity and inclusion?* https://oecdedutoday.com/coronavirus-school-closuresstudent-equity-inclusion/

OECD. (2020d). *OECD Policy Responses to COVID-19. Strengthening online learning when schools are closed: The role of families and teachers in supporting students during the COVID-19 crisis*. https://www.oecd.org/coronavirus/policy-responses/strengthening-online-learning-when-schoolsare-closed-the-role-of-families-and-teachers-in-supporting-students-during-the-covid-19-crisisc4ecba6c/

Orhan, G., & Beyhan, Ö. (2020). Teachers' Perceptions and Teaching Experiences on Distance Education Through Synchronous Video Conferencing During Covid-19 Pandemic. *Social Sciences and Education Research Review, 1*(7), 8–44. https://econpapers.repec.org/RePEc:edt:jsserr:v:7:y:2020:i:1:p:8-44

Paleodimou, A. (2017). Complementary distance school education. The case of e-twinning in kindergarten. In Minutes Proceedings of the 9th International Conference on Open and Distance Education (pp. 16–23). https://dx.doi.org/10.12681/icodl.1373

Panhellenic School Network. (2022a). *Electronic School Classroom. E-Class*. https://eclass.sch.gr

Panhellenic School Network. (2022b). *E-me Digital Education Platform. E-me*. https://e-me.edu.gr

Panhellenic School Network. (2022c). *WebEx Teleconference for Teachers*. https://webex.sch.gr/docs.php

Paraskevopoulos, M. (2005). *The contribution of Information Technologies and Communication in the Organization of the Integration Department and in Creation Personalized Programs.* http://www.etpe.eu/new/custom/pdf/etpe211.pdf

Parmigiani, D., Benigno, V., Giusto, M., Silvaggio, C., & Sperandio, S. (2021). E-inclusion: Online special education in Italy during the Covid-19 pandemic. *Technology, Pedagogy and Education*, *30*(1), 111–124. https://doi.org/10.1080/1475939X.2020.1856714

Pedagogical Institute. (2011). *Interdisciplinary Unified Curriculum Framework. The A.P.S. in Informatics*. Pedagogical Institute.

Petzold, A. M. (2020). Letter to the editor: Resources and recommendations for a quick transition to online instruction in physiology. *Advances in Physiology Education, 44*, 217-219. doi:10.1152/advan.00049.2020

Polychronopoulou-Zacharogeorga, S. (2003). *Children and adolescents with special needs and abilities* (Vol. 2). Atrapos.

Reich, J., Buttimer, C. J., Alison Fang, A., Hillaire, G., Hirsch, K., Larke, L., Littenberg-Tobias, J., Moussapour, R., Napier, A., Thompson, M., & Slama, R. (2020). *Remote Learning Guidance from State Education Agencies during the COVID-19 Pandemic: A First Look.* Massachusetts Institute of Technology - MIT Teaching Systems Lab. doi:10.35542/osf.io/437e2

Rice, M. F., & Dykman, B. (2018). The emerging research base for online learning and students with disabilities. In R. Ferdig & K. Kennedy (Eds.), *Handbook of research on K-12 online and blended learning* (pp. 189–206). ETC Press.

Scully, D., Lehane, P., & Scully, C. (2021). 'It is no longer scary': Digital learning before and during the Covid-19 pandemic in Irish secondary schools. *Technology, Pedagogy and Education*, *30*(1), 155–177. https://doi.org/https://doi.org/10.1080/1475939X.2020.1854844

Sophos, A., & Kron, F. (2010). *Effective Teaching Using Media. From primary and personal to quaternary and digital Media*. Grigoris.

Sourtzi, M., Ioakeimidou, V., Vlachos, N., Koutsospyrou, Ch., & Chatzimichailidis, V. (2013). A classroom for all. In A. Lionarakis (Ed.), Proceedings of the 7th International Conference on Open & Distance Learning: Learning Methodologies (pp. 161–169). https://doi.org/http://dx.doi.org/10.12681/icodl.649.

Stampoltzi, A., Giannoulas, A., & Kalamatianos, A. (2020). The experience of existence education of students with learning disabilities or disability during COVID-19 period: A pilot study. *Search in Education, 9*(1), 140-157. doi:10.12681/hjre.24497

Strogilos, V., Nikolaraizi, M., & Tragoulia, E. (2012). Experiences among beginning special education teachers in general education settings: The influence of school culture. *European Journal of Special Needs Education*, *27*(2), 185–199. https://doi.org/10.1080/08856257.2011.645588

Thomas, K. (2009). *"A social worker took the kids away". The power of games to help children learn.* http://archive. futurelab.org.uk/resources/publications-reports-articles/web-articles/Web-Article1507

Tsakiridou, H., & Polyzopoulou, K. (2014). Greek teachers' attitudes toward the inclusion of students with special educational needs. *American Journal of Educational Research*, *2*(4), 208–218. doi:10.12691/education-2-4-6

UNESCO. (2011). *ICTs in education for people with disabilities. Review of innovative practice.* https://unesdoc.unesco.org/ark:/48223/pf0000193655

UNESCO. (1994). *The Salamanca Statement and Framework for Action on Special Needs Education. Adopted by the World Conference on Special Needs Education: Access and Quality*. https://unesdoc.unesco.org/ark:/48223/pf0000098427

Universal Design and Development of Accessible Digital Educational Materials. (2022). *IEP*. http://www.prosvasimo.iep.edu.gr/el/

Valentine, D. (2002). Distance Learning: Promises, Problems, and Possibilities. *Online Journal of Distance Learning Administration*, *5*(3). https://www.westga.edu/~distance/ojdla/fall53/valentine53.html

Vislie, L. (2003). From integration to inclusion: Focusing global trends and changes in the western European societies. *European Journal of Special Needs Education*, *18*(1), 17–35. https://doi.org/10.1080/0885625082000042294

Whitton, N. (2010). *Learning with digital games: a practical guide to engaging students in higher education*. Routledge.

Wiggins, K. C., & Damore, Sh. J. (2006). "Survivors" or "Friends"? A Framework for Assessing Effective Collaboration. *Teaching Exceptional Children*, *38*(5), 49–56.

Williams, P. (2005). Using information and communication technology with special educational needs students: The views of frontline professionals. *Aslib Proceedings*, *57*(6), 539–553. https://doi.org/10.1108/00012530510634262

Williams, P., Jamali, R. H., & Nicholas, D. (2006). Using ICT with people with special education needs: What the literature tells us. *Aslib Proceedings*, *58*(4), 330–345. https://doi.org/10.1108/00012530610687704

Zhao, N., Zhou, X., Liu, B., & Liu, W. (2020). Guiding Teaching Strategies with the Education Platform during the COVID-19 Epidemic: Taking Guiyang No. 1 Middle School Teaching Practice as an Example. *Science Insights Education Frontiers, 5*(2), 531-539. doi:10.15354/sief.20.rp005

Zhao, Y. (2020). Tofu Is Not Cheese: Rethinking Education Amid the COVID-19 Pandemic. *ECNU Review of Education, 3*(2), 189–203. doi:10.1177/2096531120928082

Zioga, S. (2021). *Students' perceptions of distance education due to the Covid-19 pandemic* [Unpublished Master's thesis]. University of Ioannina.

Chapter 12

Inclusion of Students With Special Educational Needs and the COVID-19 Pandemic:

The Collaboration of School and Family in Distance Education Conditions

Spyridon Kazanopoulos
https://orcid.org/0000-0001-8076-7057
University of the Basque Country, Spain

Eneko Tejada
University of the Basque Country, Spain

Xabier Basogain
University of the Basque Country, Spain

Maria Mouchritsa
https://orcid.org/0000-0002-2021-7173
University of the Basque Country, Spain

ABSTRACT

With schools closed around the world during the pandemic, the use of technology and distance education has solved the problems and dysfunctions that have arisen. Students, their families, and school personnel have all been affected by the numerous challenges and barriers that have arisen because of distance education. This chapter seeks to evaluate school-family collaboration throughout the pandemic period. The study focuses on families with children who have special educational needs and disabilities (SEND) and their experiences with inclusive education. While the COVID-19 pandemic was underway, parents of children with SEND faced a variety of challenges, including a lack of resources, financial difficulties, communication difficulties, and a lack of attention from teachers. Parents believe that economic, social, and language limitations impede the effectiveness of online inclusion, whereas their digital abilities enable them to aid their children on both technical and psychological levels in overcoming distant learning difficulties.

DOI: 10.4018/978-1-6684-4735-2.ch012

INTRODUCTION

The COVID-19 pandemic has affected many parts of the world in areas directly related to human life, with education being the area that seems to be most affected after the health sector (Telli-Yamamoto & Altun, 2020). Many nations throughout the world have temporarily shuttered their schools or enforced local restrictions on schools and institutions due to the crisis. According to estimates from the United Nations Educational, Scientific, and Cultural Organization (UNESCO, 2020a), around 1.5 billion children and students have been affected by school closures, exacerbated educational inequality, and disproportionately impacted disadvantaged communities. Almost all education systems in the world were forced, in a very short time, to introduce technology as well as methods of e-government. It is noteworthy that the term referring to how quickly this learning process was implemented is "Emergency distance learning" is one (Hodges et al., 2020).

Among other things, the COVID-19 pandemic compelled the digital transformation of education. Changes that would have taken years to take place under other circumstances happened in a short period, preventing students and educators from making a smoother transition. It is a fact that the use of distance education methods has the potential to offer significant benefits, but it seems to have a controversial impact on those involved in educational activities. While the introduction of distance education strategies was impulsively reflected in the abrupt cessation of educational processes, these strategies were motivated by concerns about educational equality, inclusion, and the need to ensure that distance education content and implementation did not cause additional educational and social inequalities (Sfakiotaki, 2020). The use of technology in education has provided an immediate solution to the problems of day-to-day education that have arisen as a result of the pandemic. It has also raised barriers to the inclusion of students with Special Educational Needs (SEND), as online learning creates opportunities for some students but is not ideal for large groups of students (Zhao, 2020). As UNESCO (2020b) points out in the Global Education Monitoring Report Summary, "*In fact, the COVID-19 pandemic not only brought more inequalities to light but also contributed to deepening them, making our societies more fragile*" (p.7).

Technology was employed both at the level of school administration and in the instructional process, as well as for communication between school units and their respective parents. Schools were invited to adopt new but effective ways of communicating with all parents and students regularly, as the physical presence of both the teaching staff and the parents and students was not allowed on the school premises. Thus, school and family communication became primarily electronic because of the use of multiple means and practices made available by Information and Communication Technologies (ICT) (Kessopoulou & Tsimpidaki, 2021). Making the transition to online learning strengthened the notions of familial bonds and parental engagement in their children's education (Daub et al., 2021). The majority of educators agreed that effective communication and cooperation between teachers and parents are essential for maximizing students' learning outcomes. Instructors also showed that they were aware of cultural and language differences and the importance of being aware of different learning styles (Daub et al., 2021).

Recognizing that school and family systematic communication is an important parameter for successful collaboration between the two parts (Epstein, 2013; Solone et al., 2020; Kazanopoulos et al., 2021), the present chapter seeks to examine school-family collaboration during the pandemic period in secondary and primary education in Greece but also internationally. The study will focus on families with children with SEND and their experiences with inclusive schooling. The next section will provide a brief description of the concepts of distance learning, inclusive education, and collaboration between families and schools in the context of their integration into the conditions of Emergency Remote Teaching.

BACKGROUND

Distance Learning

Until around 2020, the phrase "Distance Learning" (DL) at school applied exclusively to a restricted sector of specialized sciences. However, in a short period, when disruptions to all levels of education were owing to the pandemic, a new landscape in education was established, with a different reality, which inevitably led to the use of DL. Over time, numerous definitions of DL have been proposed, with each researcher presenting their conceptual definition of the term. According to a study of the literature (Keegan, 2001; Moore, 1993; Sofos et al., 2015), distant education is a type of education defined by the following core characteristics:

- The presence of physical distance between the student and the instructor, almost permanently and throughout the educational process, distinguish it from traditional classroom education.
- The use of technical means—printed, audiovisual, or electronic—not only as carriers of educational content but also as a link between teacher and student.
- The ability for students to benefit from technology-supported dialogue through two-way communication, i.e., a method of using technology that is distinct from the lifelong learning process, as this technology is related to other functions.
- The absence, to a large extent, of the operation of the learning team and the use of individualized forms of teaching, which, however, do not exclude the possibility of group meetings, either face-to-face or with the use of technology.
- It is the central role of the educational organization in designing, organizing, preparing, and providing support to students that distinguish distance education from other self-teaching programs and purely personal study.
- It distinguishes it from personal study or self-teaching efforts because it assumes the existence of an educational organization that designs and implements educational materials and provides student support.

Asynchronous, Synchronous E-learning and Flipped Classroom

It is well established that the use of ICT technology tools is necessary to facilitate the process of DL. For this purpose, it is necessary to have a defined didactic and learning goal for ICT usage in education, as well as an educational design that incorporates instructional material, interactive activities, dynamic student participation, and freedom of speech. During the time of obligatory distance education in Greece and worldwide, the use of asynchronous or synchronous modes of communication predominated (Moore & Kearsley, 2012) in the educational process (asynchronous or synchronous e-learning). Simultaneously, when students gradually returned to classrooms, there was a discussion of a combined technique of the "flipped classroom" (Østerlie, 2016). According to Sofos et al. (2015), the choice of the teaching method should not be a mechanical process but should take into consideration a variety of elements, particularly the context of educational requirements and skills. The following is a brief overview of how Greece used online education both during and after the country was put on lockdown. The asynchronous and synchronous education platforms that were used in Greece will be covered. These platforms were used both during and after the mandatory distance education time.

Asynchronous E-learning

Asynchronous educational methods are those that are accessible after they have been implemented, allowing students to learn at their own pace (Collis, 1999). The asynchronous teaching method is chosen: a) when the trainees have to reflect or research a topic; b) when, due to space-time constraints, it is difficult to organize a modern meeting between all the trainees; c) when the trainees prefer or feel comfortable with self-learning; d) when the educational process is required to be segmented; e) when there are learners who have difficulty contributing to modern environments; f) when there is a need for educational material that can be referred to at any time by learners; g) when reading, listening, or attending the educational material at an individual pace is an advantage; and when the learning has to be done on demand (on-demand learning) (Sofos et al., 2015).

E- class

One of the most popular official asynchronous distance education services of the Greek Ministry of Education is the "Electronic School Classroom, E-class" (https://eclass.sch.gr) (Panhellenic School Network, 2022a), which is addressed to all teachers and students in primary and secondary education. It was part of the service ecosystem of the Panhellenic School Network from 2006 until today. It is worth mentioning that while in the school year 2014-2015 there were 6,265 available courses through e-Class in 1,365 schools across the country, in the school year 2021–2022 there was an increase of 1700% in the available online courses (11,555 courses) and an increase of 370% in the number of schools (6,454 schools across the country) that use the service systematically (Panhellenic School Network, 2022a). The E-class provides a unified digital environment that incorporates a range of learning, communication, assessment, and collaboration management tools. In addition, E-class can have electronic books, assignments, questionnaires, interactive exercises, discussions, wikis, multimedia, and communication tools. At the same time, live distance teaching and collaboration spaces can also be used.

E-me

The "E-me Digital Education Platform" (https://e-me.edu.gr) (Panhellenic School Network, 2022b) is a modern, social, and scalable digital platform that provides a complete, secure digital environment for learning, collaboration, communication, and networking for all members of the school community. At the same time, E-me has a modern and friendly environment that simulates the form of modern smart devices (tablets and mobile phones) and is at the same time secure, allowing only certified users (teachers and students) to use their Panhellenic School Network accounts. E-me provides a "space" for the following: the creation of collaborative learning environments (cells), the communication and social networking of students and teachers, the organization, storage, and exchange of files; the creation of digital educational material; and the interconnection and utilization of open resources while providing digital "tools" to support teaching and learning. The main structural feature of the platform is the "cells", which are areas of cooperation for groups of users. Each "cell" is associated with four user roles: a) the person in charge of the "cell" who has the role of administrator; b) the assistants of the "cell" with some management rights; c) the members of the "cell" and d) its followers, "cell". Each "cell" also has a wall, applications, and storage space.

Moodle

Moodle is a free, open-source software platform that has been created by a global community of users. The name is derived from the acronym: Modular Object-Oriented Dynamic Learning Environment (MOODLE), and its development began in Australia in 2002, intending to provide educators with an e-learning environment that places an emphasis on interaction and collaboration and is based on the constructivist learning model of learning. Additionally, it is fully compliant with all international e-learning standards, boasts a large number of active installations and users throughout the world, and has been translated into an extremely large number of languages, while its modular design allows for easy expansion through a large number of additional applications (plugins) and graphic design themes (Sofos et al., 2015).

Synchronous E-learning

Synchronous teaching involves the student interacting with the instructor in real-time. This method, according to Sofos et al. (2015), is chosen: a) when the trainer must observe if the trainee has acquired a skill; b) when information is shared that has value only at a specific time; c) when questions and problems must be answered immediately; d) when the "physical" presence of the instructor is required for the educational process to proceed; e) when the exchange of views and discussion between the parties involved is required in real-time; f) when there is a need to update educational material in real-time based on trainee feedback; h) when there is no time or material.

"Cisco Webex" (https://www.webex.com) (Panhellenic School Network, 2022c) is the application that educational institutions in Greece utilize to facilitate the delivery of synchronous courses in their various fields of study. It is important to note that Webex can be used on both a PC and a mobile or tablet device. Using Webex meetings is quite easy and functional. The interface is similar to that of other similar services, there are a variety of tools in a control panel from which one can choose: Start a meeting, schedule a meeting, or join a meeting. On the right-hand side, the scheduled meetings are displayed, as are recently viewed files. When scheduling a meeting, standard functions such as time, date, and duration of the meeting can be set, and the necessary people can be invited. Also, as with other services, the desired audio devices can be selected, with these settings being quite easy. On the other hand, meeting managers can record both audio and video of the meeting. Meeting participants can then download this recording or video via a link. In addition, participants can be muted. All participants can use a chat during the meeting, and hosts can share both their desktop and a specific application or files from their computer, including video files, with other people who participate in the call (Panhellenic School Network, 2022c).

Mixed Teaching Method-Flipped Classroom

A mixed type teaching method is a type of education that blends lifelong learning with the convenience of online education. In particular, there is interest in the "flipped classroom" technique (Flipped Learning Network, 2014), which is an educational method that moves lesson delivery out of the classroom (where lessons are typically monologued), allowing more time in the classroom to be devoted to interactive activities in which students are actively involved with the teaching content (Flipped Learning Network, 2014). Learners are provided some personal assistance before being given the option to study remotely the available online training materials or work independently on a project assigned to them. This educational method is implemented when direct instruction moves from the group learning space to the individual learning space. Thus, the resulting group space is transformed into a dynamic, interactive learning environment where the educator guides students as they apply concepts and engage creatively with the subject matter (Østerlie, 2016).

Using a flipped classroom technique, the practice of teaching via classroom lectures is reversed, and the practice of studying and deepening activities in the student's teaching material is conducted at home, rather than in the classroom. To supplement the classroom experience, rather than sitting in on the lesson and completing homework, the student watches the lesson from home through digital media (primarily video) while also conducting exploratory and constructive learning activities in collaboration with the teacher and his classmates during class time. One of the key findings of several studies (Nouri, 2016; Lai & Hwang, 2016; Fidalgo-Blanco et al., 2017) on the adoption of the inverted classroom model is that students' engagement in the learning process rises, regardless of whether they are high-achieving or low-performing students enrolled. Furthermore, through their active engagement, the students establish communication and teamwork skills, as a consequence of which their creativity evolves, as well as a sense of mutual support and acceptance of others. When students know what they'll learn before they start, they become more motivated to study and their performance improves, too (Gomez-Lanier, 2018).

When it comes to teaching children with SEND, one significant benefit of flipping is that these pupils get the greatest support. This is because this strategy allows the educator to spend more time working one-on-one or in small groups with children who have learning issues, which is an effective way to satisfy their needs. Inverted classrooms improve the number of time students spend interacting with instructors and other students, which benefits students with learning disabilities who need more time to engage with their instructor to learn. This alteration to the traditional sequence will allow for more diversity within the class as a result of this shift (Altemueller & Lindquist, 2017).

At the end of this section, it should be highlighted that the overall planning framework should put focus on interaction, collaboration, and complementarity between synchronous and asynchronous methods of education. Additionally, current methods of education, such as distant learning, teleconferencing, and other similar approaches, should not be seen as a transfer of knowledge from the physical classroom to a digital one in any manner. All these practices should not serve the purpose of teaching, as is the case in traditional education, but rather serve the purpose of communication, interaction, support, and participation (Alasona, 2021).

Inclusive Education and Students with SEND.

At the educational level, "inclusion" describes the procedures adopted to support students with SEND to be incorporated into the school curriculum (Ainscow, 2005; Angelides et al., 2009; Carter & Kennedy, 2006). It is a global educational policy that is part of the effort to restore "*social justice*" within the school environment, with the ultimate goal of evaluating each student as a "single contributor" (Carlson et al., 2012; DePauw & Doll-Tepper, 2000). The goal of the inclusion process is to achieve the greatest possible interaction between students, which will help with the educational process and develop their personalities and abilities. A key prerequisite for achieving the above-mentioned goal is to create appropriate conditions in the school environment that will allow adaptations to educational tools and programs to meet the needs of all students (Booth et al., 2006). If a student faces difficulties that hinder his learning process, then, it is considered preferable to identify the problem in the context of learning strategies applied in general and in the operation of the school rather than the student himself (Sharma et al., 2012).

The advantages of adopting inclusion programs are many, as they enhance teaching techniques (enriching them) while broadening student horizons (perceptions, attitudes, preconceptions) in tolerating diversity and increasing social awareness (Mortier et al., 2010; Spencer-Cavaliere & Watkinson, 2010). Through this process, students with disabilities gain a more positive image of themselves and are motivated by their peers, while the school itself acquires the humanitarian character it ought to have (Polychronopoulou, 2003; Vogler et al., 2000). The ultimate goal of "inclusive education" is the creation of a single school and joint teaching, at all levels of education for students with and without SEND (Johnston et al., 2003; Leiter, 2007). As a result, it is critical to provide the essential framework that removes or at least reduces any barriers to learning and engagement while also eliminating any social exclusion (Nutbrown et al., 2007). It is an inalienable right of every student to be an active member of the school he attends, to be a member of the community, and to do so without restrictions in an educational system that must serve his individual needs (Polychronopoulou, 2003).

Inclusion is achieved in three specific ways: The first is its integrated form, which includes students with and without a disability in the mainstream classroom, who receive direct support from the general teacher (Neely-Barnes et al., 2010). The second involves the simultaneous presence of two pedagogues in the classroom, special and general, and the third refers to part-time education, during which the pupil attends the general classroom, as well as courses in inclusion or reinforcement teaching (Polychronopoulou, 2003). Perhaps the greatest benefit of this process is the right of all students to individualized teaching, while the implementation of corresponding co-education programs enhances the quality of education provided, through co-teaching, cooperation, and acceptance of each other, while at the same time improving relationships between school community members (Anderson et al., 2007).

Successful student inclusion necessitates adherence to specific rules regarding the assessment of each student to determine whether or not they can participate (Breitenbach et al., 2013), appropriate strategies for program implementation, and a high level of commitment from participants (Fox et al., 2004; Hart & Whalon, 2011; Oliver & Barnes, 2010). Furthermore, an important factor for success is the attitude of teachers, who can influence all members of the school community and have the ultimate responsibility for including students with disabilities (Avramidis & Norwich, 2002). So, the decision to use these programs should be made together by everyone in the educational and school community. The advantages of adopting inclusion programs are many, as they enhance teaching techniques (enriching them) while broadening student horizons (perceptions, attitudes, preconceptions) in tolerating diversity and increasing social awareness (Mortier et al., 2010; Spencer-Cavaliere & Watkinson, 2010). Through this process, students with disabilities gain a more positive image of themselves and are motivated by their peers, while the school itself acquires the humanitarian character it ought to have (Polychronopoulou, 2003; Vogler et al., 2000).

Inclusive Education in Greece

Based on current Greek legislation, inclusive education is widely implemented in Greece through a variety of models. The most prominent model of providing educational services for children with disabilities, though, is a typical model of co-teaching, which in Greece is called *Parallel Support* (PS). According to Greek Law (Law for Special Education and Training of Students with Disabilities or Special Educational Needs, 2008), children with special educational needs and/or disabilities (SEND) have the right to attend general school by receiving support services from special education teachers, which are related to the type and severity of the child's diagnosis. In other words, it is the coexistence and co-teaching of all children, regardless of individuality and educational needs (Liodakis, 2000). To provide PS to a student, he or she must have a report from Greece's official diagnostic center, "Educational and Counseling Center" (KESY), which is responsible for diagnosing and integrating students with disabilities into special education structures, as well as assisting teachers in resolving problems. Parents' requests for PS are submitted to the headmaster of the school, who then sends them to the Ministry of Education.

Students with SEND can attend mainstream school classes with PS by special education teachers, depending on the type and degree of disability. Parallel support is provided to those who can attend the classroom program if they have individual support and to students with severe educational needs when there is no special school or integration department in their area of study. High-functioning autistic students can attend general school supported by their classroom teacher and with support from a special education teacher. PS for these students is terminated only after the opinion of the KESY and the consent of the parents. The goal of the program is for the student to become more and more independent so that the teacher doesn't have to stay for the whole class time (Law for Special Education and Training of Students with Disabilities or Special Educational Needs, 2008).

Teacher-parent Collaboration in the Context of Inclusion

It is undeniably true that the family plays a critical role in a child's spiritual, emotional, and social development. The child's growth and psychosocial adjustment begin in the family and are impacted by the family's cohesiveness and parental conduct. Other support variables, most notably the school, are incorporated afterward (Babalis & Xanthakou, 2008).

Furthermore, the family's characteristics - socioeconomic status, cultural level, and dynamics-influence not only the child's psychology and self-image formation but also the formation of the pedagogical relationship, as the child's perceptions of his family environment influence and often determine his behavior in the school environment (Mylonakou-Keke, 2009). A school that strives for the greatest possible psychosocial adjustment of the student both at home and at school, for example, might encourage dialogue and collaboration with parents. In addition, Epstein (1995) describes six different types of parental involvement in the education process: a) parental activities aimed at creating a positive learning environment at home, b) parent-teacher communication about the school curriculum and children's progress, c) parental involvement in school activities and voluntary contributions to the school, d) involvement of parents in preparing children for school and learning at home in general, e) involvement of parents in decision-making boards and school administration, and f) involvement of parents in seeking access to social services aimed at improving learning opportunities.

Working together with families of children who have impairments or special educational needs is critical to the child's growth and development, as well as the success of school-based practices. Parental involvement in the lives of these children is quite vital, and their collaboration with the school and with everyone involved in the educational process is critical to the success of inclusive educational programs. Research has shown that most teachers and parents want to communicate and work together (Sheridan & Kratochwill, 2008). However, the process of parity and collaboration between schools and parents or caregivers is frequently difficult (Syriopoulou-Delli et al., 2016). Several studies on the relationship between parents of children with SEND and professionals (Angell et al., 2008; Haines et al., 2013; Staples & Dilberto, 2010) have found that teachers frequently do not understand the system and family experiences of children's abilities and needs, making it difficult to apply collaborative principles. Furthermore, collaboration in special education processes is challenging due to the multiple stakeholders typically involved, the wide variety of needs and cultural backgrounds represented by students with disabilities and their families, and the lack of adequate preparation for collaborative skills (Syriopoulou-Delli et al., 2016).

Because their opinions are not heard, many parents feel unwanted and uncomfortable engaging in their children's education. They may also regard themselves as passive beneficiaries of professional choices (Solone et al., 2020). Numerous studies show that parents are poorly prepared to respond to special education jargon because they do not fully understand the terms or issues discussed in meetings with professionals (Francis et al., 2016; Friend & Cook, 2016), and they are unprepared to meet their children's educational needs (Friend & Cook, 2016). The lack of adequate information and skills from professionals and educators on how to set the scene for healthy family involvement seems to be another major element that appears to be impeding the achievement of effective collaborations. Finally, a significant barrier to effective parent-teacher communication is a lack of time, which especially affects working parents who find it difficult to find the right time to be active in their children's education(Kazanopoulos et al., 2021).

MAIN FOCUS OF THE CHAPTER

Distance Learning: ICT Technologies and Students with SEND

While ICT may be a beneficial tool for learners with SEND, it is critical to assess individual needs and adjust technology appropriately on a student-by-student basis, since assistive technology solutions must be tailored to the learner's unique circumstances (Abed, 2018). Students with SEND have the opportunity to learn about topics in several ways via the use of information and communication technology (ICT), which helps them build social skills and increase communication and collaboration with their classmates and teachers. The appropriate use of ICT, on the other hand, assists these pupils in becoming more self-sufficient, and it also has a significant influence on their cognitive, emotional, and communication abilities (Aggelopoulou, 2011). If ICT is to be successfully integrated into education (Nam et al., 2013), the student must be viewed as an active participant in the development and comprehension of knowledge.

It should be noted that even before the era of pandemic and mandatory DL, synchronous e-learning platforms such as Cisco Webex were being used in attention-deficit/hyperactivity disorder (ADHD) adolescent support programs (Sibley et al., 2017), as well as in support programs for parents of children with autism to help them improve their behavioral skills (Sibley et al., 2017; Subramaniam et al., 2016). In addition, the same platform is used for both video conferencing services and distance psychoeducational support services because of how many groups can join in, how easy it is to integrate presentation content into the platform, and how easy it is for people who want to use it to get around.

Educational technology has progressed, but it has also posed challenges for students with disabilities, since online learning may benefit certain students, but it is unlikely to benefit vast numbers of children (Zhao, 2020). Even before the pandemic, students with SEND had an increased risk of being denied access to resources, including suitable schooling for their non-disabled classmates. In times of emergencies and crises, such as the current pandemic, these children are at a disadvantage (Kuper et al., 2020). In a nationwide survey in Germany (Letzel et al., 2020), including students, parents, and teachers, it was revealed that during online courses throughout the pandemic period, differentiated instruction was not utilized to include students with specific educational needs, with teachers also indicating heightened stress, anxiety, and anger over the unpredictability and difficulties of the current situation. Among other things, a lack of internet access, a lack of staff to assist students with disabilities, and a lack of digitally accessible materials were found to be the main obstacles to the effectiveness of DL, while only 21% of teachers believe that they have the appropriate support training to meet the needs of students with disabilities (Letzel et al., 2020).

Distance Learning and Teacher-parent Collaboration

Distance Learning courses challenged the conventional notion of learning taking place in a physical area (such as a school), and the home became the new learning environment (León-Nabal et al., 2021). During the COVID-19 pandemic, interactions between students and their families were more crucial. The involvement of families is essential for the efficiency of online inclusive initiatives. Therefore, inclusion strategies are difficult to adopt if families do not cooperate(Parmigiani et al., 2021). When schools were closed and the DL was a part of their everyday educating and learning process, parents were called upon to help, in many circumstances, their children. As a sign of support for this process, UNESCO released instructions that took into account the activities of parents in individual processes and the prospective engagement of their children (Huang et al., 2020). Parents' educational level and the amount of time they devote to their children's schooling have a substantial impact on their children's ability to learn (Heineck & Anger, 2010). In a study by Bonal and González (2021) in more than 30,000 families in the region of Catalonia in Spain, it was observed that parents who had a university education helped their children more than those who had only a basic education. Nevertheless, it was highlighted that the parents' socioeconomic status influenced the family and extracurricular activities, which had a significant positive effect on academic achievement.

To carry out the DL process while also dealing with the psychological effects of staying at home due to COVID-19, parents, and schools communicate with each other continuously. The educational organization was faced with a new situation that had been formed without prior knowledge or strategy. The administration of each school was called upon to implement distance education and enforce the law. In this context, it was necessary to inform parents and students, record the lack of digital media in the student population, and ensure the supply of students with the appropriate tools where necessary, to resolve questions, identify their stakeholder groups, and guide the implementation of measures (Kessopoulou & Tsimpidaki, 2021). Before the pandemic, the connection between families and schools was mediated by the regulated use of written messages and appointments to settle problems or address inadequacies, respectively. This connection has evolved in response to the new scenario, as the use of mobile applications and devices for parenting discussions and information has led the child to act as an active protagonist (León-Nabal et al., 2021).

Parents' digital abilities assisted them in supporting their children on both a technical and psychological level to face the challenges of the DL, but they also acted as advocates for their children's well-being (Drakopoulou, 2020). Surveys that studied parental worries regarding the long-term impact of distance education on their children's academic performance (e.g. learning gaps, poor performance, test failure) captured a high degree of concern (Adnan & Anwar, 2020; Vuorikari et al., 2020). In terms of pre-school education, pre-pandemic research has shown that effective communication between pre-school teachers and parents is essential for ensuring a long-term commitment to pre-school education (Yildirim, 2021). In the research by Adnan and Anwar (2020), during the COVID-19 pandemic, the majority of parents said that they solely participated in activities assigned by their children's instructors, while some stated that they participated in activities assigned by their children as well as additional support activities. Pre-school instructors use the telephone and social networking apps (WhatsApp, video calling, Facebook, and Instagram) to communicate with parents and students. A lot of parents believed that the COVID-19 pandemic had resulted in more parental dedication and enhanced student-parent relationships, while also believing that children learn more effectively at home when there is open communication between the educator and the parents. Parents generally think that the COVID-19 outbreak has had negative consequences on their children's socialization, primary school preparedness, emotional development, the interaction between teachers and students, face-to-face education, and academic success. Lack of resources, financial difficulties (situation), poor self-esteem, communication difficulties, housekeeping (personal), and attention are only a few of the difficulties that parents face while providing pre-school education during the pandemic (Adnan & Anwar, 2020).

Collaboration of Teacher and Parent of Children with SEND in Distance Education Conditions

In the field of special education, collaboration and communication between school and family are regarded as crucial for the development of the child, and it has various advantages for all stakeholders: family, school, and educators/specialists. During the COVID-19 pandemic, interactions between students and their families were more crucial since the involvement of families is essential for the efficiency of online inclusive initiatives. Therefore, inclusion strategies are difficult to adopt if families do not cooperate (Parmigiani et al., 2021). According to the findings of Asbury et al., (2021), parents of children with SEND believe that it is critical to maintain communication with the school and teachers throughout the family, not only to maintain contact and routine with the child during his or her forced stay at home but also to ensure the child's smooth reintegration into the school context.

Furthermore, according to Parmigiani et al. (2021), interactions between school professionals and families are crucial to the effective integration of children with SEND in DL contexts. It is difficult to create an effective inclusion environment when families do not display a desire to work with teachers (partly owing to the parents' incapacity to organize their children's activities). In the absence of family cooperation, some students are completely excluded from online activities, mostly the younger students and those with severe impairments who are unable to handle the activities on their own. Moreover, the economic, social, and linguistic barriers hinder the efficacy of online inclusion because all these factors are related to technology limits (lack of devices and/or connectivity) (Parmigiani et al., 2021).

According to the findings of Letzel et al. (2020), parents have stated that the technological tools that their children have at home are sufficient for them to carry out homeschooling activities successfully. It was noted, however, that the existing homeschooling environment does not ensure that all pupils have equal access to educational opportunities. In addition, parents declare that teachers aren't meeting the needs of kids with special needs in the classroom.

Another research (Colizzi et al., 2020) found that during the COVID-19 pandemic, the educational community actively assisted the families of children with disabilities. In these tough and unexpected conditions, direct (video chats, telephone conversations) and indirect (messages) connections between the school and the family seemed to be beneficial for the vast majority of families that participated. On the contrary, it has been shown that a lack of communication with the school environment is connected with the onset of behavioral issues in children with SEND (Colizzi et al., 2020).

The COVID-19 pandemic is having an additional and unprecedented impact on families as a result of the application of social distance and isolation measures as a result of the pandemic's outbreak. In particular, this is of concern to family caregivers since families that have a relative who has Intellectual and Developmental Disabilities (IDD) are likely to have numerous additional responsibilities. Initial accounts from healthcare services and families concerning the pandemic's impact have been mixed. As a result of social isolation, some therapists are reporting less problematic behavior in people with IDD, which may be due to lowered expectations and a quieter lifestyle on the part of the individuals. In addition, some families are finding that living a simpler lifestyle with more opportunities for good engagement with their children can be beneficial to them (Rose et al., 2020).

In contrast, a large-scale survey of 6720 parents from seven European countries on the effects of the pandemic on their children's education revealed that most parents of children with SEND reported receiving no or insufficient support during homeschooling. Parents of children with mental health conditions reported significantly more negative experiences with homeschooling (Majoko & Dudu, 2020). According to most parents who responded to the study, additional aid for homeschooling was either non-existent or inadequate for 63 percent of children who had mental health issues. As a result, these children are at risk of slipping even farther behind their peers in terms of academic performance, which has a higher potential for progressing to depression (Powell et al., 2020).

According to Carrión-Martnez et al. (2021), homeschooling was considered a feasible alternative to traditional teaching by many parents of SEND children, who noted that relationships with specialists remained positive throughout the lockdown and that students showed considerable gains in both knowledge and behavior. In addition, because of communication barriers among teachers, many parents sought assistance from other families who were in a similar situation. It is worth noting that in the case of children with Autism Spectrum Disorder (ASD), any kind of assistance from the community, but particularly from families, is vital for their homeschooling since families with similar experiences often help peer families of children with ASD (Majoko & Dudu, 2020).

CONCLUSION AND FUTURE RESEARCH DIRECTIONS

COVID-19 pandemic, which was a significant health crisis, resulted in several changes in schools while also underlining the need for ICT in all aspects of the educational process during the mandatory DL period. ICT was crucial in facilitating contact between the school and the family during this time frame since the physical presence of teaching personnel, parents, and children were prohibited on the school compound. However, as the review of the literature indicates, in educational reality, technology seems to have created barriers for impaired students throughout the pandemic period. While online education may assist certain children, it is ultimately more difficult to benefit a significant number of young people, and children with SEND face a greater risk of resource denial.

According to the findings of the study, interactions between students and their families were particularly important during the COVID-19 outbreak. Distance learning methods have shattered the conventional knowledge of in-person learning, while parents' educational level and time commitment to their children's education have been critical to the educational process's efficacy under these crucial circumstances. The findings revealed that interactions between students and their families were especially critical during the pandemic. Distance learning approaches have shattered the form of knowledge about in-person learning, while the educational level and time commitment of parents to their children's education have proven vital to the educational process's success in these critical situations.

Further study on best practices in school-family engagement during times of school malfunction and crises, whether caused by natural disasters or pandemics, or other potential emergencies, will be possible as a result of this review. Furthermore, it is considered critical to perform large-scale quantitative and qualitative research on a Pan-Hellenic scale in order to effectively represent the general nature of collaboration in this era, as well as the significance of ICT infrastructure. Future studies may also approach the problem from the perspective of parents and students, to get an understanding of their views on how collaboration with the school should be handled in the case of an outbreak. This would allow for a more comprehensive examination of the issue.

REFERENCES

Abed, M. G. (2018). Teachers' Perspectives Surrounding ICT Use amongst SEN Students in the Mainstream Educational Setting. *World Journal of Education*, *8*(1), 6. doi:10.5430/wje.v8n1p6

Adnan, M., & Anwar, K. (2020). *Online learning amid the COVID-19 pandemic : Students ' perspectives*. Academic Press.

Aggelopoulou, D. (2011). Pedagogical utilization of new technologies and educational software for students with/ or without special educational needs. In E. Papanis, P. Giavrimis, & A. Viky (Eds.), *Research and Educational Practice in Special Education* (pp. 187–215). Sideris.

Ainscow, M. (2005). Developing inclusive education systems: What are the levers for change? *Journal of Educational Change*, *6*(2), 109–124. doi:10.100710833-005-1298-4

Alasona, N. (2021). *ICT and remote methods in border areas: the case of children with learning disabilities* (No. 50070) [Doctoral dissertation, National Kapodistrian University of Athens]. National Archive of Doctoral Dissertations.

Altemueller, L., & Lindquist, C. (2017). Flipped classroom instruction for inclusive learning. *British Journal of Special Education*, *44*(3), 341–358. doi:10.1111/1467-8578.12177

Anderson, C., Klassen, R., & Georgiou, G. (2007). What teachers say they need and what school psychologists can offer. *School Psychology International*, *28*(2), 131–147. doi:10.1177/0143034307078086

Angelides, P., Constantinou, C., & Leigh, J. (2009). The role of paraprofessionals in developing inclusive education in Cyprus. *European Journal of Special Needs Education*, *24*(1), 75–89. doi:10.1080/08856250802596741

Angell, M. E., Stoner, J. B., & Shelden, D. L. (2008). Trust in Education Professionals: Perspectives of Mothers of Children With Disabilities. *Remedial and Special Education*, *30*(3), 160–176. doi:10.1177/0741932508315648

Asbury, K., Fox, L., Deniz, E., Code, A., & Toseeb, U. (2021). How is COVID-19 Affecting the Mental Health of Children with Special Educational Needs and Disabilities and Their Families? *Journal of Autism and Developmental Disorders*, *51*(5), 1772–1780. doi:10.100710803-020-04577-2 PMID:32737668

Avramidis, E., & Norwich, B. (2002). Teachers' attitudes towards integration/inclusion: A review of the literature. *European Journal of Special Needs Education*, *17*(2), 129–147. doi:10.1080/08856250210129056

Babalis, T., & Xanthakou, G. (2008). School class and socialization of the student. *Education Sciences*, (3), 55–64.

Bonal, X., & González, S. (2021). Educación formal e informal en confinamiento: Una creciente desigualdad de oportunidades de aprendizaje. *Research in Sociology of Education*, *14*(1), 44–62. doi:10.7203/RASE.14.1.18177

Booth, T., Ainscow, M., & Kingston, D. (2006). *Index for inclusion: Developing play, learning, and participation in early years and childcare*. Centre for Studies on Inclusive Education.

Breitenbach, M. M., Armstrong, V. L., & Bryson, S. E. (2013). The implementation of best education practices for a student severely affected by autism. *International Journal of Inclusive Education*, *17*(3), 277–294. doi:10.1080/13603116.2012.676087

Carlson, L., Hemmings, B., Wurf, G., & Reupert, A. (2012). The instructional strategies and attitudes of effective inclusive teachers. *Special Education Perspectives*, *21*(1), 7–20.

Carrión-Martínez, J. J., Pinel-Martínez, C., Pérez-Esteban, M. D., & Román-Sánchez, I. M. (2021). Family and school relationship during COVID-19 pandemic: A systematic review. *International Journal of Environmental Research and Public Health*, *18*(21), 11710. Advance online publication. doi:10.3390/ijerph182111710 PMID:34770223

Carter, E. W., & Kennedy, C. H. (2006). Promoting Access to the General Curriculum Using Peer Support Strategies. *Research and Practice for Persons with Severe Disabilities*, *31*(4), 284–292. doi:10.1177/154079690603100402

Colizzi, M., Sironi, E., Antonini, F., Ciceri, M. L., Bovo, C., & Zoccante, L. (2020). Psychosocial and behavioral impact of COVID-19 in autism spectrum disorder: An online parent survey. *Brain Sciences*, *10*(6), 341. Advance online publication. doi:10.3390/brainsci10060341 PMID:32503172

Collis, B. (1999). *Tele-Learning in a Digital World - The Future of Distance Learning*. International Thompson Computer Press.

Daub, A. C., Villanueva, S., Soares, M. C., & Huber, T. (2021). Educators ' Experiences With Teaching During COVID-19 : Journey of a Participatory Action Research Inquiry Team Educators ' Experiences With Teaching During COVID-19 : Journey of a Participatory Action Research Inquiry Team. *Journal of Multicultural Affairs*, *6*(2).

DePauw, K. P., & Doll-Tepper, G. (2000). Toward progressive inclusion and acceptance: Myth or Reality? The inclusion debate and bandwagon discourse. *Adapted Physical Activity Quarterly; APAQ*, *17*(2), 135–143. doi:10.1123/apaq.17.2.135

Drakopoulou, E. (2020). *Inclusive Education and the Impact of COVID-19 on learners with disabilities*. https://www.edf-feph.org/education-policy/

Epstein, J. (1995). School- family- community partnerships: Caring for the children we share. *Phi Delta Kappan*, *76*(9), 701–712.

Fidalgo-Blanco, A., Martinez-Nuñez, M., Borrás-Gene, O., & Sanchez-Medina, J. J. (2017). Micro flip teaching – An innovative model to promote the active involvement of students. *Computers in Human Behavior*, *72*, 713–723. doi:10.1016/j.chb.2016.07.060

Flipped Learning Network. (2014). *Definition of Flipped Learning.* Retrieved from Retrieved March 10, 2022, from https://flippedlearning.org/definition-of-flipped-learning/

Fox, S., Farrell, P., & Davis, P. (2004). Factors associated with the effective inclusion of primary-aged pupils with Down's syndrome. *British Journal of Special Education*, *31*(4), 184–190. doi:10.1111/j.0952-3383.2004.00353.x

Francis, G. L., Blue-banning, M., Turnbull, A. P., & Haines, S. (2016). Culture in Inclusive Schools: Parental Perspectives on Trusting Family-Professional Partnerships. *Education and Training in Autism and Developmental Disabilities*, *51*(3), 281–293.

Friend, M., & Cook, L. (2016). *Interactions: Collaboration skills for school professionals* (7th ed.). Pearson.

Gomez-Lanier, L. (2018). Building collaboration in the flipped classroom: A case study. *International Journal for the Scholarship of Teaching and Learning*, *12*(2), 1–9. doi:10.20429/ijsotl.2018.120207

Haines, S. J., McCart, A., & Turnbull, A. P. (2013). Family engagement within early childhood response to intervention. In V. Buysse & E. Peisner-Feinberg (Eds.), *Handbook on response to intervention (RTI) in early childhood* (pp. 313–324). Brookes.

Hart, J. E., & Whalon, K. J. (2011). Creating Social Opportunities for Students With Autism Spectrum Disorder in Inclusive Settings. *Criminal Justice and Behavior*, *46*(5), 1071–1092. doi:10.1177/0093854818771721

Heineck, G., & Anger, S. (2010). The returns to cognitive abilities and personality traits in Germany. *Labour Economics*, *17*(3), 535–546. doi:10.1016/j.labeco.2009.06.001

Hodges, C. B., Moore, S. L., Lockee, B. B., Trust, T., & Bond, M. A. (2020). The Difference Between Emergency Remote Teaching and Online Learning. *Educational Review*.

Huang, R., Tlili, A., Chang, T.-W., Zhang, X., Nascimbeni, F., & Burgos, D. (2020). Disrupted classes, undisrupted learning during COVID-19 outbreak in China: Application of open educational practices and resources. *Smart Learning Environments*, *7*(1), 19. doi:10.118640561-020-00125-8

Johnston, S. S., McDonnell, A. P., Nelson, C., & Magnavito, A. (2003). Teaching Functional Communication Skills Using Augmentative and Alternative Communication in Inclusive Settings. *Journal of Early Intervention*, *25*(4), 263–280. doi:10.1177/105381510302500403

Kazanopoulos, S., Mouchritsa, M., Tejada, E., & Basogain, O. (2021). Collaboration between In-Service School Teachers and Families in the Context of Inclusive Education : A Review of the Recent Literature. *Journal of Education and Practice*, *12*(6), 47–53. doi:10.7176/JEP/12-6-05

Keegan, D. (Ed.). (1993). *Theoretical Principles of Distance Education* (1st ed.). Routledge.

Kessopoulou, M., & Tsimpidaki, A. (2021). Electronic communication between school and family during the COVID-19 pandemic. *Research in Education*, 137–160.

KuperH.Morgon BanksL.BrightT.DaveyC.ShakespeareT.DickinsonH.WalesS. (2020). *Disability-inclusive COVID-19 response: What it is, why it is important, and what we can learn from the United Kingdom's response*. doi:10.12688/wellcomeopenres.15833.1

Lai, C.-L., & Hwang, G.-J. (2016). A self-regulated flipped-classroom approach to improving students' learning performance in a mathematics course. *Computers & Education, 100*, 126–140. doi:10.1016/j.compedu.2016.05.006

Law: Special Education and Training of Students with Disabilities or Special Educational Needs, Government Gazette 199 / A. (2008). https://www.e-nomothesia.gr/kat-ekpaideuse/n-3699-2008.html

Leiter, V. (2007). "Nobody's just normal, you know": The social creation of developmental disability. *Social Science & Medicine*, *65*(8), 1630–1641. doi:10.1016/j.socscimed.2007.06.006 PMID:17655995

León-Nabal, B., Zhang-Yu, C., & Lalueza, J. L. (2021). Uses of Digital Mediation in the School-Families Relationship During the COVID-19 Pandemic. *Frontiers in Psychology, 12*, 12. doi:10.3389/fpsyg.2021.687400 PMID:34248793

Letzel, V., Pozas, M., & Schneider, C. (2020). Energetic Students, Stressed Parents, and Nervous Teachers: A Comprehensive Exploration of Inclusive Homeschooling During the COVID-19 Crisis. *Open Education Studies*, *2*(1), 159–170. doi:10.1515/edu-2020-0122

Liodakis, D. (2000). *Educational programs for the blind.* Atrapos.

Majoko, T., & Dudu, A. (2020). Parents' strategies for home educating their children with Autism Spectrum Disorder during the COVID-19 period in Zimbabwe. *International Journal of Developmental Disabilities*, *0*(0), 1–5. doi:10.1080/20473869.2020.1803025 PMID:35937168

Moore, M. G. (1993). Theory of transactional distance. In D. Keegan (Ed.), *Theoretical principles of distance education* (pp. 22–38). Routledge.

Moore, M. G., & Kearsley, G. (2012). *Distance education: A systems view of online learning*. Wadsworth Cengage Learning.

Mortier, K., Hunt, P., Leroy, M., Van de Putte, I., & Van Hove, G. (2010). Communities of practice in inclusive education. *Educational Studies*, *36*(3), 345–355. doi:10.1080/03055690903424816

Mylonakou-Keke, H. (2009). *Family and Community School Collaboration, Theoretical Approaches and Practical Applications*. Papazisis.

Nam, C. S., Bahn, S., & Lee, R. (2013). Acceptance of Assistive Technology by Special Education Teachers: A Structural Equation Model Approach. *International Journal of Human-Computer Interaction*, *29*(5), 365–377. doi:10.1080/10447318.2012.711990

Neely-Barnes, S. L., Graff, J. C., Roberts, R. J., Hall, H. R., & Hankins, J. S. (2010). "It's our job": Qualitative study of family responses to ableism. *Intellectual and Developmental Disabilities*, *48*(4), 245–258. doi:10.1352/1934-9556-48.4.245 PMID:20722475

Nouri, J. (2016). The Flipped Classroom: For Active, Effective and Increased Learning—Especially for Low Achievers. *International Journal of Educational Technology in Higher Education, 13*(33), 1–10. doi:10.118641239-016-0032-z

Nutbrown, C., Clough, P., Nutbrown, C., & Clough, P. (2007). *Inclusion and exclusion in the early years : conversations with European educators Inclusion and exclusion in the early years : conversations with European educators. 6257.* doi:10.1080/0885625042000262479

Oliver, M., & Barnes, C. (2010). Disability studies, disabled people and the struggle for inclusion. *British Journal of Sociology of Education, 31*(5), 547–560. doi:10.1080/01425692.2010.500088

Østerlie. (2016). Flipped Learning in Physical Education : Why and How? *Physical Education and New Technologies*, 166–176. https://ntnuopen.ntnu.no/ntnu-xmlui/bitstream/handle/11250/2405451/Østerlie-2016-Flipped Learning in Physical Edu %28002%29.pdf?sequence=1

Panhellenic School Network. (2022a). *Electronic School Classroom*. E-Class. Retrieved March 10, 2022, from https://eclass.sch.gr

Panhellenic School Network. (2022b). *E-me Digital Education Platform*.E-me. Retrieved March 10, 2022, from https://e-me.edu.gr

Panhellenic School Network. (2022c). *WebEx Teleconference for Teachers*. Retrieved March 10, 2022, from https://webex.sch.gr/docs.php

Parmigiani, D., Benigno, V., Giusto, M., Silvaggio, C., & Sperandio, S. (2021). E-inclusion : online special education in Italy during the Covid-19 pandemic E-inclusion : online special education in Italy during the Covid-19. *Technology, Pedagogy and Education, 30*(1), 111–124. doi:10.1080/1475939X.2020.1856714

Polychronopoulou, S. (2003). *Children and adolescents with disabilities and abilities. Contemporary trends in education and support*. Route.

Powell, V., Riglin, L., Hammerton, G., Eyre, O., Martin, J., Anney, R., Thapar, A., & Rice, F. (2020). What explains the link between childhood ADHD and adolescent depression? Investigating the role of peer relationships and academic attainment. *European Child & Adolescent Psychiatry, 29*(11), 1581–1591. doi:10.100700787-019-01463-w PMID:31932968

Rose, J., Willner, P., Cooper, V., Langdon, P. E., Murphy, G. H., & Stenfert Kroese, B. (2020). The effect on and experience of families with a member who has Intellectual and Developmental Disabilities of the COVID-19 pandemic in the UK: Developing an investigation. *International Journal of Developmental Disabilities, 0*(0), 1–3. doi:10.1080/20473869.2020.1764257 PMID:35309704

Sfakiotaki, K. K. (2020). Education during a pandemic: International practices. In *1st International Online Training Conference From the 20th to the 21st Century in 15 Days. Attitudes-Perceptions-Scenarios-Perspectives-Proposals* (pp. 451–461). Hellenic Documentation Center.

Sharma, U., Loreman, T., & Forlin, C. (2012). Measuring teacher efficacy to implement inclusive practices. *Journal of Research in Special Educational Needs, 12*(1), 12–21. doi:10.1111/j.1471-3802.2011.01200.x

Sheridan, S. M., & Kratochwill, T. R. (2008). *Conjoint behavioral consultation*. Springer.

Sibley, M., Comer, J., & Gonzalez, J. (2017). Delivering Parent-Teen Therapy for ADHD through Videoconferencing: A Preliminary Investigation. *Journal of Psychopathology and Behavioral Assessment*, *39*(3), 467–485. doi:10.100710862-017-9598-6 PMID:28989230

Sofos, A., Costas, A., & Paraschou, B. (2015). Distance Education & Technology. In *Online distance education* (pp. 145–194). Kallipos, Open Academic Publications. https://repository.kallipos.gr/handle/11419/185

Solone, C. J., Thornton, B. E., Chiappe, J. C., Perez, C., Rearick, M. K., & Falvey, M. A. (2020). Creating collaborative schools in the united states: A review of best practices. *International Electronic Journal of Elementary Education*, *12*(3), 283–292. doi:10.26822/iejee.2020358222

Spencer-Cavaliere, N., & Watkinson, E. J. (2010). Inclusion understood from the perspectives of children with disability. *Adapted Physical Activity Quarterly; APAQ*, *27*(4), 275–293. doi:10.1123/apaq.27.4.275 PMID:20956835

Staples, K. E., & Diliberto, J. A. (2010). Guidelines for successful parent involvement: Working with parents of students with disabilities. *Teaching Exceptional Children*, *42*(6), 58–63. doi:10.1177/004005991004200607

Subramaniam, S., Brunson, L., Cook, J., Larson, N., Poe, S., & St. Peter, C. (2016). Maintenance of Parent-Implemented Discrete-Trial Instruction during Videoconferencing. *Journal of Behavioral Education*, *26*(1), 1–26. doi:10.100710864-016-9258-z

Syriopoulou-Delli, C. K., Cassimos, D. C., & Polychronopoulou, S. A. (2016). Collaboration between teachers and parents of children with ASD on issues of education. *Research in Developmental Disabilities*, *55*, 330–345. doi:10.1016/j.ridd.2016.04.011 PMID:27235770

Telli-Yamamoto, S. G., & Altun, D. (2020). The Coronavirus and the rising of online education. *Journal of University Research*, *3*(1), 25–34. doi:10.32329/uad.711110

UNESCO. (2020a). *COVID-19 Educational disruption and response*. https://en.unesco.org/covid19/educationresponse

UNESCO. (2020b). *Global Education Monitoring Report Summary 2020: Inclusion and education. All means all*. https://bit.ly/2020gemreport

Vogler, E. W., Koranda, P., & Romance, T. J. (2000). Including a Child with Severe Cerebral Palsy in Physical Education: A Case Study. *Adapted Physical Activity Quarterly; APAQ*, *17*(2), 161–175. doi:10.1123/apaq.17.2.161

Vuorikari, R., Velicu, A., Chaudron, S., Cachia, R., & Di Gioia, R. (2020). How Families Handled Emergency Remote Schooling during the COVID-19 Lockdown in Spring 2020: Summary of Key Findings from Families with Children in 11 European Countries. JRC Science for Policy Report. Publications Office of the European Union. doi:10.2760/31977

Yıldırım, B. (2021). Preschool Education in Turkey During the Covid-19 Pandemic : A Phenomenological Study. *Early Childhood Education Journal*, *49*(5), 947–963. doi:10.100710643-021-01153-w PMID:33519174

Zhao, Y. (2020). Tofu Is Not Cheese: Rethinking Education Amid the COVID-19 Pandemic. *ECNU Review of Education*, *3*(2), 189–203. doi:10.1177/2096531120928082

Chapter 13
Distance Vocational Education and Training in the Pandemic:
Adaptations and Challenges for Learners and Trainers in Europe – How the Pandemic Affected Distance Vocational Education and Training

Christos Lalos
University of Alicante, Spain

ABSTRACT

The COVID-19 pandemic has brought unprecedented challenges to all types and levels of learning, including vocational education and training. The chapter attempts to provide a preliminary analysis regarding the transition to ex distance education as a consequence of the closure of schools. Based on inputs from 14 informants, members of the Cedefop Ambassadors network for addressing early withdrawal from vocational education and training, covering five Member States and two non-EU countries, the work sheds light on aspects of this in order to highlight the challenges that trainees face in risk of early departure, but also their trainers, as well as the measures taken adopted for their support. Cedefop published a study in English, which the authors translated and summarized in the present work. The study shows that there is no digital integration without social integration. Vulnerable learners are less likely to participate in distance education, while their detachment from the learning process can lead to their early withdrawal from vocational education and training.

DOI: 10.4018/978-1-6684-4735-2.ch013

INTRODUCTION

The Covid-19 pandemic posed unprecedented challenges at all types and levels learning, including vocational education and training. An entire generation of Vocational Education and Training students experienced its cessation education and training in an unprecedented way due to traffic ban measures and avoiding social contacts that have been implemented both in Europe and globally. Educational institutions were invited to organize and offer direct digital education and training, while at the same time they had to mobilize teachers and trainers in this direction.

All of these were aimed at ensuring "learning and training anywhere, anytime ", an idea that is at the heart of the concept of lifelong learning, but is far removed from traditional Vocational practices Education and Training that are strongly entrenched in his physical presence trainee in a specific institution of Vocational Education and Training. With schools remaining closed for more than two months during the first phase of the pandemic, in the spring of 2020, in more than 190 countries, 90% of the world student population was affected, according to UNESCO estimates (1.57 billions of children and young people).

According to UNICEF (2020), 99% of the educated population under the age of 18 worldwide (2.34 billion) live in one of these countries, with some form of travel restriction and are affected therefore from the closure of schools due to Covid-19. However, the socio-economic impact of Covid-19 is being felt more strongly than the most vulnerable learners across Europe. Many of them live in poverty conditions without digital devices and / or without internet access at home or live in remote areas where there is a shortage of teachers or school materials. In addition, there are many challenges that the Vocational Education and Training teachers and trainers in the effort to deal with the current crisis.

The effects, possibly independent of this level or type of education, appear more pronounced in Vocational Education and Training, as here an important component of learning is based on work, which s discontinued after the companies that offer apprenticeships have closed in many countries (Cedefop, 2020b).

The purpose of this article is to provide a summary of the preliminary findings from a small-scale inquiry based on the answers of its ambassadors Cedefop for Dealing with Early Vocational Training. The next section briefly presents the research questions as well as its limitations. The following sections compose the main findings that extracted from the informants' answers and which have been presented in more detail in a relevant Cedefop report (2020a). The conclusions highlight the key messages while suggesting fields further research.

DATA COLLECTION

This work is based on preliminary information received from fourteen ambassadors from seven European countries: five EU Member States (Germany, Greece, Portugal, Romania and Spain) and two non-EU countries (Turkey and the United Kingdom). The information were collected in April - May 2020, a period during which all seven countries already had develop measures to continue the courses in order to deal with the interruption caused by the Covid-19 crisis and the closure of schools. The full text of research results has been published as a report by Cedefop (2020a). This paper attempts to summarize the findings of this report.

The Questions

The report was drawn up around two central themes for which input was requested of the Cedefop Ambassadors Network to address early withdrawal from Vocational Education and Training. They were asked two sets of questions regarding how the closure of schools affected the trainees who are at risk of early retirement, as well as how teachers and Vocational Education and Training instructors were supported in teaching in new e-learning environments. These two topics are presented in detail in Table 1.

The attempt to collect this preliminary information was not intended to an inventory of measures, policies or practices designed, developed or implemented in the countries concerned. Instead, its purpose was to understand how crisis management and, therefore, reflection on needs and challenges for teachers and Vocational Education and Training and for trainees who are at risk of leaving early.

Table 1. Reference questions and questions source: Cedefop 2020a

1 Questions about the impact of school closures on students at risk of leaving early.
1.1 How is the closure of schools, as part of the government's measures against Covid-19, affect trainees at risk of leaving early? 1.2 Support measures have been taken for them in your country or region trainees at risk of early retirement? 1.3 You know good practices for ensuring equal access for all learners of Vocational Education and Training in distance education (including students with a less favorable socioeconomic background and disabilities).
2 Questions for teachers and trainers of Vocational Education and Training.
2.1 Teachers and trainers of Vocational Education and Training have the necessary technical and pedagogical skills to integrate them digital devices in teaching? 2.2 Supported by vocational training in distance education during duration of the pandemic? 2.3 There are other effective professional resources for learning to use digital devices available to teachers and trainers of Vocational Education and Training.

Compensating for the Negative Impact on Trainees at Risk Early Retirement from Vocational Education and Training

Cedefop network informants gave us rich examples of initiatives promoted by governments and specific educational institutions for support of Vocational Education and Training trainees at risk of early retirement, including students with less favored socio-economic background, of immigrants and those of ethnic origin minorities, students with disabilities but also those with special educational needs. Some of these activities are summarized in Table 2.

Table 2. Initiatives to support students at risk of leaving early vocational education and training. Source: Cedefop 2020a

1 What activities were developed to support students at risk of early departure?
1.1 Ensuring equal access to distance education for all Vocational Education and Training trainees with its free provision necessary equipment as well as free unlimited internet access. 1.2 Providing training opportunities for learners regarding development digital skills. 1.3 Translation of educational material into languages spoken by ethnic groups minorities, refugees and immigrants, as well as in semantics for trainees with hearing problems. 1.4 Monitoring the participation of learners in distance education. 1.5 Provision of personalized remote support to trainees at risk of early withdrawal from Vocational Education and Training and their parents, both in academic and mental health matters

Equal access to distance education is important for all Vocational Education and Training, but especially for most vulnerable, who either belong to groups with less favorable socio-economic status background, whether they are students with disabilities. All countries examined paid efforts to provide internet access and the necessary equipment for ex distance education. The Greek government entered into an agreement with the companies telecommunications to provide unlimited free access to online platforms e-learning for all Vocational Training trainees and Training.

Donations and funding were also made to strengthen public Vocational Education and Training schools with necessary digital equipment, which will be used by students through borrowing. Another initiative, the "Learning at Home" website is an information center for all educational services provided by educational structures. In addition, the Ministry of Digital Governance gathered, at one point, at the Digital Academy Citizens, educational content for the general public, creating an innovative platform for collective learning, in which educational institutions are invited to assist.

The Romanian Ministry of Education has developed a digital platform for the Relevant project Curriculum, Open Education for All - CRED, offering various types of digital in order to support teachers and students to continue their education at home at no cost. In addition, the initiative of the Ministry of Reaction for education managed to identify digital material that students and educators need in order to continue online courses. NGOs and other organizations also funded students or schools in rural areas that had the appropriate equipment to have access to online courses.

Respectively, in Spain, the Ministry of Education and Vocational Training, along with some technology companies, provided digital devices and internet access for trainees at premature risk one month after providing the same support to students who do not were in danger. As most students at risk were not enrolled in the formal education system, but in non-formal educational institutions education, some of them set up the Spanish Second School Association Opportunity, by granting them access to online courses.

They received, also laptops and internet access, but also economical and emotional support. In Portugal, similar agreements were reached with private companies, in order to provide free access to additional training content. The Digital Literacy Integration Program was initially offered in libraries, parishes and municipal facilities. It is now offered to all people who want to acquire a broad climate of digital skills in order to participate and groups at risk of exclusion. In addition, a new platform was created with special Vocational Education and Training material in order to facilitate teachers and trainers to maintain systematic contact, to establish knowledge they have already acquired and develop new skills to complement their knowledge.

NGOs and other international organizations also contributed to their support trainees at risk of early withdrawal. In Turkey, the professional high schools that work with universities conduct their courses in virtual rooms, through the online education systems provided by each university. In Greece, distance education courses are provided for trainees with hearing problems and, in cooperation with UNICEF, remote control instructions education were translated into eleven different languages spoken by refugees and immigrants living in Greece.

Apprenticeship and Internship During the Pandemic

A significant difficulty, which was mentioned by all our informants, concerns continuation of the practical part of the Vocational Education and Training programs during the curfew and closure of businesses. While the Theoretical courses can usually be taught and studied online, the practical part can not be carried out effectively, e.g. due to lack of access to tools, materials and equipment. In all seven countries from which information was collected, Vocational Education and Training and Apprenticeship providers integrate online platforms to facilitate learning and assessment.

Many have already switched to online internships, while others plan evaluations using online platforms. Others take advantage of options for innovative, digital pedagogical approaches, such as simulators, augmented / virtual reality or artificial intelligence for practicing specialists practical skills. Online learning solutions are utilized in the apprenticeships that engineering, information technology, finance and insurance.

The apprentices who were still going to the companies, had it right, occasionally, in cooperation with the schools, to compensate for its part training that was to take place at the school. Several applications and websites have been used that connect trainees and trainers in the workplace to ensure the continuation of education.

There is a possibility of teleworking, especially for apprenticeships in information technology. Work-based experience is promoted through simulated businesses, while platforms facilitate communication with partners dual training.

Offering Personalized Support to Trainees at Risk of Early Departure

The global crisis has intensified and strengthened the digital, social, emotional, cultural and economic inequalities already faced by many Vocational students Education And Training And Their Families. The provision of personalized psychological support can prevent learners from being released from learning. In Romania, the first line of psychological counseling was created for Covid-19, free of charge for teachers, parents and students. Guidance is also provided at Spain, in the context of second chance schools, especially for younger students (16 to 21 years old), with personalized telephone sessions, during which they are resolved issues at the academic and personal level as well as at the health level. Communication and coordination with social workers and between teachers is carried out on a daily basis (Cedefop, 2020c).

Similar support measures were adopted in Portugal, where schools were instructed for the implementation of distance education in students with special educational needs, which included support measures for parents and students, promoting learning and prosperity.

In England and Wales, some institutions had to remain open and adopt appropriate measures to provide education to children whose parents work in critical positions and in children and young people belonging to vulnerable groups, who were supported by the social welfare system or have identified as vulnerable by educational institutions and local authorities.

For vulnerable people who do not have access to a social worker, the national program Families First in Wales, aims to improve results for children and young people (including effective participation in education and training), focusing on prevention and providing level support family and not individual.

In Germany, the so - called "transition guidance" supports trainees at school in the completion of general secondary education or (assisted) Vocational Education and Training or other form of upper secondary education. In collaboration with each student, the facilitator (coach) prepares a plan transition. To ensure the continuation of personalized support throughout of the crisis, the transition mediators have adapted their services, directing young people as much as possible to telephone services guidance.

Support for Vocational Education teachers and trainers and Training in taking on new roles In the context of the global crisis caused by Covid-19 and its closure schools, the continuation of learning can only be ensured thanks to digital skills, he flexibility and creativity of teachers and trainers to develop and use creative solutions with online material. In a profession that is practiced mainly in its traditional form, through living, where personal interaction and proximity is essential, social distancing certainly plays new roles and challenges for Vocational Education teachers and trainers and Training. Online learning environments call them to show high quality digital teaching skills and confidence in using online solutions conferences.

They also need to be vigilant about increased cyberbullying and protect their learners from disconnecting from the "real world ", paying attention to the time they spend on the internet. The trainers Vocational Education and Training must work with employers and social partners to share their material online or to produce new digital learning tools (Psifidou, 2020a).

Unfortunately, not all Vocational Training teachers and trainers and Training prepared for this process. According to the OECD, the recent TALIS 2018 research (OECD, 2020) showed that the use of information technologies and communication (ICT) for teaching purposes was the second highest field professional development, for which teachers (18%) reported a high need. However, only 56% of teachers in OECD countries had participated in training for the use of ICT for didactic purposes, as part of their initial education or training, and only 43% of teachers felt well or very well prepared for the use of technologies in education when they started teaching.

The findings of TALIS research may explain to some extent why teachers and Vocational Education and Training instructors face significant difficulties as they turn physical classrooms into digital learning environments by overnight. According to our informants, some initiatives that aimed at addressing these obstacles are those presented in Table 3.

Table 3. Initiatives to support teachers and trainers vocational education and training. Source: Cedefop, 2020a

What activities were implemented to support teachers and trainers of Vocational Education and Training?
2.1 Distance learning modules for the development of digital skills and pedagogical e-learning practices.
2.2 Equipment of Vocational Education and Training schools with necessary digital devices.
2.3 necessary digital devices.
2.3 Caring for the well-being of teachers and trainers of Vocational Education and Training.

Taking care of the well-being of teachers and Vocational trainers Education and Training According to the World Health Organization, the teaching profession is one of the most anxious. This has a variety of consequences, such as absences from work, occupation abandonment, illness, emotional exhaustion and stress.

While the Covid-19 crisis pushes our society to change, creating new challenges and roles for teachers and trainers of Vocational Education and Training, threatens along with their well-being, which is vital and can have significant impact on learners' learning and well-being.

Given the changes required to slow the spread of Covid 19, the new conditions of work for teachers may increase their discomfort as the hours workload and the complexity of teaching are increasing significantly. The teachers are called to change their work environment overnight and to go to virtual rooms and workplaces. So they often struggle to respond to the new demands that have been imposed on them and to overcome the new challenges that now they have to face and need more than ever support and larger investments in their space. Some of the challenges mentioned most often are those presented below in Table 4.

Table 4. Challenges faced by teachers and trainers of vocational education and training. Source: Cedefop, 2020a.

What challenges do teachers and Vocational Education and Training face?
2.1 Lack of access to equipment and internet connection for distance learning.
2.2 Lack of digital skills and competencies for effective use of training platforms.
2.3 Lack of experience in creating digital teaching content.
2.4 Lack of experience in e-learning and other effective distance learning pedagogy in Vocational Education and Training, especially for the teaching of practical courses.
2.5 Concerns about privacy, copyright and data protection issues. Heads of Vocational Education and Training - both directors Schools as well as immediate supervisors - seem to have an important role to play a role in caring for the well-being of teachers and trainers of Vocational Education and Training.

Countries that have given more autonomy in Vocational Education and Training institutions and directors enjoy significant benefits for organizing distance learning (Psifidou, 2020b).

The leadership that supports autonomy in Vocational schools Education and Training during Covid-19 may include: Understanding the needs of teachers and trainers for effective providing distance education and tackling the problems that arise, inclusion of teachers 'and trainers' views in the procedures school-level decision-making, maintaining an open dialogue at a distance with teachers about the various duties Research has shown that when teachers consider their school principals are more supportive of autonomy, they report more positive relationships with students and colleagues, greater adaptability, greater prosperity at work and less emotional exhaustion. Therefore, the behaviors of leaders who support autonomy is an important way of support for teachers' experiences of social support and adaptability.

Recent studies (Collie et al., 2019) have shown that when teachers consider that their school principals are more supportive of autonomy, indicate greater resilience in the workplace, which means ability, effectively address, common challenges at work, which it acquires of particular importance in addressing the challenges posed by Covid-19.

CONCLUSION

The pandemic forced all European Vocational Training Institutions and Training to operate with unpredictable, unplanned and unexpected ways. Therefore, they were asked to organize quickly, digitally or remotely education and training programs, while at the same time they had to mobilize teachers, educators and of course students to preserve continuity of learning processes. The extraordinary situation of the pandemic created great pressures not only in the health system but also in the education system, forcing it to implement ad hoc solutions often posed by both teachers and students, outside their comfort zone.

The crisis and dealing with it by closing schools they seem to have acted as catalysts for the digitization of schools and the transition in distance education. Innovative distance learning processes that ensure "learning and education anywhere, anytime" is, for many, new and quite distant compared to traditional and widely adopted learning of Vocational Education and Training practices which are developed on the basis of physical presence of the trainee, in a specific institution of Vocational Education and Training, specific hours and days. Vocational Education and Training teachers now need more than ever further develop technical and pedagogical skills at a distance e-learning environments.

They must be supported with the necessary material and appropriate training to improve its effectiveness and experience e-learning as a whole. Some countries train teachers, trainers, facilitators and consultants for the development of teaching material, for acquisition of knowledge in effective e - learning methodologies and for conducting an online evaluation, while some platforms offer presentations and online education to users. This crisis can provide an opportunity to focus on conservation efforts and creating a workforce of teachers and Vocational trainers of Highly qualified Education and Training.

Some governments see an opportunity for to grant greater autonomy to educational institutions, in order to promote public-private partnerships and provide them, not just the necessary techniques and pedagogical skills to integrate digital devices into education, but also transversal skills, such as flexibility, adaptability, social support and responsibility. Finally, the crisis has once again shown that students come from less favored groups are less likely to participate in the processes distance training and therefore an increased number should be expected departures.

The most vulnerable are most at risk of being affected by the crisis. Further research should continue to explore the reactions of its sector of Vocational Education and Training in the Covid-19 crisis. In the next period, as countries will make efforts to return to the new regularity, it will be possible to assess how the closure of schools, as part of governments' efforts to tackle Covid-19, affected students from less-favored groups and increased of their early retirement rates, as well as how teachers and Vocational Education and Training educators face this challenge adapting their practices and role.

REFERENCES

Cedefop. (2020a). *Digital gap during Covid-19 for VET learners at risk in Europe. Synthesis report.* https://www.cedefop.europa.eu/bg/toolkits/vet-toolkit-tackling-early-leaving/resources/digitalgap-during-covid-19-vet-learners-risk-europe

Cedefop. (2020b). *How are European countries managing apprenticeships to respond to the Covid-19 crisis? Synthesis report based on information provided by Cedefop community of apprenticeship experts.* https://www.cedefop.europa.eu/files/cedefop_community_apprenticeship_experts_synthesis_ho_are_european_countries_managing_apprenticeships_to_respond_to_the_coronavirus_crisis.pdf

Collie, R. J., Bostwick, K. C., & Martin, A. J. (2019). Perceived autonomy support, relatedness with students, and workplace outcomes: An investigation of differences by teacher gender. Educational Psychology. *An International Journal of Experimental Educational Psychology*, *40*(3), 253–272.

OECD. (2020). *TALIS 2018 Results (Volume II): Teachers and School Leaders as Valued Professionals.* TALIS, OECD Publishing. doi:10.1787/19cf08df-en

Psifidou, I. (2020a). Challenges and support for VET Teachers and Trainers during Covid-19. In *Croatian Presidency Conference Teachers and Trainers for the Future: Towards the 'New Normal'.* Ministry of Science and Education.

Psifidou, I. (2020b). New roles for VET Teachers and Trainers. *Directors' General for VET (DGVT) online meeting "Paving the way for a better future VET - towards 2030".*

UNICEF. (2020). *Protecting the most vulnerable children from the impact of coronavirus: An agenda for action.* Available here: https://www.unicef.org/coronavirus/agenda-for-action

Chapter 14
Therapeutic and Learning Benefits of Reading During COVID-19 Among Spanish Secondary Students

Juan-Francisco Álvarez-Herrero
https://orcid.org/0000-0002-9988-8286
Universidad de Alicante, Spain

ABSTRACT

During the confinement due to COVID-19, the educational centers tried to cope as much as possible with the continuity of the teaching-learning processes. In this research, it was tried to verify if the implementation of a proposal that promoted reading among secondary school students of a science subject, characteristic to improve their learning as well as benefit their mental health. The comparison of the results obtained in a test before and after carrying out the proposal confirmed that there was an improvement in learning and a perception of therapeutic effects of reading in this difficult situation. It is necessary to continue carrying out proposals of this type, even without being subjected to situations of anxiety and stress, in order to improve both learning and the mental health of students.

INTRODUCTION

The promotion of reading is not exclusive to the areas of languages. Also, from the areas of science, reading should be encouraged among the students. And this must be done from an early age, it is not necessary to wait for the stage of primary or secondary studies. With the promotion of reading from these areas of science, not only is it possible to improve the reading competence of the students, but it also favors an improvement in motivation and interest in learning these subjects. Reading manages to transfer students to the history of science, to learn first-hand about the life and work of scientists, and with adapted texts or using comics and illustrated albums, they can even achieve the acquisition of learning in scientific content more or less complex.

DOI: 10.4018/978-1-6684-4735-2.ch014

The confinement caused by the COVID-19 pandemic throughout the world, and more specifically in Spain between March and June 2020; led to educational institutions having to adapt the teachings from a totally face-to-face modality to an online one. This fact of not being present in the classrooms supposed a double aspect of reading among the students. On the one hand, having to make greater use of digital technologies and the fact that there was no greater control and monitoring of what students read and how they read; it implied a greater abandonment of reading and that the students opted for other more comfortable practices such as watching series, interaction on social networks in which the image fundamentally prevails (YouTube, Instagram, Tik Tok, etc.) or playing online from various platforms or from the Internet itself. But, on the other hand, having more time at home, not having technological devices or having to share them with the rest of the members of a family, as well as dedicating themselves to other more analogical tasks that would allow them to rest from technology digital; led to the students also finding in reading a way to escape or even therapy in the face of the situation that was being experienced with confinement.

For this reason, this confinement caused by the COVID-19 pandemic was an excellent opportunity to promote reading among students. And the research presented here tries to verify if the promotion of reading scientific texts during confinement allowed improving and increasing the taste for reading among secondary school students. Likewise, it was wanted to verify if this practice allowed to be an excellent resource for the improvement of the motivation and learning of sciences among the students.

BACKGROUND

In recent years, and as a result of the COVID-19 pandemic, there have been contradictory data about people's reading habits. And if you pay attention to what happened worldwide with reading during confinement, you see that although there are cases in which it seems that the percentage of readers and time dedicated to reading increased (Sun et al., 2021), there are cases in which this increase only occurred in the first weeks (Reimer et al., 2021), and in other cases it can be affirmed that the number of readers and time dedicated to reading has decreased considerably (Ardington et al., 2021).

In the particular case of Spain, the reading competence of Spaniards continues to give stagnant values and well below the average of the rest of the OECD countries, in its latest report: Skills Outlook 2021: learning for life (OECD, 2021). And if 57% of Spaniards read frequently during the state of alarm, the reading rate hardly grew in 2020 (Morales, 2021). The Spanish recognize reading as the third resource, behind watching television and talking on the phone, that helps the most in quarantine; but it goes to ninth place when asked about the activities they have carried out in quarantine (Conecta, 2020). Another study carried out among the adult population carried out by the University of Valencia and the University of Salamanca (ERI-Lectura, 2020), concludes that, individually, between 39.9 and 47. 9% had a reading frequency similar to before the pandemic, while between 8.8 and 27.4% decreased. On the other hand, the greatest increases occurred in social reading (Instagram, Facebook, WhatsApp, etc.) with 46.1%, and 45.3% of the sample increased their leisure reading frequency (novels, comics, magazines or blogs) during confinement.

In the specific case of young people, 80% of them recognize that reading has been of great help to better cope with the confinement situation (Fundación SM, 2021).

If observed within the educational field, contradictory studies are also found, in which although it is observed that the pandemic has come to reflect low results in students in reading habits (Aziz et al.,

2021). Thus, although it seems that there is progress in the promotion of reading, later, the academic results are lower than those of a normal academic year, without a pandemic (Clark et al., 2021; Lewis et al., 2021; Locke et al., 2021; Maldonado & De Witte, 2022; Schult et al., 2021; Tomasik et al., 2021). But, on the other hand, a good use of reading during this period of confinement, with for example the daily reading of books by the students, it has also served to mitigate the devastating effects that a confinement of the characteristics that has been suffered can have on the learning and development of the different literacies (Bao et al., 2020). It would be worth analyzing before what type of reading is what has led to these results, or although both recreational and academic have been contemplated, perhaps that is the reason for such contradictory results.

The promotion of academic reading among students has been contemplated many times from those areas of languages that are taught in schools (Baker, 2'18; De Naeghel et al., 2012). It seems that reading is only recommended by schools to their students, from those areas that in turn study literature. And that the areas of letters are at odds with the areas of science, when it turns out that the interconnection that exists between them is very great. But actually, reading and reading comprehension are two actions that are not alien, or should not be alien, to all areas of the formal training of students. For example, in learning mathematics, it is very helpful to know how to read mathematical textbooks, and with this there is an improvement in the learning of both mathematics and in the development of a reading capacity that tends to be more orderly, reflective and active (Guo, 2021). Hence, it is very important to work on the reading of all kinds of texts in all kinds of academic areas, either in a disciplinary way or in a transversal way. The areas of science, due to the usual presence in their texts of numerous technical terms, as well as operators and mathematical formulas, seem inappropriate to encourage reading among students. However, if properly oriented and with a careful selection of texts, whether original or adapted, an improvement in learning can be achieved. Science, technology, engineering and mathematics (so-called STEM areas), they are indisputable partners of reading and writing (Wilson-López & Gregory, 2015). Reading facilitates the understanding of STEM texts and this allows a better interpretation of these disciplines and with it, an improvement in their learning (Freeman et al., 2022).

Reading in a digital medium and not in print is also a concept that is generating a lot of controversy. To what extent do students begin to consider reading print as something boring, compared to reading digitally? And, does digital reading really make it easier or harder for students to pay attention to words and the ideas behind them? And with respect to print reading, is there a better understanding when it is reading in print or when it is digital? In this sense, there are studies with contradictory results (Baron, 2017; Kaufman & Flanagan, 2016; Mangen et al., 2013; Pardede, 2019). The contradictions become such that even the students under study, although they prefer and believe they perceive a better understanding in the digital text,

Reading is and should continue to be a means of acquiring learning, which is why it is so important to influence it from the earliest educational stages (Ruiz-Bejarano, 2019). And since people learn to read, they should acquire a reading habit that lasts throughout their lives (Petscher et al., 2020), as is the case with learning, which must be produced continuously as long as it exists.

And what about science readings in secondary education? At this stage, reading is still a much-needed activity among students. And a good reading skill helps improve performance in all areas, and more specifically improves learning in subjects such as mathematics and science (Zhu, 2021). This task of promoting reading from science areas can be carried out from various practices, all of them very interesting and with excellent results in improving reading skills and student learning in these areas. Thus, for example, one of them involves proposing complementary readings to the students that they can already find in their textbook. These can be either original scientific books or with rigor and accepted scientific terminology, or adapted texts or that even resort to comics or illustrated albums to more easily generate interest among students. In the end, reading these texts becomes a support for science teaching and can become the inspiration for that student who ends up being an excellent scientist or engineer (Broemmel et al., 2021). There is talk of the need to incorporate reading as another discipline, or at least, to train science teachers in reading strategies that allow the understanding of scientific texts and that are capable of transferring them to their students (Mawyer & Johnson, 2019). Students will be able to learn from the reading of specific texts of the subject, in this case science, allowing their understanding and that increasingly more complex and appropriate texts can be presented at each level as they advance in their academic training (Roldán, 2019). In addition, this understanding of what is read must be reached by using the art of questioning, that is, subjecting students to questions that confirm that there has been a correct understanding of the text they have read (Santos, 2019).

The reading of science texts with high school students should be at these ages, directed or at least comparing true information with that other false or contradictory. Strategies should be given so that students, in addition to improving their reading process and reading comprehension, also do so in identifying true information from that other that is false or contradictory (Keck et al., 2015). This critical reading is also the basis for effective science learning (Norris et al., 2009).

In this study, far from considering whether today's young high school students read more or less, whether they read or not in schools, whether the readings that are carried out are done from the areas of science or from those of letters, or if what is read is preferred and better understood through digital reading or through reading printed text; What it seeks is to verify whether, through a proposal to read scientific texts carried out during the home confinement experienced as a result of the COVID-19 pandemic, it caused a greater dedication to reading among secondary school students and if this had an effect. therapeutic and healing, in addition to generating an improvement in the learning of said students.

MAIN FOCUS OF THE CHAPTER

This chapter deals with an experience carried out during confinement with Compulsory Secondary Education (ESO) students from an educational center in Alcoi (Alicante), Spain; with which it was first investigated what use of free reading they were making and in a second phase and after two brief interventions, it was verified if reading had acquired a greater prominence, even becoming a way of escaping from the problem caused by the confinement.

The research was carried out with 71 students in the 3rd and 4th years of ESO. 43 women (60.6%) and 28 men (39.4%), aged between 14 and 17 years. All of them are students from an educational center located in an expansion area of the town of Alcoy (Alicante), and with a low- or middle-class family profile.

It was carried out between the months of March and June 2020, the entire time in which teaching was completely online, as both teachers and students were confined to their homes. For this, the resources offered by Google for Education were used: Google Classroom, Google meet, Google Docs, etc.

In its realization, two phases were differentiated (Figure 1), with two and three actions respectively. The first phase was carried out at the end of April, after almost a month and a half of confinement, and was more exploratory or investigative to discover the reality of the students. And a second phase that was carried out between May and June, and that was of direct intervention on the students and collection of the final results to be able to compare with the initial ones.

Figure 1. Investigation phases and actions
Source: own elaboration

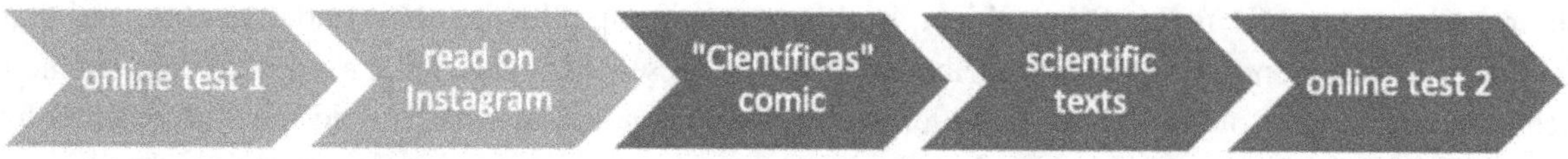
online test 1
read on Instagram
"Científicas" comic
scientific texts
online test 2

First Phase

In this first phase, at the end of April and after the Easter holidays, two actions were carried out with the idea of collecting information.

Online test 1

First, an online test (online test 1) was given to the students asking about the type of activities they carried out mostly in their free time (not study or academic work) in the month and a half that they had been in confinement. They were given different closed options, but also the possibility of indicating in open answers those that were not contemplated.

The first question of the questionnaire read as follows:

- Indicate up to a total of three actions to which you have dedicated the most leisure time or your free time during these weeks of confinement. (In case you mark others, indicate which other activities you are referring to).

    1. Watch multimedia content (cinema, television, content on platforms such as Netflix, Amazon Prime, HBO, etc.)
    2. Browse the Internet (watch YouTube videos, blogs, web pages)
    3. Social Networks (Instagram, Tik Tok, Twitter, Facebook, etc.)
    4. Instant messaging (WhatsApp, telegram, etc.)
    5. Games online or on video consoles
    6. Board games, family games
    7. Listen to music
    8. Reading (Novels, comics, newspapers, magazines, etc.)
    9. Cook
    10. Exercise tables, exercise bike, yoga,
    11. Crafts (drawing, painting, knitting, sewing, etc.)
    12. Talk with family members

13. Talking on the phone with family and friends
14. Others

Other questions related to reading during this first part of confinement present in the test were:

- What average weekly time have you dedicated to reading?
- What kind of readings have you mostly done?
    1. novels
    2. comics
    3. journals
    4. newspapers
    5. finger reading
- What sensations have you experienced when you read?

The results obtained in the first question can be seen in Table 1.

Table 1. Main activities in which students spent their free time on the first phase

Activity	Man (28)		Woman (43)		Overall (71)	
	n	%	n	%	n	%
Social media	24	85.7	40	93.0	64	90.1
Instant messaging	17	60.7	30	69.7	47	66.2
View media content	16	57.1	21	48.8	37	52.1
Surfing the Internet	12	42.8	19	44.2	31	43.6
Listen to music	4	14.3	7	16.3	11	15.5
Online games	8	28.6	0	0	8	11.2
Talk to family members	2	7.1	4	9.3	6	8.4
Cook	0	0	4	9.3	4	5.6
Read	0	0	2	4.6	2	2.8
Crafts	0	0	1	23	1	1.4
Physical exercise	1	3.6	0	0	1	1.4
Others (play an instrument)	0	0	1	23	1	1.4

Source: own elaboration

In the results obtained (Table 1) it was found that the use of social networks, instant messaging (mainly through WhatsApp), as well as viewing multimedia content and browsing the Internet, occupy the first four places with difference rest of activities. In the case of reading, only two students include it among their three main activities carried out in their free time in this first phase of confinement.

Regarding question 5 of the test, the weekly average time of the 71 students turned out to be 1 hour and 17 minutes, detecting that in the case of men it was less, 48 minutes, and in the case of women greater, 1 hour and 46 minutes. Regarding the type of reading they did, 47 students (66.2%) stated that it was digital reading, 11 indicated novels (11.2%), 10 read comics (14.1%) and only 3 students confessed to reading newspapers (1) or magazines (2), the remaining 4.2%.

Question 7, being open and giving rise to a multitude of qualitative answers, these were grouped into different categories, being summarized as follows: fun (39, 54.9%), adventure (17, 23.9%), curiosity/learning (9, 12.6%), being informed (5, 7%), escaping from reality (1, 1.4%).

Read on Instagram

On the other hand, a small experience was also carried out that consisted of the publication on the social network Instagram in the teacher's profile, of an image in which a blank notebook with a pen appeared, and which was accompanied by a brief text in which invited the students who read it to send an email to the teacher indicating that they had read it. These networks fundamentally based on the use and social interaction with images mean that, on many occasions, the text that accompanies the images goes completely unnoticed. Given that the 71 students have a profile on Instagram and that they all follow the teacher's account, this experience served to verify that only a small percentage of them (26.7%) read the text that accompanied the image. Although almost all (68, 95.8%) gave a "Like" to said photo, very few were those who wrote an email to the teacher (19 students), thereby indicating that they had read the text.

Second Phase

Given the poor results that reading had obtained in the first phase, in the second phase of this research, action was taken to allow students to discover in reading an excellent resource not only for learning, but also as therapy. before the moments that were being lived.

"Científicas" Comic

The first action that was carried out with the students was to provide them with the comic "Científicas", a comic available in pdf and online (http://institucional.us.es/cientificas/comic/), which brought the students closer to the life and work of women scientists. After their reading and in small groups of 5 students, they carried out a research project on one of the female protagonists of the comic in which they delved deeper into her life and work. To work online and in groups, they used the tools that the Google Suite for Education offers (Google Meet, Google Docs and Google Slides, mainly), and thus work was carried out on the life and work of:

- Hypatia of Alexandria
- Ada Lovelace
- Marie Curie
- Rosalind Franklin
- Hedy Lamarr

Scientific texts

The second action that was carried out was to present short texts adapted from scientists, related to the contents that were being worked on. Thus, for example, texts adapted from: Semmelweis, Mendel,

Darwin, Asimov, etc. were presented. From the reading of these texts, the students were asked to carry out various activities that delved into the learning of their lives and works, focusing on the contents that about their works are dealt with in the curriculum of these secondary education courses.

Online test 2

At the end of this second phase of the investigation and before the end of the classes, the questionnaire from the first phase was passed again about what actions they dedicated more time to during this other phase of confinement and in which on this occasion greater interest was shown in knowing the answers that had been given in question 7 of the questionnaire, about how they had felt regarding a greater use and role of reading in their teaching-learning process during this stage.
The results obtained in the first question can be seen in Table 2.

Table 2. Main activities in which students spent their free time on the second phase

Activity	Man (28)		Woman (43)		Overall (71)	
	n	%	n	%	n	%
Social media	25	89.3	41	95.3	66	92.9
Instant messaging	17	60.7	31	72.1	48	67.6
View media content	14	50.0	16	37.2	30	42.2
Surfing the Internet	13	46.4	15	34.9	28	39.4
Read	3	10.7	7	16.3	10	14.1
Listen to music	2	7.1	6	13.9	8	11.2
Talk to family members	3	10.7	5	11.6	8	11.2
Board games, family games	2	7.1	4	9.3	6	8.4
Online games	4	14.3	0	0	4	5.6
Cook	0	0	2	4.6	2	2.8
Crafts	0	0	1	23	1	1.4
Physical exercise	1	3.6	0	0	1	1.4
Others (laya n instrument)	0	0	1	23	1	1.4

Source: own elaboration

In the results obtained (Table 2), it was found that the use of social networks, instant messaging (mainly through WhatsApp), as well as viewing multimedia content and browsing the Internet, continue to occupy the first four places and with different from other activities. Although their percentages have decreased compared to the first phase of confinement, they are still well above the rest of the activities. On the other hand, in the specific case of reading, this has come to occupy fifth place (when in the previous phase it was in ninth place). Although it is not a notable increase, it is significant, since it is verified that it has gone from being named only twice, to being so a total of ten times. In addition, if before there were only two women, now we see that, of the 10 people, 3 are men and 7 are women. If it is observed that other activities have been more affected, such as listening to music, cooking and online games, which have come to have a lower number of responses, and although there are others that maintain the same results obtained previously, it is observed that board games or family games appear this time, when they did not appear in the first test.

Regarding question 5 of the test, the weekly average time of the 71 students, this time turned out to be much higher compared to the previous phase, and thus an average time of 2 hours and 23 minutes was obtained, almost doubling the time invested in reading in the first phase. But, detecting again that in the case of men this reading time was still less, 1 hour and 27 minutes, and in the case of women it was also still longer, 3 hours and 19 minutes. Regarding the type of reading they did, significant changes were also observed, since digital reading was reduced, but the reading of novels and comics increased considerably. Thus, 29 students (40.8%) continued stating that their reading was digital, 22 indicated novels (30.9%), 17 read comics (23.9%) and again, only 3 students confessed to reading newspapers (1) or magazines (2), the remaining 4.2%. Therefore, in the reading of novels, the number of students who recognized their reading in this second phase of confinement doubled and its explanation lies in the intervention made of a proposal that motivated the academic reading of scientific texts.

But really, the most illuminating results of online test 2 were obtained in question 7. Again, and as it was an open question, with a multitude of qualitative answers, these were grouped into different categories, being summarized this time. thus: fun (29, 40.8%); curiosity/learning (17, 23.9%); escape from reality/therapeutic purposes (15, 21.1%); adventure (9, 12.6%); and being informed (1.7%). Both reading as a way of learning, and reading for therapeutic purposes or to escape from a reality that at that time was still very hard (full confinement due to the COVID-19 pandemic), have increased their response percentages very significantly. poured by students.

All these results show that, after the intervention carried out in the second phase, the students began to dedicate more free time to reading, including it among the 5 activities that they most frequently carried out in this period of confinement and both these readings and those derived from the The interventions carried out are considered by the students as very therapeutic and comforting. Likewise, it has also been seen how the effect of these academic readings has also led to an increase in the number of students who have gone on to read novels and comics, in preference to digital reading. It is true that this may also be due to the presence of digital fatigue that was suffered in this period, where the dependence on screens meant that in the last moments of confinement, people decided to carry out other types of activities that did not involve the use of screens; but it can be affirmed that this increase is mainly caused by the proposal carried out with the students, since otherwise, said students could have derived in other types of actions that were not reading, and that is not verified in the results of the first question of the questionnaire (Table 2). For all these reasons, we come to the conclusion that reading, well proposed and with actions that lead to its rediscovery, is an excellent resource not only in improving student learning, but also as a therapeutic resource in a situation that generates stress and anxiety such as the confinement suffered.

SOLUTIONS AND RECOMMENDATIONS

It is necessary to activate proposals and actions that promote reading in all educational stages, and this must be promoted from initiatives that are motivating and close to students, and always more from contagion than from imposition. Only by reaching students in this way will a positive attitude towards reading prevail, compared to the great competitor represented by the consumption of digital audiovisual content, social networks or recreational elements such as online games. Reading does not understand ages or areas or subjects of knowledge. In other words, reading can and should be encouraged at any age and from any subject of knowledge. Reading has the exceptional advantage that, for its consumption, it is not essential to have a screen, since the printed text can be counted on. Faced with a situation such as the one experienced throughout the world with home confinement, between March and June 2020 at least in Spain, and which gave rise to a dependency and need to consume digital resources, both for leisure and to continue with the processes of teaching-learning in the educational world; There have been many difficulties experienced and those that have had to be faced. The most important has been the one that has affected people's mental health, and here it has been seen how the secondary school students participating in this research have been able to find in reading, first academically and then in reading that has been done in his free time, an excellent therapeutic resource that has allowed him to escape from the harsh reality and reconcile his academic and family life without too many problems. Reading and writing literature have also been proven in other studies (Acim, 2021; Dera, 2021; Sharma, 2021), which has been a healing therapy in this confinement. Although during confinement, there has been an increase in digital reading (Vyas & Tandel, 2020), being able to count on printed text (books, comics, magazines and newspapers) has also been a considerable advantage in being able to deal with the digital fatigue that began to appear in the final moments of confinement. People, and students and teachers in particular, suffered from this digital fatigue, after several months in which the means to follow the normal development of teaching-learning processes was none other than the use of screens and technological devices, which, after so many hours of exposure,

For all these reasons, reading, whether digital or printed, should be considered an excellent resource that fosters an increase in interest and motivation to want to learn, and therefore, thus becomes an excellent didactic resource. But at the same time, as has been seen here, it is an excellent therapeutic resource, which manages to immerse the reader in other worlds, being able to live adventures, realities and situations that can go beyond the most immediate reality and with it, allow that the person can avoid real situations or experiences that may be harmful to their mental health, as is also recommended in other studies (Singh et al., 2020). And in this way, avoid reading texts and news that provide information about the pandemic or the difficult situations experienced, because they only bring greater stress and anxiety (Gunawan et al., 2020; Magson et al., 2021). Didactic proposals must be established in which reading is treated at any age, from any area of knowledge, and with a multitude and variety of activities that encourage its implementation beyond academic time, encouraging that, in their free time, the students also use it for these same purposes. It is sad to see how sometimes, and when careful and continuous use of reading is not made among the students, when a student is asked to read aloud, it is verified that said student reads frankly badly for not having maintained a taste for reading and continuity in reading throughout their training. This also requires that educational centers, of any stage and specialty, they must implement a careful and effective quality reading plan, which goes beyond reading work with the students only from the language areas, and also goes beyond checking if they read academic texts or other types of texts, as well as verifying it orally. Collective readings, reading aloud in class, analysis and oral approaches in class should be considered, since reading, beyond improving and increasing the lexicon, also promotes good diction, in addition to comprehension and expression, both oral and written. In these proposals, there is also room for digital resources and tools, which, as always, can favor and improve interest in reading, since these devices and resources alone motivate their use. But always, from the attentive look of making good use of said devices, a use that does not reach the situation of an addiction to them, or a rejection or fatigue when abusive and continued use of these is made. At present, a problem is also being found in those augmented reality mobile applications, applications made with the good intention of serving and bringing reading closer to people with some type of visual or hearing impairment, but in the hands of people without any disability. They can be counterproductive for a good development of reading skills.

It is also advisable to work towards a culture where reading is promoted from families, from a family environment in which reading and shared readings between parents and children are given importance (Vuong et al., 2021). In this way, reading is also encouraged beyond being for academic or learning purposes, and getting closer to being considered by the student as a resource that empowers him and allows him to continue growing as a person. Self-esteem is also favored, and as this research has already shown, good mental health.

FUTURE RESEARCH DIRECTIONS

Given the results obtained in this research and the ideas obtained from its analysis, it is necessary to continue working in this line of designing, creating and putting into practice proposals to promote reading, both academic and recreational, both digital and printed text, and that they are from any age and subject of knowledge. As has been justified and argued, this must be done while contemplated in the center's reading plan, and where said plan is not the exclusive task of only the language areas, but of all the areas of the student's curriculum. These proposals must also contemplate numerous and varied activities, which are linked and contextualized with the realities of the students, so that in this way they are not alien to them and encourage the taste for reading to spread. Activities that pursue more the analysis of whether there is a development of reading competence, comprehension and expression, both oral and written. They must be activities that encourage the student reader to want to continue being readers, and not as sometimes happens, that this type of activity and also the proposed readings, achieve the opposite effect to the desired one, that the students abandon their reading habits, end up hating the reading and look for mechanisms and strategies to cheat academically tests or activities that seek to verify if it is being read and that it is being understood from said reading.

It is also intended to analyze the reading plans of various educational centers and of a specific educational stage, which could well be secondary, since it is the one that has the most possibilities of neglecting the development of the student's reading competence.

Likewise, and whether with or without a pandemic, the healing and therapeutic role that reading can have beyond experiencing difficult situations such as the one experienced with confinement by COVID-19 should continue to be analyzed and verified. Thus, we must continue investigating the sensations and perceptions of reading students, be it in any context, reality, type of reading, etc.

And finally, an important field of research is also opened in digital reading compared to reading printed text, since it remains to be seen whether the levels of comprehension of one are better than those of the other and if this is enough to justify one opposite. to the other, knowing that digital reading, by requiring technology, makes it more attractive to students.

CONCLUSION

At this point, as has been seen, in situations of stress and anxiety in adolescents who live under the pressure of home confinement, reading, although it is not initially found as an activity among those preferred by them; Well directed and motivated, it can be an excellent resource not only for improvement and interest in learning, but also as an outlet and refuge from dramatic and disconcerting situations. It has been found that thanks to reading proposals that are motivating for students, it is possible to increase the time they dedicate to reading in their leisure or free time, as well as the approach to printed text, whether novels or comics.

For this reason, whether in situations of stress or without it, we should continue betting on proposals to promote reading among our students of any subject and stage, and do it in an integrated way, from the coordination of the entire teaching team of an educational center, and taking into account that they must be proposals contextualized and attractive to the interests, motivations and realities of the students. Only in this way will positive results be achieved that allow us to continue caring for our students' reading skills.

REFERENCES

Acim, R. (2021). Lockdown poetry, healing and the COVID-19 pandemic. *Journal of Poetry Therapy, 34*(2), 67–76. doi:10.1080/08893675.2021.1899629

Ardington, C., Wills, G., & Kotze, J. (2021). COVID-19 learning losses: Early grade reading in South Africa. *International Journal of Educational Development, 86*, 102480. doi:10.1016/j.ijedudev.2021.102480

Aziz, R., Susanto, D., Safitri, S. I., Mazida, L. I., & Wijaya, T. (2021). Literacy learning problems: Developing the character of reading fondness in elementary school students during the covid-19. *Premiere Educandum: Jurnal Pendidikan Dasar dan Pembelajaran, 11*(2), 243-253. doi:10.25273/pe.v11i2.10221

Baker, S. (2018). Shifts in the treatment of knowledge in academic reading and writing: Adding complexity to students' transitions between A-levels and university in the UK. *Arts and Humanities in Higher Education, 17*(4), 388–409. doi:10.1177/1474022217722433

Bao, X., Qu, H., Zhang, R., & Hogan, T. P. (2020). *Literacy loss in kindergarten children during COVID-19 school closures*. Academic Press.

Baron, N. S. (2017). Reading in a digital age. *Phi Delta Kappan, 99*(2), 15–20. doi:10.1177/0031721717734184

Broemmel, A. D., Rearden, K. T., & Buckner, C. (2021). Teachers' choices: Are they the right books for science instruction? *The Reading Teacher, 75*(1), 7–16. doi:10.1002/trtr.1998

Clark, A. E., Nong, H., Zhu, H., & Zhu, R. (2021). Compensating for academic loss: Online learning and student performance during the COVID-19 pandemic. *China Economic Review, 68*, 101629. doi:10.1016/j.chieco.2021.101629

Conecta. (2020). *La lectura en tiempos de COVID-19*. https://www.editoresmadrid.org/wp-content/uploads/2020/05/LA-LECTURA-EN-TIEMPOS-DE-COVID-19.pdf

De Naeghel, J., Van Keer, H., Vansteenkiste, M., & Rosseel, Y. (2012). The relation between elementary students' recreational and academic reading motivation, reading frequency, engagement, and comprehension: A self-determination theory perspective. *Journal of Educational Psychology, 104*(4), 1006–1021. doi:10.1037/a0027800

Dera, J. (2021). Evaluating poetry on COVID-19: Attitudes of poetry readers toward corona poems. *Journal of Poetry Therapy, 34*(2), 77–94. doi:10.1080/08893675.2021.1899630

ERI-Lectura. (2020). *Hábitos lectores durante el confinamiento por la covid-19.* https://roderic.uv.es/handle/10550/74797

Freeman, C., Mack, T., & Collins, T. (2022, January). Oral Presentation: Intersections: Reading STEM in Tennessee Elementary Schools. *16th Annual Tennessee STEM Education Research Conference*, 36.

Fundación, S. M. (2021). *Anuario Iberoamericano sobre el Libro Infantil y Juvenil 2021*. Fundación SM. shorturl.at/ckmBF

Gunawan, J., Juthamanee, S., & Aungsuroch, Y. (2020). Current mental health issues in the era of Covid-19. *Asian Journal of Psychiatry*, *51*, 102103. doi:10.1016/j.ajp.2020.102103 PMID:32361675

Guo, J. (2021). The Analysis of the Status Quo and Promotion Strategies of Mathematical Reading of Lower Grade Students. *Science Insights Education Frontiers*, *10*(S1), 24. doi:10.15354ief.21.s1.ab054

Kaufman, G., & Flanagan, M. (2016). High-low split: Divergent cognitive construal levels triggered by digital and nondigital platforms. In *Proceedings of the 2016 CHI Conference on Human Factors in Computing Systems* (pp. 2773-2777). ACM. 10.1145/2858036.2858550

Keck, D., Kammerer, Y., & Starauschek, E. (2015). Reading science texts online: Does source information influence the identification of contradictions within texts? *Computers & Education*, *82*, 442–449. doi:10.1016/j.compedu.2014.12.005

Kurata, K., Ishita, E., Miyata, Y., & Minami, Y. (2017). Print or digital? Reading behavior and preferences in Japan. *Journal of the Association for Information Science and Technology*, *68*(4), 884–894. doi:10.1002/asi.23712

Lewis, K., Kuhfeld, M., Ruzek, E., & McEachin, A. (2021). *Learning during COVID-19: Reading and math achievement in the 2020-21 school year.* Center for School and Student Progress. https://www.nwea.org/research/publication/learning-duringcovid-19-reading-and-math-achievement-in-the-2020-2021-school-year

Locke, V. N., Patarapichayatham, C., & Lewis, S. (2021). *Learning Loss in Reading and Math in US Schools Due to the COVID-19 Pandemic*. Academic Press.

Magson, N. R., Freeman, J. Y., Rapee, R. M., Richardson, C. E., Oar, E. L., & Fardouly, J. (2021). Risk and protective factors for prospective changes in adolescent mental health during the COVID-19 pandemic. *Journal of Youth and Adolescence*, *50*(1), 44–57. doi:10.100710964-020-01332-9 PMID:33108542

Maldonado, J. E., & De Witte, K. (2022). The effect of school closures on standardised student test outcomes. *British Educational Research Journal*, *48*(1), 49–94. doi:10.1002/berj.3754

Mangen, A., Walgermo, B. R., & Brønnick, K. (2013). Reading linear texts on paper versus computer screen: Effects on reading comprehension. *International Journal of Educational Research*, *58*, 61–68. doi:10.1016/j.ijer.2012.12.002

Mawyer, K. K., & Johnson, H. J. (2019). Eliciting preservice teachers' reading strategies through structured literacy activities. *Journal of Science Teacher Education*, *30*(6), 583–600. doi:10.1080/1046560X.2019.1589848

Morales, M. (2021, February 26). El confinamiento llevó a un máximo histórico el índice de lectura entre los españoles. *El País*. https://elpais.com/cultura/2021-02-26/el-confinamiento-llevo-a-un-maximo-historico-el-indice-de-lectura-entre-los-espanoles.html

Norris, S. P., Falk, H., Federico-Agraso, M., Jiménez-Aleixandre, M. P., Phillips, L. M., & Yarden, A. (2009). Reading science texts—epistemology, inquiry, authenticity—a rejoinder to Jonathan Osborne. *Research in Science Education*, *39*(3), 405–410. doi:10.100711165-008-9118-5

OECD. (2021). *OECD Skills Outlook 2021: Learning for Life*. OECD Publishing. doi:10.1787/0ae365b4-

Pardede, P. (2019). Print vs Digital Reading Comprehension in EFL. *Journal of English Teaching*, *5*(2), 77–90. doi:10.33541/jet.v5i2.1059

Petscher, Y., Cabell, S. Q., Catts, H. W., Compton, D. L., Foorman, B. R., Hart, S. A., Lonigan, C. J., Phillips, B. M., Schatschneider, C., Steacy, L. M., Terry, N. P., & Wagner, R. K. (2020). How the science of reading informs 21st-century education. *Reading Research Quarterly*, *55*(1), S267–S282. doi:10.1002/rrq.352 PMID:34007089

Reimer, D., Smith, E., Andersen, I. G., & Sortkær, B. (2021). What happens when schools shut down? Investigating inequality in students' reading behavior during Covid-19 in Denmark. *Research in Social Stratification and Mobility*, *71*, 100568. doi:10.1016/j.rssm.2020.100568

Roldán, L. Á. (2019). Reading, understanding and learning in secondary education: Approaches and perspectives. *Psicologia USP*, *30*. Advance online publication. doi:10.1590/0103-6564e20180126

Ruiz-Bejarano, A. M. (2019). Del placer de la lectura al deseo de leer: el aprendizaje del buen lector. *Revista complutense de educación*, *30*(3), 863-878. doi:10.5209/rced.59489

Santos, S. C. (2019). Art of Questioning (Aq): A Tool in Improving the Reading Comprehension of the BSED-1 Majors in English and Science at Holy Child Jesus College. *Ascendens Asia Journal of Multidisciplinary Research Abstracts*, *3*(8).

Schult, J., Mahler, N., Fauth, B., & Lindner, M. A. (2021). Did students learn less during the COVID-19 pandemic? reading and mathematics competencies before and after the first pandemic wave. doi:10.31234/osf.io/pqtgfosf.io/pqtgf

Sharma, D. (2021). Reading and rewriting poetry on life to survive the COVID-19 pandemic. *Journal of Poetry Therapy*, *34*(2), 95–108. doi:10.1080/08893675.2021.1899631

Singer, L. M., & Alexander, P. A. (2017). Reading across mediums: Effects of reading digital and print texts on comprehension and calibration. *Journal of Experimental Education*, *85*(1), 155–172. doi:10.1080/00220973.2016.1143794

Singh, S., Roy, D., Sinha, K., Parveen, S., Sharma, G., & Joshi, G. (2020). Impact of COVID-19 and lockdown on mental health of children and adolescents: A narrative review with recommendations. *Psychiatry Research*, *293*, 113429. doi:10.1016/j.psychres.2020.113429 PMID:32882598

Sun, B., Loh, C. E., & Nie, Y. (2021). The COVID-19 school closure effect on students' print and digital leisure reading. *Computers and Education Open*, *2*, 100033. doi:10.1016/j.caeo.2021.100033

Tomasik, M. J., Helbling, L. A., & Moser, U. (2021). Educational gains of in-person vs. distance learning in primary and secondary schools: A natural experiment during the COVID-19 pandemic school closures in Switzerland. *International Journal of Psychology*, *56*(4), 566–576. doi:10.1002/ijop.12728 PMID:33236341

Vinterek, M., Winberg, M., Tegmark, M., Alatalo, T., & Liberg, C. (2022). The Decrease of School Related Reading in Swedish Compulsory School–Trends Between 2007 and 2017. *Scandinavian Journal of Educational Research*, *66*(1), 119–133. doi:10.1080/00313831.2020.1833247

Vuong, Q. H., La, V. P., Nguyen, T. H. T., Nguyen, M. H., Vuong, T. T., Vuong, H. M., & Ho, M. T. (2021). Impacts of parents and reading promotion on creating a reading culture: Evidence from a developing context. *Children and Youth Services Review*, *131*, 106311. doi:10.1016/j.childyouth.2021.106311

Vyas, P., & Tandel, B. (2020). The impact of lockdown due to Covid-19 in 2020 on reading habits of academic staff of state open universities: a study. *The Journal of Higher Education*, *12*(1), 28–37. doi:10.37867/TE120104

Wilson-Lopez, A., & Gregory, S. (2015). Integrating literacy and engineering instruction for young learners. *The Reading Teacher*, *69*(1), 25–33. doi:10.1002/trtr.1351

Zhu, Y. (2021). Reading matters more than mathematics in science learning: An analysis of the relationship between student achievement in reading, mathematics, and science. *International Journal of Science Education*, *44*(1), 1–17. doi:10.1080/09500693.2021.2007552

Chapter 15
Challenging Picturebooks and Domestic Geographies:
A Multimodal Learning Path to Discuss the Consequences of the COVID-19 Lockdowns in the Classroom

Margarida Castellano Sanz
Universitat de València, Spain

ABSTRACT

The COVID-19 pandemic has brought new ways of facing the world and its multiple realities. Picturebooks, as a crossover genre, help in the process of understanding new contexts while offering literature as therapy. The new challenges of the 21st century require the implementation of methodologies that focus both on words and on other modes of representation to construct knowledge, and to this end, literacy education through challenging picturebooks involves paying attention to the diverse pedagogical demands of a global, aesthetic, and multimodal world. This chapter supports the notion of visual literacy as a multi-dimensional concept and proposes the approach to different picturebooks dealing with neighbours and neighbourhoods through the pedagogy of the multiliteracies, in order to enhance the transformation of the self and the global and local understanding of the current world. A learning path for teachers is designed according to the four knowledge processes: experiencing, conceptualizing, analyzing, and applying.

INTRODUCTION

The main goal of this chapter lies in the introduction of challenging picturebooks as a resource to talk with both young and also experienced readers about the SARS-Co V-2 pandemic and its consequences upon mental health. As Verònica Orazi (2022) stated, the spreading of Covid-19 has not only brought restrictions in people's daily lives, social interactions, leisure activities and ways of working, but also psychological implications, which is a type of repercussion less evident than others (Brooks, Webster, Smith et al., 2020). More than two years after the first lockdown in southern Europe (March 2020), the

DOI: 10.4018/978-1-6684-4735-2.ch015

pandemic still demands concern and interventions in various spheres of everyday life, such as supporting people in quarantine to cope with isolation, confinement, new liquid realities and other limitations (Brooks, Webster, Smith et al., 2020). Through the interpretation of different multimodal texts, mainly around visual literacy and picturebooks, this chapter offers a learning path based on the Pedagogy of the Multiliteracies for teachers to guide students to discuss the implications of the lockdown and the pandemic in their everyday lives. In this sense, we are approaching this crossover genre (Beckett, 2012) with a twofold goal: on the one hand, analyzing the different possibilities for the transformation of the self and, on the other hand, reading aesthetic images and other multimodal texts to help the reader understand an uncommon situation. The main interest of this learning path is to share readings that help children dealing with ambivalent emotions and behavior (Ommundsen, 2022), as well as offering texts upon which readers are left restless and questioning their reality, as a way to acquire knowledge about ambiguity and polysemy in art and life (Bajour, 2009).

Decoding the world through images becomes an important literacy project. Marnie Campagnaro states that children live immerse in images: "They grow up interacting with images and visual screens long before they learn to read. In toddlers, visual precedes verbal alphabetization" (2022, p. 79). In fact, children recognize the world and its daily objects before they can name them, so "if this awareness is combined with a literary, iconographic, aesthetic, and sociocultural expertise, this way of gaining knowledge in childhood can generate effective educational outcomes" (Campagnaro, 2022, p. 79). Our questions here are: what does it happen when the situation is so unfamiliar, such as during the lockdown periods in 2020? How does children literature help coping with awkward contexts? How do literature and the reading of picturebooks help expressing feelings? How has the physiognomy of neighborhoods been affected by the pandemic?

CHALLENGING PICTUREBOOKS FOR A CHANGING WORLD

Since Janet Evans edited the collection *Challenging and Controversial Picturebooks* in 2015, the term 'challenging picturebooks' has been widely discussed. Maria Nikolajeva (2014) states that "[c]omplex picturebooks are beneficial for young readers' cognitive-affective development because they offer the brain something to work on (p.214; see also Kümmerling-Meibauer and Ommundsen, 2022). In fact, reading different kinds of picturebooks enables young readers to develop a sophisticated visual competence and aesthetic literacy, as several recent studies show (Arizpe and Style, 2003; Beckett, 2018; Campagnaro and Dallari, 2013; Kümmerling-Meibauer, 2014; Druker and Kümmerling-Meiebauer, 2015; Evans, 2015). Also, regarding experienced readers may find interesting facing challenging picturebooks, since some of the aspects of this genre is that they can be "highly sophisticated, in cognitive, aesthetic, and critical terms" (Farrar et al., 2022, p.46). So that, challenging picturebooks can be seen challenging in terms of:

1. A scholastic challenge, regarding expectations about literacy through the form, format and modalities employed traditionally in this genre.
2. A connection with emotionally demanding themes or topics.

For this reason, picturebooks read for the sake of reflecting personal and collective experiences during the lockdown can also been considered challenging: because they assume an introspection in what we understand to be our immediate reality (our house, our neighbours, our habits) and, also, different abstract feelings (the fear, the loneliness, the confusion, the bewilderment, etc.). Orazi describes the swift in the perception of time and space after the Coronavirus pandemic and the subsequent lockdowns: "whereas previously there was an outdoor space and an indoor space, during quarantine the circumstances changed, and the individual found himself living in a single space" (2022, p.1). To understand this mono-space in which individuals were confined and to reflect upon the different stages of the different lockdowns becomes a challenge for teachers, which may find in the multimodal texts offered in this chapter useful resources.

What is it about the challenge provided by such texts, then? As Farrar, Arizpe and McAdam state "It can be seen as reflective of many of the concerns and themes that are characteristic of directions in contemporary literacy theory" (2022, p.43). In this sense, challenging picturebooks help putting together the pieces of a puzzle, which represents multimodality in the 21st century. The nature and diversities of contemporary picturebooks act as 'training fields' (Nikolajeva, 2014, p.94) for the multiliteracies that are now a key feature of communication in current societies (New London Group, 1996).

LITERACY AND ITS DIMENSIONS

A main feature of nowadays literacy is that it is multidimensional. Paesani et al. state "one becomes literate. Literacy is a process, not a product" (2016, p.12). In this sense, Kern (2000) and Kucer (2014) talk about the three dimensions of literacy: the cognitive, the conceptual and the sociocultural, which are complementary and distributed in an equity ratio.

- The cognitive or personal dimension is involved with identity, values, attitudes and previous knowledge (Kucer, 2014). Kern (2000) emphasises that literacy is a reflective process in which written words, visual texts and context elements are linked by the readers' previous knowledge and their sociocultural context. Readers become meaning-makers, since their task is to create and link, not just acquiring passively the knowledge (Reyes-Torres and Portalés-Raga, 2020). As a consequence, the learning path proposed has as main objective to connect readers with their cognitive strategies through the analyses of a multimodal text and, in this way, to start the process of creation of meaning, by using previous knowledge and self experiences.

- Conceptual or linguistic dimension, according to Kucer (2015, p.4): "focuses on the multimodal communication systems [...] through which meaning is conveyed". Readers identify, learn and use the text's features and symbols to create new meanings. In this sense, the selection criteria of multimodal texts is of utmost importance.

The sociocultural and aesthetic dimension focuses on the text and the reader's cultural context. The reason for this double focalization (text-reader) is to offer readers the opportunity to interpret whatever multimodal source and to exchange points of view in a discussion with other readers. This dimension takes into account "the social identities and how various groups use literacy to negotiate and critique their transactions with the world" (Kucer, 2015, p.4). It implies providing the readers/students with opportunities to interact, discuss and accepting different points of view.

To sum up, these three dimensions show that the process of meaning making does not depend solely on cognitive elements, but also on conceptual and sociocultural. This is the reason why reading the picturebooks selected for this learning path has a very different response depending upon the personal experiences during the lockdown. In other words: in the process of decoding the selected picturebooks, what the reader understands, how the reader transmits the significance and how the reader interacts with it, is mediated by the cognitive, the conceptual and the sociocultural dimensions of the multiliteracy (Reyes-Torres and García Perera, 2022).

THE PEDAGOGY OF THE MULTILITERACIES

Recent researches such as the ones by Kern (2000), Westby (2010), Cope and Kalantzis (2015) or Reyes-Torres, Portalés-Raga and Torres (2021) point out that the meaning of literacy has changed over the last decades and it is no longer used exclusively to describe the ability to decode and encode written language. Nowadays, literacy is a multidimensional, dynamic process that integrates the comprehension and the production of a wide variety of texts, which help creating and/or transforming knowledge (Kucer, 2014; Serafini, 2014; Paesani et al., 2016; Warner and Dupuy, 2018). The development of multimodal theories (Kress and Van Leeuwen, 2001) has helped to shift awareness of the range of available representational modes and processes away from the traditional, towards a far broader range that includes visual, gestural, and speech (Farrar et al., 2022). As a result of this shift in the concept of literacy and the growing interest in the process of meaning-making, in 1996 the New London Group (NLG) named this new concept after *Multiliteracies.* Their goal was to establish:

A more contemporary view of literacy that reflect multiple communication forms and a context of cultural and linguistic diversity within a globalized society. Thus, multiliteracies was defined as the multiple ways of communicating and making meaning, including such modes as visual, audio, spatial, behavioral, and gestural (Pilgrim and Martínez, 2013, p.62).

Taking into account the saturation of images we are faced to in the current world, NLG was interested in mediating the process of creation of knowledge and the guidelines to the acquisition of multiliteracies. The *Meaning Design* and the *Knowledge Processes Framework* (1.Experiencing; 2.Conceptualizing; 3.Analysing and 4.Applying) are key concepts for the Pedagogy of the Multiliteracies. These processes constitute 4 pedagogical actions that serve as a guide for teachers to develop learners' literacy without any linear hierarchy or sequence, as "elements of each of these pedagogical acts may occur at any time during the learning process" (NLG, 1996, p.85):

- Experiencing engages learners in meaningful lessons that incorporate both spontaneous reflection and lived experiences. This allows them to immerse themselves in the text. Learning activities should initially be grounded in questions and tasks that are meaningful to students.
- Conceptualizing draws students' attention towards specific concepts and explicit instructions on how form produces meaning. The goal is to enable learners to gain conscious or metacognitive awareness and control over what they are learning and prepare them for competent participation.
- Analyzing aims to reflect on the author's writing, discuss any given message from another perspective and how it might relate to particular cultures, social contexts and/or ideologies (Reyes-Torres and Portalés-Raga, 2020). Students must recognize how the social/cultural context influences the selection of particular text and how these factors influence comprehension in designing.
- Applying allows learners to elaborate their own interpretations based on what they have learned. According to Cope and Kalantzis (2015, p.32), "knowledge is not (just) the stuff that ends up in our minds. It is what we do and make. Learning is a consequence of a series of knowledge ac-

tions." In essence, it is the transfer of new knowledge to other situations and the production of new designs.

A New Pedagogical Approach Based on Multimodality

The vast majority of texts young readers face currently can be considered multimodal, since they are composed by symbols and signals to facilitate its comprehension: graphics, diverse typographies, illustrations, pictures, colours, information hierarchy, etc. Readers live and learn in a multimodal environment that demands and advances visual and verbal literacies and social competences (Arizpe and Styles, 2016; Kümmerling-Meibauer et al., 2015; Mackey, 2002). Reading together multimodal texts and paying attention to the stories and images can be seen as the most effective way to become active listeners, which is a prerequisite to becoming a good reader and an active citizen (Arizpe et al., 2018; Serafini, 2014; Torr, 2008; Jewitt, 2008; Kress, 2003).

Much has been written about the powerful relationship between words and images in picturebooks (Nodelman, 1999; Nikolajeva and Scott, 2000; Salisbury, 2005; Van der Linden, 2007; Salisbury and Styles, 2012; Beckett, 2012; Ramos, 2017), to end up confirming that picturebooks require their readers to think multimodal by extracting and assembling meaning from both words and pictures (Nikolajeva, 2003; Farrar et al., 2022), rather than "assuming the pictures to be in the service of the words" (Lewis, 1990, p.141). This idea may confront traditional approaches to picturebooks, schooled into privileging words over images (Meek, 1988; Millard and Marsh, 2001; Farrar et al., 2022). By reading together the interaction between text and image (2015) and by situating them socially and culturally, the reader delves into challenging picturebooks' practices that support a critical pedagogy of multiliteracies.

In the learning path proposal described in the following section, we will show how reading and decoding picturebooks dealing with neighbours and neighbourhoods may help managing pandemic isolation and open new possibilities for the transformation of the self. Understanding literature as therapy also helps in the acquisition of personal and social skills, as well as the acquisition of a broad linguistic knowledge (Menke and Paesani, 2019).

In this sense, a learning path based on the Pedagogy of the Multiliteracies (NLG, 1996) combined with Paesani's reading stages (2016) has been designed and put into practice with 1st year pre-service teachers from the Universitat de València and the Universidade de Aveiro during the academic year 2021-2022. The main goal of the learning path was to offer a guide to future teachers on how picturebooks help children into becoming competent and confident readers (Ommundsen, 2022) while also challenging picturebooks may help them coping with uncommon situations. Specifically, the learning path offers diverse multimodal texts that can be analysed under the perspective of personal and social implications during the lockdown periods. Since the learning path was conceived for primary or high-school students, with minor adaptations, the applying stage designed is related with the elaboration of a new picturebook entiled "My neighbourhood" and based on basic linguistic skills together with the creation of creative characters.

All in all, we present with this chapter a learning path starting in an emblematic *topos* in children's literature: the home; a domestic scenario that has acquired a different meaning after the pandemic and its different lockdowns. A mono-space, as revised by Orazi (2022), where life ran also in a mono-time, where all neighbours were connected by same kind of experiences. The aim of the learning path is to analyze the domestic geographies, starting from the private domains and amplifying to complete neighbourhoods, as spaces of personal characterization and psychological, social and cultural evolution:

The home is intended primarily as a physical place where the family comes together, and where the protagonists' primary needs are generally met. The home is also a place of memories and knowledge acquisition. It is capable of revealing the attitudes of the characters, their lifestyles, translating them into words and images. The home can reveal the quality of human relations within its walls and outside the family circle (Campagnaro, 2019, p.9).

The selection criteria of picturebooks chosen to design the learning path are divided into primary sources and secondary ones. As a primary source, our proposal is to analyse *Neighbors* by Kasya Denisevich (2020), in terms of visual literacy and its poetics of displacement. As secondary sources we propose the following picturebooks: *Chez moi, chez toi* by Marianne Dubuc (2020); *Gràcies. Història d'un veïnat*, by Rocío Bonilla (2021), and *The Neighbours* by Einat Tsafarti (2017). Other picturebooks worth mentioning that have also ben taken into account and which offer an exquisite multiliteracies' knowledge are *Tão, tão grande* by Catarina Sobral (2016) - a revision of Kafka's *Metamorphoses* through the personal changes taking place inside the protagonist's room-; *Malacatú* by María Pascual de la Torre (2018) - a linguistic *divertimento* set on a domestic ordinary context and dealing with everyday's hygienic habits-; *Ma maison* by Läetitia Bourget and Alice Gravier (2018) - an accordion-style book which shows the protagonist's path from the forest to his/her home, which let students talk about the need of nature in our lives-; *Outside In* by Deborah Underwood (2020) - written with an exquisite lyrical language, a celebration of nature which is also a stirring invitation to find the wonder that awaits us all- and, when dealing with intercultural understanding, the artwork Madlenka, by Peter Sís (2000) - a contemporary classic and an approach to differences and similarities among cultures living together in a same place-. The main goal was offering different graphic books, rich in themes and formats, which contained nowadays' personal journeys, geographical journeys, spatial journeys, intercultural journeys and chronological journeys, under the same topic. In Figure 1 we can observe the different covers' illustrations, which act as paratexts (Genette 1987) regarding the pre-information given. The analyses of these covers by means of a process of exploratory observation and descriptive strategies referred as *slow looking* (Tishman, 2018, p.8) is essential to create a learning context in which students are willing to participate, look carefully, develop opinions, express themselves and consider multiple viewpoints (Reyes-Torres and Portalés-Raga, 2020, p.104).

Figure 1. Picturebooks analyzed in the Learning path

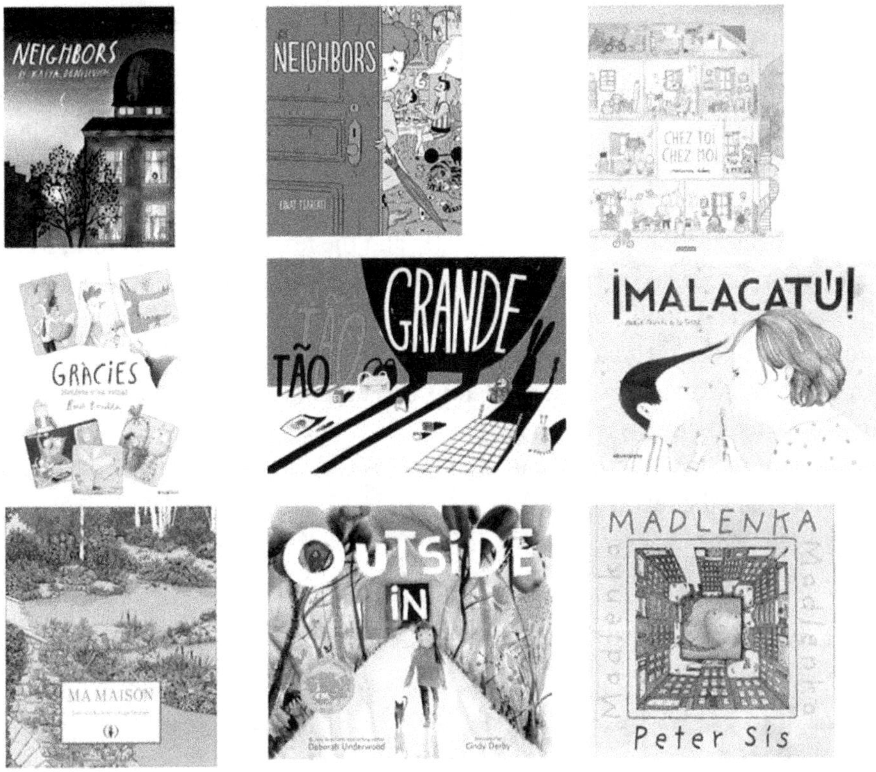

The Pedagogy of the Multiliteracies helps organising didactic sequences based on an interdisciplinary and a communicative approach. Taking these elements into account, the specific goals of the learning path presented were:

1. To offer an innovative methodology to deal with the reading of picturebooks, which can stimulate a rich discussion on a specific topic. In this case, the covid-19 pandemic, the cartographies of home and the lockdown.
2. To guide readers to construct meaning through the implementation of the four-knowledge processes framework: experiencing, conceptualizing, analyzing and applying.
3. To analyze the process of meaning-making while promoting reading, observation, discussion, reflection and critical thinking, as a way to release previously untapped thoughts and emotions.
4. To connect the actions described with personal experiences during the lockdown and using them to create new knowledge, through the elaboration of a new picturebook.

As will be shown, the resources selected fulfil the goals stated and confer special attention to the process of autonomous meaning making, personal interest and the responding to texts based on reader-based theories.

Reader-based Theories: Decoding Picturebooks

Two of the most influential researchers in reader-based theories are Louise Rosenblatt and Wolfgang Iser. Rosenblatt, very much influenced by Dewey, explored the relationship between the reader and the text and noted that "a novel or poem or play remains merely ink spots on paper until the reader transforms them into a set of meaningful symbols" (1938, p.25). It is the reader, therefore, who brings background information, previous experience, and a whole range of sociocultural issues to the text (Evans, 2016). Rosenblatt described this type of interaction as "transaction" and the term "reader response theory" was used to describe these interactions between the reader and the text. In her later work, Rosenblatt stated: "The relation between reader and text is not linear. It is a situation, an event at a particular time and place in which each element conditions the other" (1978, p.16). In relation with this, Iser saw reading as an interaction between the text and the active reader (Evans, 2016, p.55), due to the gaps or 'indeterminacies' in a text: no text can describe all details and authors frequently leave things unsaid - often deliberately in picturebooks, Evans adds.

In looking at the way readers respond to picturebooks, Evans (1998) depicted the relationship between the author, the reader, and the text (Figure 2).

Figure 2. The relationship between the author, the reader, and the text (Evans 1998, xv).

Reader's previous experience, textual knowledge and sociocultural background
Reader response: reader's ability to interact with and respond to text
Polysemic nature of the text to include intertextuality and 'gap'.

Bearing this scheme in mind, the learning path offers classroom situations to link the texts selected with personal experiences and actual opportunities to discuss and share those experiences.

In Figure 3 below, we present a template to design the lesson plan by establishing the contents (linguistic, artistic and sociocultural) together with the aims for each pedagogical act, the type of tasks, and the characteristics of the resources that work well for each stage. As already mentioned, in this case the process of meaning making focuses on the topic of the confinement and the students' memories. That is what we refer to as the *critical axis*: the lockdown, its implications and the possibilities for the transformation of the self. Other key factors that are important in order to design the learning path are being acquainted with the linguistic and cognitive level of the students, the number of participants and the timing of the class period.

Regarding the learning contents, these are related with these 3 dimensions of literacy:

- the linguistic aspects
- the sociocultural interaction that takes place
- the artistic engagement through the decoding of the text and the images.

Figure 3. Template using the KPF combined with Paesani's Reading Stages.

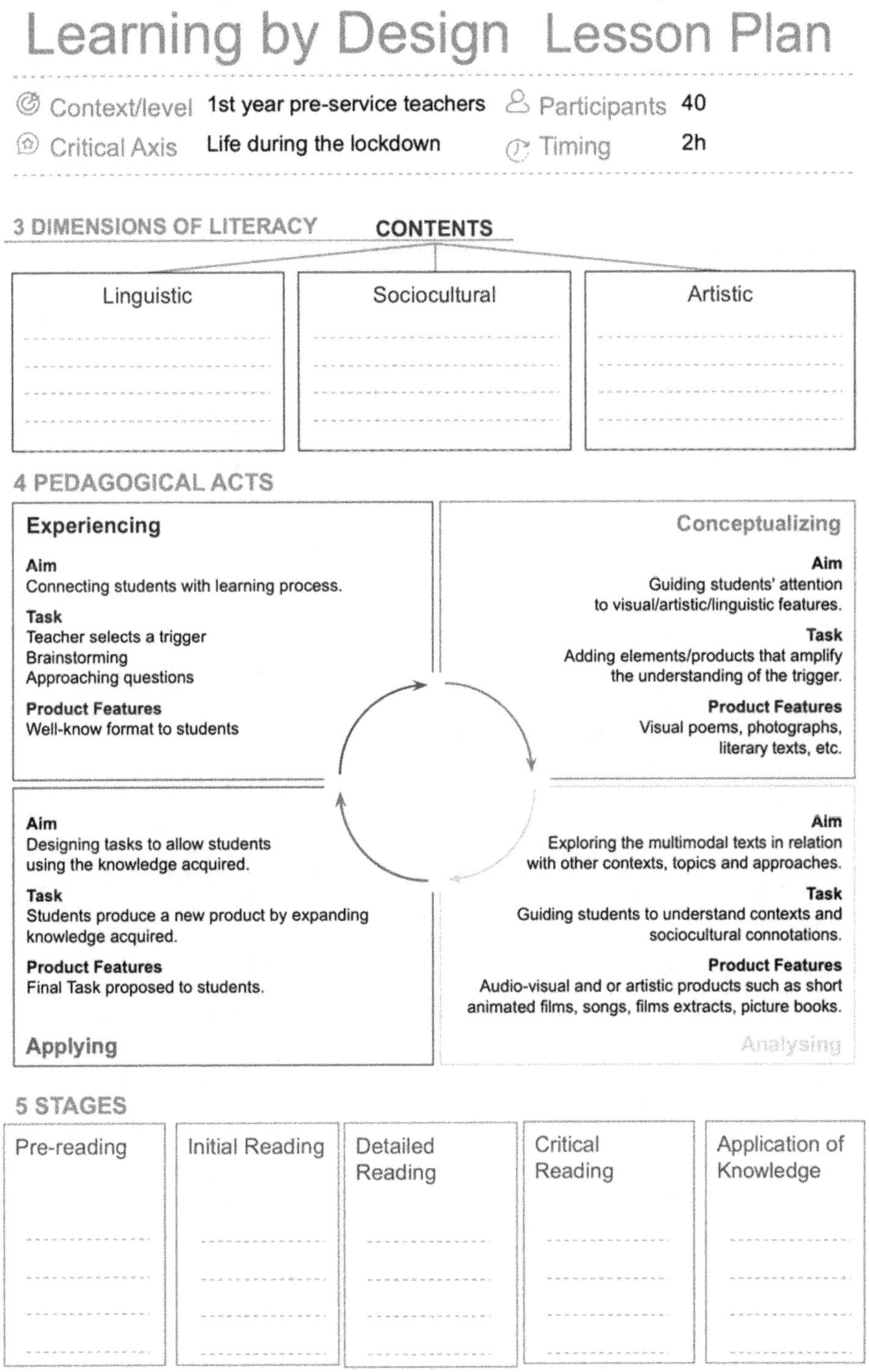

The selection of resources becomes paramount, as they may help students acquiring not only the vocabulary to express their thoughts, but also the sociocultural interaction and its critical axis. Combining the four acts - experiencing, conceptualizing, analyzing and applying- can engage students actively in the process of expressing interpretations and feelings, so that they also develop their multiliteracies. To that end, in this case the learning-path has also taken into account the reading model proposed by Paesani et al. (2016) that consists of five stages: (1) Pre-reading: It aims to catch the interest of the students and making use of their previous knowledge to connect with the text that is going to be discuss. (2) Initial reading: It aims to guide students to understand the most important information. (3) Detailed reading: It consists of guiding students to elaborate an interpretation of the text paying attention to the linguistic or visual elements that the author and/or illustrator have used (4) Critical reading: This phase aims to relate the linguistic and visual meaning with social, cultural, historical or ideological purposes. (5) Application of knowledge: readers make use of their interpretations to carry out other tasks (Paesani et al., 2016).

In the following table (Figure 4), each stage incorporates various pedagogical acts in order to involve students in the process of designing meaning through the different actions. Although the order of the phases is conceived as a fixed sequence that responds to the "Learning by design" approach -seen above- (NLG, 1996), the order of the acts can vary depending on the interests and needs of teachers.

Figure 4. Paesani's reading model combined with the Learning by Design approach (NLG).

Stage	Pedagogical act according to KPF	Multiliteracies
1. Pre-reading	**Experiencing**: Multimodal text/image as a trigger. **Conceptualizing**: Introduction to the topic **Analysing**: co-relating text and image to start creating meaning	Language Use Cultural Knowledge Multimodal text decoding Problem Solving Art's appreciation
2. Initial Reading	**Experiencing**: guided reading **Conceptualizing**: introducing key literary and/or visual elements. **Analysing**: interacting with image and/or text.	Language Use Cultural Knowledge Multimodal text decoding Problem Solving Art's appreciation
3. Detailed Reading	**Experiencing**: oral and group's reading **Conceptualizing**: identifying literary and/or visual elements represented in a multimodal text. **Analysing**: Attention and interpretation of specific topic in co-relation with text and/or images.	Language Use Cultural Knowledge Multimodal text decoding Problem Solving Art's appreciation Intertextual connections
4. Critical Reading	**Analysing**: training students to reach a new perspective. **Analysing**: adding a critical approach to the selected topic.	Language Use Cultural Knowledge Problem Solving Art's appreciation Intertextual connections
5. Knowledge Application	**Applying**: use of knowledge acquired **Applying**: decoding language and images	Language Use Cultural Knowledge Problem Solving Art's appreciation Intertextual connections Multimodal text creation

PRACTICAL EXPERIENCE

Next, an actual lesson plan based on the Pedagogy of the Multiliteracies and Paesani's reading stages has been designed and implemented with pre-service teachers (1st year) from the Universitat de València and Universidade de Aveiro, during the academic year 2021-2022. However, the learning path has been designed to be applied in Primary and Secondary Education with minor adaptations. These are the sic multimodal texts selected:

(1) A BBC reel entitled *The reality of confinement with a four-year-old*, by Pol Mallafré and Anna Pazos[1]; (2) Catalan Newspaper *Diari Ara*'s frontpage: an illustration to commemorate lockdown Book's Day in 2020 and The New Yorker's cover, December 2020, an illustration entitled *Love Life*, by Adrian Tomine; (3) Picturebook *Neighbors* by Kasya Denisevich as main source to analyse images and text; (4) supporting picturebooks, to analyse stories of different neighbourhoods, mainly under a child's point of view: *The neighbours*, by Einat Tsarfati; *Gràcies. Història d'un veïnat*, by Rocío Bonilla; *Your house, my house*, by Marianne Dubuc; *Madlenka* by Peter Sís and (5) Images and gifs taken from the IG account @abstractsunday (artist Christoph Niemann), dealing with single characters, which will be used to inspire new creations done by students (6) the poem "My neighbours and friends" by Ellen Bailey, used as the starting lines of student's picturebook creation.

It goes without saying how essential it is to reflect beforehand on the resources that we are going to use, so teachers can design the learning path properly and play a key role as mediators.

Combining the KPF with Paesani's Reading Stages

As stated in Figure 4, since one of the main goals of the lesson plan was to explore cognitively challenging picture books as a way to learn and talk about a specific topic (the covid-19 pandemic and its lockdown) in the classroom, we have combined different multimodal texts according to the Knowledge Processes Framework and Paesani's reading stages, in order to draw a intuitive and complete lesson plan. So that, the above mention texts were offered to students in the following order:

- Stage 1. Pre-reading. The born-digital text selected to begin is a video that acts as a trigger in the sense that students can recognize the format, while they may also get surprised because of the content and the context. The video is extracted from the BBC playlist *Lockdown Diaries. Stories from people around the world during pandemic*, and it shows the reality of confinement with a four-year-old girl. By watching this video, we engage students in experiencing, conceptualizing and analyzing as they start to brainstorm on the topic and attempt to come up a title for it. Questions we can ask are: Have you ever been in that situation? Who was it? Do you share any of the experiences with the protagonists?
- Stage 2. Initial reading. We use two illustrations: cover illustration for the Catalan Newspaper Diari Ara on Sant Jordi's Day (Book's Day) 2020 by Mari Fouz (Figure 5) and The New Yorker Illustration December 2020 by Adrian Tomine, Love Life (Figure 6). We ask students to talk about any ideas that come to their mind and to connect the images in any possible way with the previous video. Once they see that both images address the topic of life during lockdown, we can ask them about their own perception. What is the relation between the illustrations and the words/ title? In the first image, what is the relation between the building and the verbs "to read, to love". And in the 2nd illustration, why is it entitled "Love life"? Why do they have in common the verb

"to love"? Also, moving towards a more personal tone, to reflect on students' own experiences: Did days go by quickly or slowly during the pandemic? How did it differ the lockdown depending on different contexts, such as big cities vs. small villages? Do you feel represented by any of the images?

Figure 5. Mari Fouz's cover illustration for Diari Ara on Sant Jordi's Day 2020

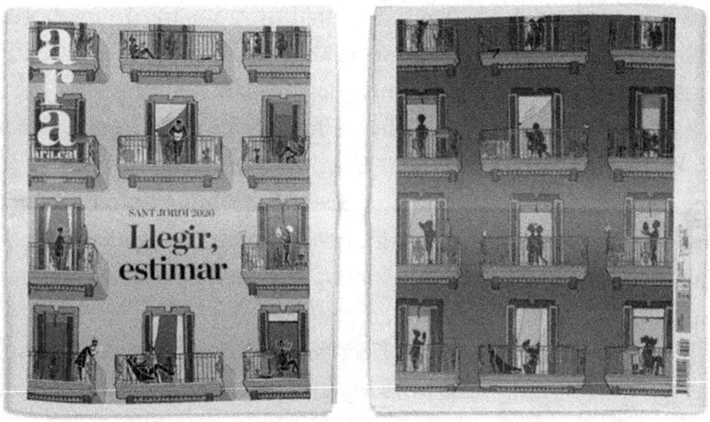

Figure 6. Adrian Tomine's New Yorker Illustration, Love Life. December 2020.

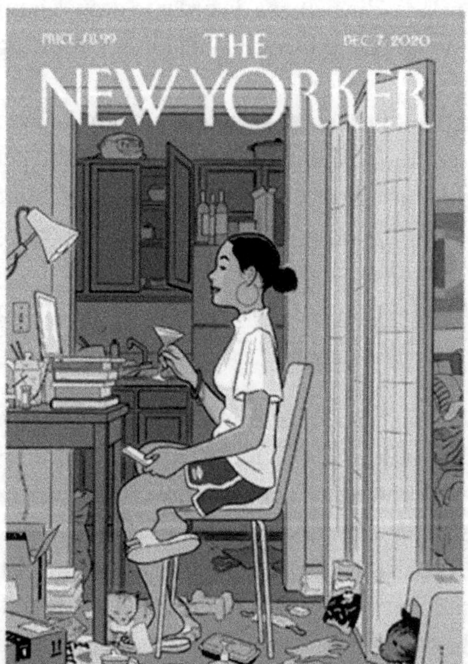

- Stage 3. Detailed reading. We show students different picturebooks, starting with *Neighbors* by Kasya Denisevich and paying attention to both elements of literature and visual elements (Reyes-Torres and Portalés-Raga, 2020): story and plot, tone, character, language style on the one hand, and elements (color, shape, line, texture) or principles (global rules of perception and composition) on the other hand. Special interested is paid to two central illustrations, that occupy both pages, giving the picturebook the sense of graphic book (Van der Linden, 2015), since the importance is given to the image and the text is intertwined within the image. These central illustrations describe the inside of a building with all its inhabitants under the point of view of the reader and, the next one, under the point of view of the girl-protagonist: her sociocultural context and her knowledge of the world being described here (Figures 7 and 8):

Figure 7. Neighbors by Kasya Denisevich under the reader's point of view.

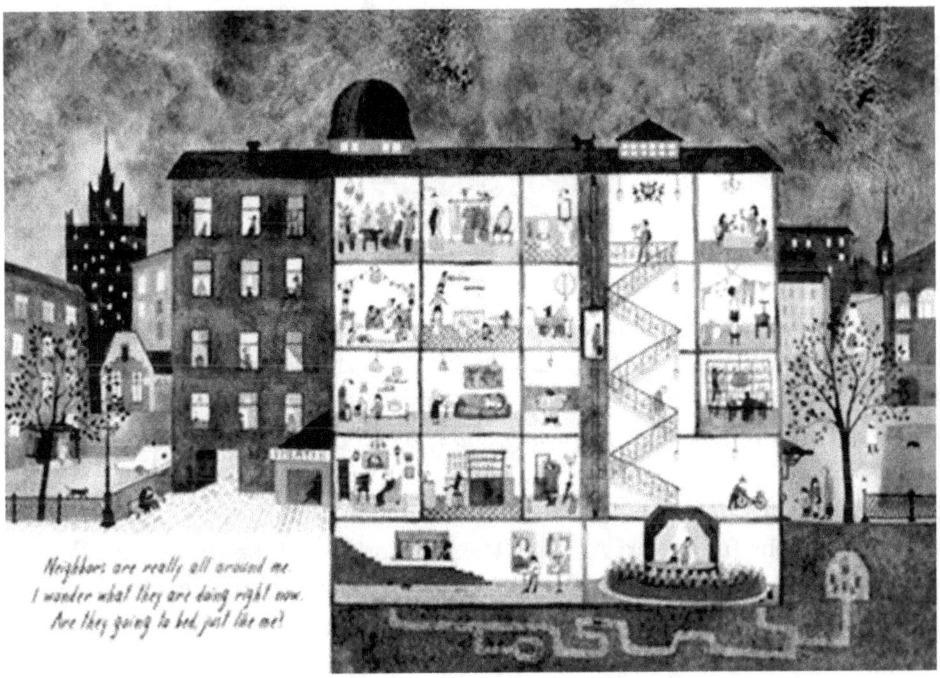
Neighbors are really all around me.
I wonder what they are doing right now.
Are they going to bed, just like me?

Figure 8. Neighbors by Kasya Denisevich under the protagonist point of view.

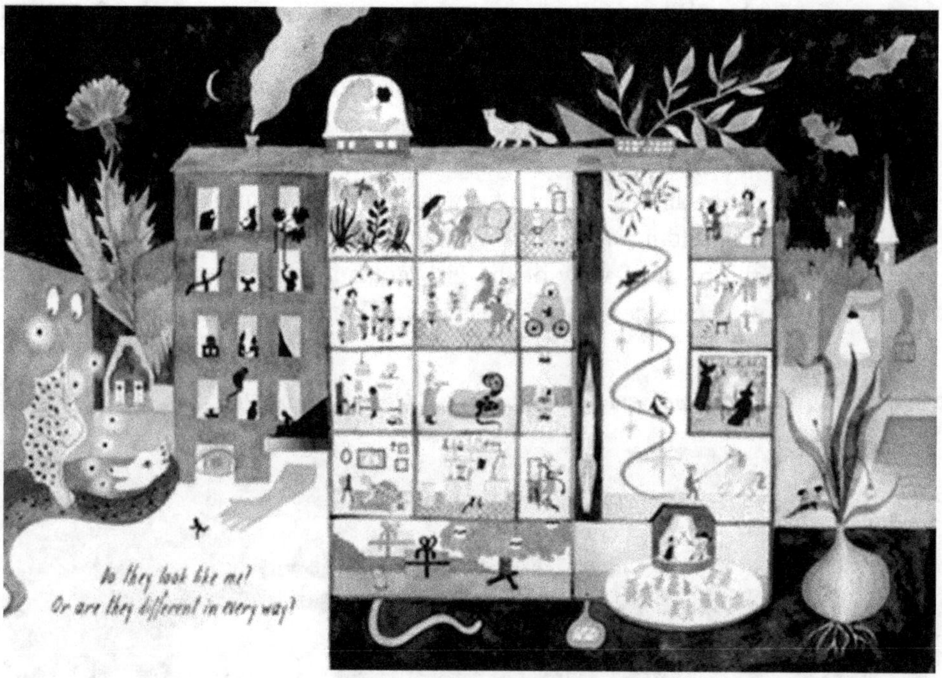
Do they look like me?
Or are they different in every way?

- Stage 4. Critical Reading. Once Denisevich's picturebook is read and interpreted, differents picturebooks dealing with the same topic are offered, so that they can share views and discuss in small groups of 3-4 people. The list of picturebooks, as established before, were: *The neighbours*, by Einat Tsarfati; *Gràcies. Història d'un veïnat*, by Rocío Bonilla; *Your house, my house*, by Marianne Dubuc; *Madlenka* by Peter Sís. Students are encouraged to find points in common among the different picturebooks with the one analysed in class and, also, with the previous texts: the cover illustrations from Diari Ara and The Newyorker and the BBC video. We ask students to exchange their perspectives and, also, students write a short reflection in which they need to establish three types of connection: a) text-to-self (how does the topic relate to their current or past life?); b) text-to-text (how is this picture book similar to other books or videos they have read or watched?); c) text-to-world (how does this picture book remind them of the real world and or real experiences?).
- Stage 5. Knowledge application. After all the previous tasks, students have already developed their own views. Now it is the moment to use them to produce a piece of creative, artistic writing: a new picture book under the title "My neighbours". We present students some images taken from the IG account @abstractsunday (artist Christoph Niemann), showing different characters that are going to belong to the same neighbourhood. The first stanzas from the poem "My neighbours and friends" by Ellen Bailey serves as starting point and model to follow in the students' creations, which also have to be stanzas following the ABBA or ABAB pattern. After that, students are encouraged to create, in small groups, a character - by means of ordinary, daily objects brought to class- and also the text -stanza-. By means of ICT tools, all images and texts are included into a

same digital presentation and, in the end, we get the image of a neighbourhood, somehow mediated by their own knowledge of their neighbourhoods and /or societies.

Throughout the whole lesson, we ask students to work in small groups, or independently so that they can exchange their ideas and ask questions that may arise. In the meantime, we keep records of the comments they make and their interaction. At the end, we show some examples of the final tasks they have produced. The study is based on an interpretative paradigm, which seeks to analyze and understand the data provided by the participants (Creswell, 2009).

RESULTS

The data gathered has generated findings in three different areas according to the objectives initially established: First, how implementing the Pedagogy of Multiliteracies enhances the meaning-making process by implementing the four curricular components: experiencing, conceptualizing, analyzing and applying. Second, how by means of structuring the texts according to Paesani's reading stages has helped developing critical thinking and reflecting upon personal and social experiences lived during the lockdowns and reflected through children's literature. Finally, the last aim was to promote students' multiliteracies in order to be able to work with a variety of multimodal texts, which enriches their future task as teachers.

In this case, some sample productions from the Applying stage of the Knowledge Processes Framework are offered. These creations were done after a whole session discussing the implications of the lockdown for the students, as well as for children. The main idea was to reflect upon how Covid-19 pandemic has achieved in getting people closer to its neighbours or, even, in getting to know them. Bearing this idea in mind, students from a degree in Education from the Universitat de València (Figure 9) and from the Universidade de Aveiro (Figure 10) have created a new neighbourhood where peculiar characters live.

Overall, the learning path designed was effective for students to work not only multiliteracies' skills, but also creative and artistic ones. If with previous stages we managed to talk openly about topics related to the pandemic: life under lockdown, privacy of freedom, mental health, need for nature, living in a rush, etc., our last intention was to connect all these thought with children's multiliteracy education. As mentioned before, by promoting the necessary skills and selecting different texts, teachers will be able to guide in the decoding and the production of a variety of multimodal texts.

In this case, out of ordinary objects and simple linguistic guidelines, students managed to create a new picturebook which showed different cultural and social features. As we can see in Figure 9, students from the Universitat de València made use of literary figures such as the 'madwoman in the attic' (who "yells and screams like a lunatic") together with current popular characters from TV serials, such as *The Bridgerton's* ("The Opera singer"). It is interesting also to mention some very contextual features, such as the one related to peering behind a door ("Peephole girl") or a current issue related, mainly, to social networks: pretending to be ("The just married couple").

On the other hand, it is worth mentioning, in the case of students from the Universidade de Aveiro, that they managed to give a real name to all neighbours and, also, to establish relations among them, especially sentimental ones, by using verbs such as "namorar" or "apaixonar-se" (to fall in love) or "ficar com raiva" (to get angry). Also, the figure of a person who represents the indiscretion in a neighbourhood is presented ("Dona Lourdes, a cusca"), as well as other literary and ethnographic figures, such as the witch ("A bruxa").

Figure 9. Applying stage. Students' picturebook "My neighbours". Pre-service teachers, UV.

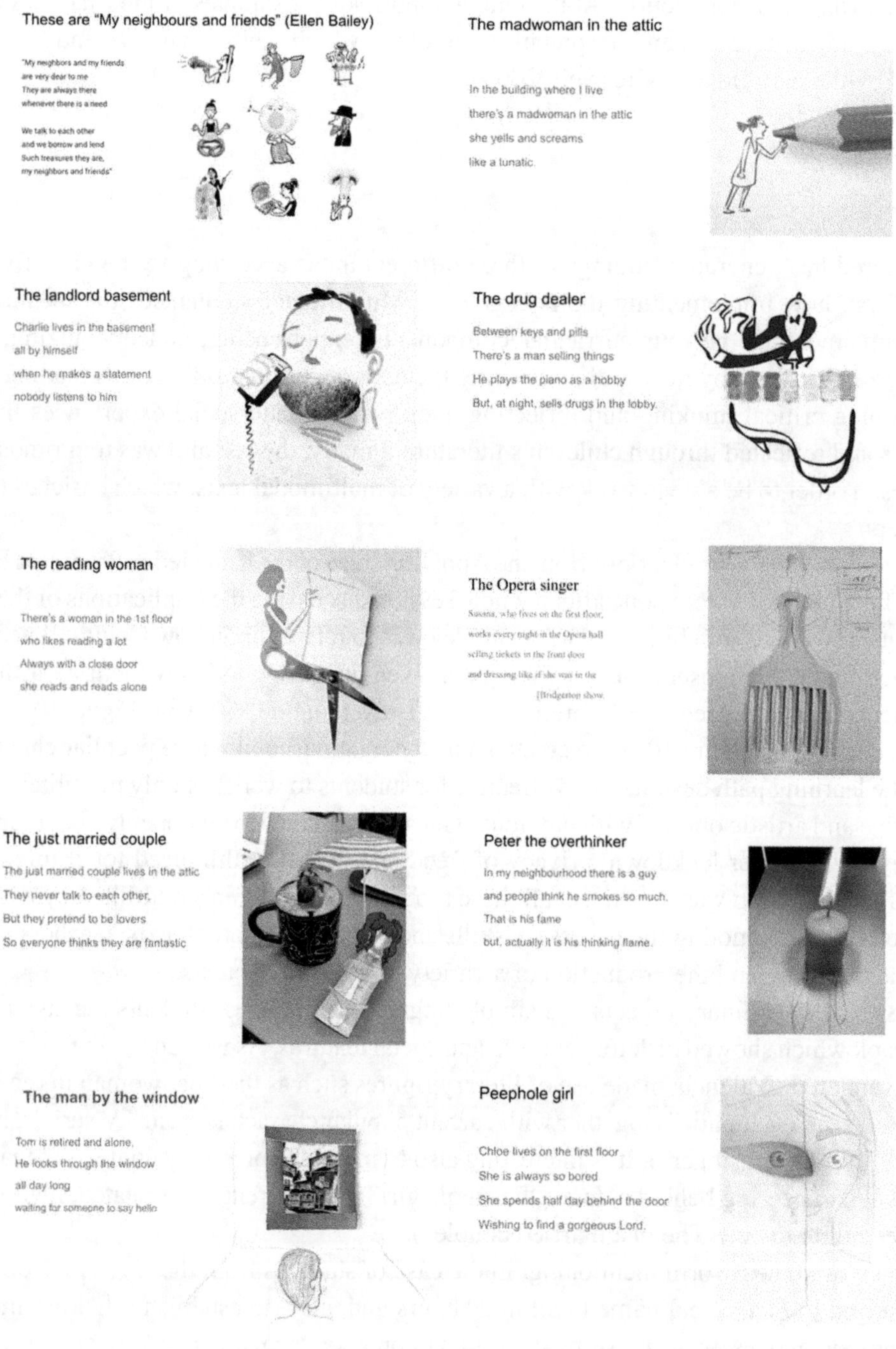

Figure 10. Applying stage. Students' picturebook "My neighbours". Pre-service teachers, UA.

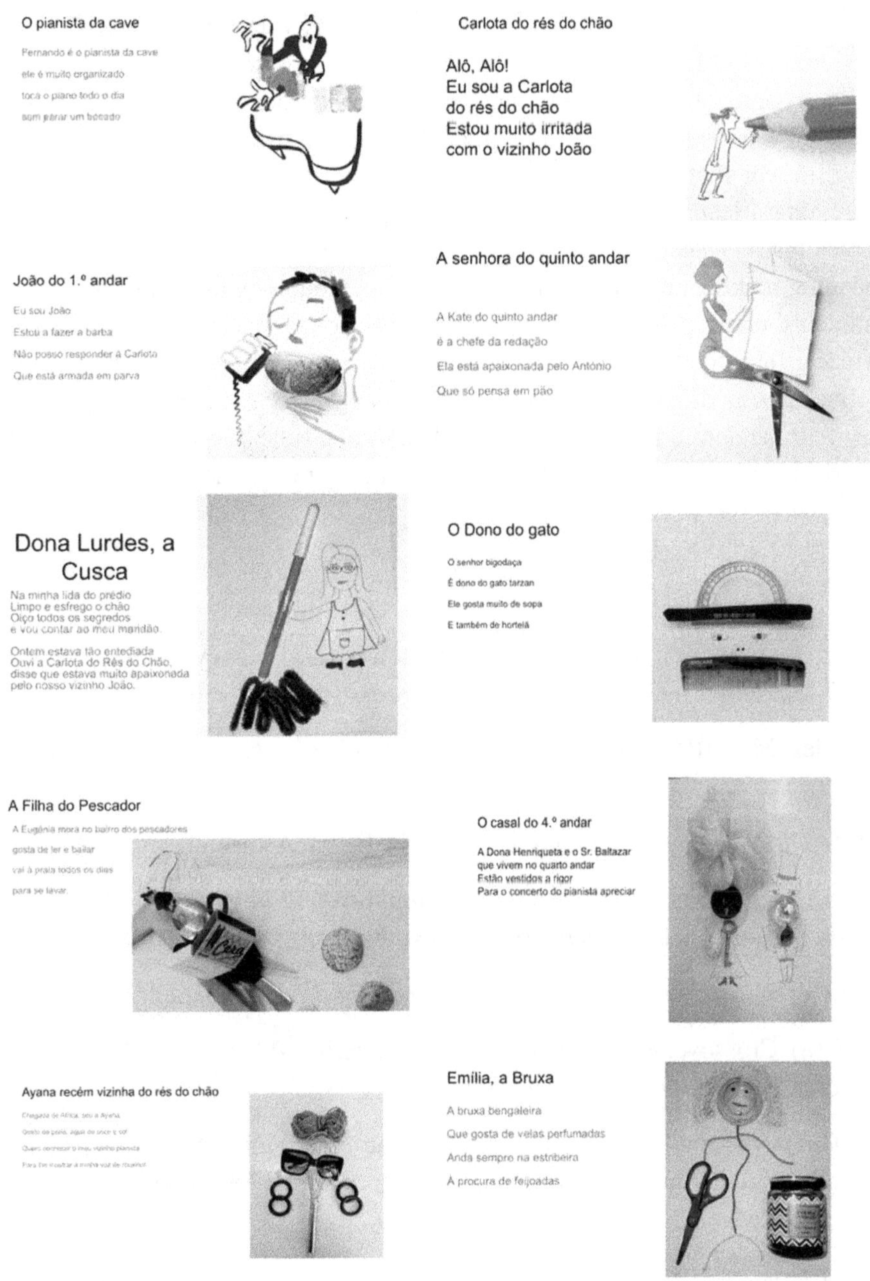

CONCLUSION

Dealing with challenging picturebooks and other complementary multimodal texts offers a wide range of opportunities to guide students to improve not only their literary competences, but also to become multiliterate and to reflect about life and the world. This chapter is expected to guide teachers to design lesson plans by using different types of texts that integrate different modes of representation, with special emphasis on picturebooks as a crossover genre. Nevertheless, there are several limitations in this study that can be addressed in future research. Due to the fact that the investigation was carried out in a 2 hour-session, it would be interesting to carry it out in a longer period of time and keep further record of all the work students do. Likewise, another possibility to enrich this research is implementing the same methodology across different levels, since the learning path provided has been designed to be implemented in different contexts with minor adaptations.

All in all, creating a learning path using challenging picturebooks by following the Pedagogy of the Multiliteracies places teachers as "designers" and students as "co-designers" in a complementary multimodal meaning-making process. In this sense, this methodology facilitates the co-construction of meaning and students' proactive engagement and natural curiosity in learning. As it has been shown, the picturebooks selected around the topic of lockdowns, domestic geographies, neighbours and neighbourhoods are effective multimodal artefacts through which a deep reflection of personal and social situations during the Covid-19 pandemic can be done and. At the same time, these crossover, multimodal texts help students to develop a natural bond with creativity, literature and mental health.

REFERENCES

Arizpe, E., Farrar, J., & McAdam, J. (2018). Picturebooks and Literacy Studies. In B. Kümmerling-Meibauer (Ed.), *The Routledge Companion to Picturebooks* (pp. 371–380). Routledge.

Arizpe, E., & Styles, M. (2016). *Children Reading Picturebooks. Interpreting Visual Texts* (2nd ed.). Routledge.

Bajour, C. (2009). *Oír entre líneas* [Hearing between the lines]. Asolectura.

BBC Playlist. (n.d.). *Lockdown Diaries. Stories from people around the world during pandemic.* Retrieved from: https://www.bbc.com/reel/playlist/world-in-lockdown

Beckett, S. L. (2012). *Crossover Picturebooks. A Genre for All Ages.* Routledge.

Beckett, S. L. (2018). Crossover Picturebooks. In B. Kümmerling-Meibauer (Ed.), *The Routledge Companion to Picturebooks* (pp. 209–2019). Routledge.

Beckett, S. L. (2022) Crossing Boundaries of Age, Culture, and Time with Challenging Picturebooks. In Exploring Challenging Picturebooks in Education. International Perspectives on Language and Literature Learning. Routledge.

Bonilla, R. (2021). *Gràcies. Història d'un veïnat* [Thank you. History of a neighborhood]. Animallibres.

Bourget, L. (2018). *Ma Maison* [My home]. Éditions Les Grands Personnes.

Brooks, S. K., Webster, R. K., Smith, L. E., Woodland, L., Wessley, S., Greenberg, N., & Rubin, G. J. (2020). The psychological impact of quarantine and how to reduce it: Rapid review of the evidence. *Lancet, 395*(10227), 912–920. doi:10.1016/S0140-6736(20)30460-8 PMID:32112714

Campagnaro, M. (2019). Do Touch! How Bruno Munari's Picturebooks Work. *Revista di Storia dell'Educazione, 6*(1), 81-96.

Campagnaro, M. (2022). Picturebooks and aesthetic Literacy in Early Childhood Education. In *Exploring Challenging Picturebooks in Education. International Perspectives on Language and Literature Learning* (pp. 79–98). Routledge.

Campagnaro, M., & Dallari, M. (2013). Incanto e racconto nel labirinto delle figure [Enchantment and story in the labyrinth of figures]. In Albii illustrati c relazione educativa. Trento: Erickson.

Cope, B., & Kalantzis, M. (2000). *Multiliteracies. Literacy Learning and the Design of Social Futures.* Routledge.

Cope, B., & Kalantzis, M. (2015). *A Pedagogy of Multiliteracies. Learning by design.* Palgrave and Macmillan.

Cortijo Ocaña, A., & Martines, V. (Eds.). (2022). Handbook of Research on Historical Pandemic Analysis and the Social Implications of COVID-19. IGI Global.

Creswell, J. W. (2009). *Research Design. Qualitative, quantitative and Mixed Methods Approaches.* Sage.

Denisevich, K. (2020). *Neighbors.* Chronicle Books.

Dewey, J. (1938). *Experience and Education.* Kappa Delta Pi.

Druker, E., & Kümmerling-Meibaucr, B. (Eds.). (2015). *Children's Literature and the Avant-Garde.* John Benjamins. doi:10.1075/clcc.5

Dubuc, M. (2020). *Chez moi, chez toi* [At home, at home]. Casterman.

Evans, J. (1998). *What's in the Picture? Responding to Illustrations in Picture Books.* Sage.

Evans, J. (Ed.). (2015a). *Challenging and Controversial Picturebooks: Creative and Critical Responses to Visual Texts.* Routledge. doi:10.4324/9781315756912

Evans, J. (2015b). Picturebooks as Strange, Challenging and Controversial Texts. In J. Evans (Ed.), *Challenging and Controversial Picturebooks: Creative and Critical Responses to Visual Texts* (pp. 3–32). Routledge. doi:10.4324/9781315756912-12

Evans, J. (2016). Who am I Why I am here? and Where do I come from? Responding to Philosophical Picturebooks. *Education 3-13, 44*(1), 53-67. doi:10.1080/03004279.2015.1109815

Farrar, J., Arizpe, E., & McAdam, J. (2022). Challenging Picturebooks and Literacy Studies. In *Exploring Challenging Picturebooks in Education. International Perspectives on Language and Literature Learning* (pp. 43–56). Routledge.

Genette, G. (1987). *Seouils* [Seoul.]. Seouil.

Hall, N., Larson, J., & Marsch, J. (Eds.). (2003). *Handbook of Early Childhood Literacy.* Sage. doi:10.4135/9781848608207

Jewitt, C. (2008). Multimodality and Literacy in School Classrooms. *Review of Research in Education, 32*(2), 241–267. doi:10.3102/0091732X07310586

Kern, R. (2000). *Literacy and language teaching.* Oxford University Press.

Kress, G. (2003). *Literacy in the New Media Age*. Routledge.

Kress, G. (2009). *Multimodality: A Social Semiotic Approach to Contemporary Communication*. Routledge. doi:10.4324/9780203970034

Kress, G., & Van Leeuwen, T. (2001). *Multimodal discourse: The modes and media of contemporary communication*. Arnold Publishers.

Kucer, S. (2014). *Dimensions of Literacy: A Conceptual Base for Teaching, Reading and Writing in School Settings*. Routledge. doi:10.4324/9780203428405

Kucer, S. (2015). Literacy: Varied, Dynamic and Multidimensional. *Journal of Family Strengths*, *15*(2), 1–35.

Kümmerling-Meibauer, B. (Ed.). (2014). *Picturebooks: Representation and Narration*. Routledge. doi:10.4324/9780203582275

Kümmerling-Meibauer, B. (Ed.). (2018). *The Routledge Companion to Picturebooks*. Routledge.

Kümmerling-Meibauer, B., Meibauer, J., Nachtigäller, K., & Rohlfing, K. J. (Eds.). (2015). *Learning from Picturebooks: Perspectives from Child Development and Literacy Studies*. Routledge. doi:10.4324/9781315866710

Lewis, D. (1990). The Constructedness of Texts: Picture Books and the Metafictive. *Signal*, *62*, 31–46.

Lewis, D. (2001). *Reading Contemporary Picturebooks: Picturing Text*. Routledge Falmer.

Mackey, M. (2002). *Literacies across Media: Playing the Text*. Routledge Falmer.

Meek, M. (1988). *How Texts Teach What Readers Learn*. Thimble Press.

Menke, M. R., & Paesani, K. (2019). Analysing Foreign Language Instructional Materials through the Lens of Multiliteracies Framework. *Language, Culture and Curriculum*, *32*(1), 34–49. doi:10.1080/07908318.2018.1461898

Millard, E., & Marsh, J. (2001). Sending Minnie the Minx Home: Comics and Reading Choices. *Cambridge Journal of Education*, *31*(1), 25–38. doi:10.1080/03057640123853

Mociño-González, I. (2019). Libro-objeto y poesía: construyendo significados a través de los sentidos [Book-object and poetry: constructing meanings through the senses]. In R. Tabernero Sala (Ed.), *El objeto libro en el universo infantil. La materialidad en la construcción del discurso* (pp. 89–108). Prensas de la Universidad de Zaragoza.

New London Group. (1996). A Pedagogy of Multiliteracies: Designing social futures. *Educational Review*, *66*(1), 60–93.

Nikolajeva, M., & Scott, C. (2000). The Dynamics of Picturebook Communication. *Children's Literature in Education*, *31*(4), 225–239. doi:10.1023/A:1026426902123

Nikolajeva, M., & Scott, C. (2003). Verbal and Visual Literacy: The Role of Picturebooks in the Reading Experience of Young Children. In *Handbook of Early Childhood Literacy* (pp. 235–248). Sage. doi:10.4135/9781848608207.n20

Nikolajeva, M., & Scott, C. (2014). *Reading for Learning: Cognitive Approaches to Children's Literature*. John Benjamins. doi:10.1075/clcc.3

Nodelman, P. (1999). Decoding the Images: Illustration and Picture Books. In P. Hunt (Ed.), *Understanding Children's Literature* (pp. 128–139). Routledge.

Ommundsen, A. M. (2022). Cognitively Challenging Picturebooks and the Plesures of Reading. Explorative Learning from Picturebooks in the Classroom. In *Exploring Challenging Picturebooks in Education. International Perspectives on Language and Literature Learning* (pp. 99–121). Routledge.

Ommundsen, A. M., Haaland, G., & Kümmerling-Meibauer, B. (Ed.). (2022). Exploring Challenging Picturebooks in Education. International Perspectives on Language and Literature Learning. Routledge.

Orazi, V. (2020a). COVID19 – Literatura, interculturalitat, TIC, entrenament conductal i gestió de l'estrés durant la pandèmia per Coronavirus [COVID19 – Literature, interculturality, ICT, behavioral training and stress management during the Coronavirus pandemic]. In *Coneixement en temps de pandèmia*. Universitat d'Alacant. Seu Universitària de La Nucia. Retrieved from https://www.youtube.com/watch?v=PqVAi9-E2ro&fbclid=IwAR3dbgxgJylCSYOqTbn-BBv80WdVT0XdC-s8KYRHhgy7VRYnbex9PTZc_fQ

Orazi, V. (2022). Literature, Language, Art in/and Highher Education in Times of Covid-19 in the Paniberian Context. *eHumanista. Journal of Iberian Studies*, *21*, 1–6.

Paesani, K., Allen, H. W., & Dupuy, B. (2016). *Multiliteracies Framework for Collegiate Foreign Language Teaching*. Pearson.

Pascual de la Torre, M. (2018). *Malacatú*. Barcelona: A buen paso.

Pilgrim, J., & Martínez, E. (2013). Defining Literacy in the 21st Century: A guide to Terminology and Skills. *Texas Journal of Literacy Education*, *1*(1), 60–69.

Ramos, A. M. (2017). *Aproximações ao livro objeto: das potencialidades criativas às propostas de leitura* [Approaches to the object book: from creative potential to reading proposals]. Tropelias & Companhia.

Reyes-Torres, A., & García-Perera, A. (2022). Influence of Positive Student-Teacher Interaction on the Meaning-Making Process in Virtual Learning: A Study in the Primary English Class. In C. N. Giannikas (Ed.), *Transferring Language Learning and Teaching From Face-to-Face to Online Settings* (pp. 165–188). IGI Global. doi:10.4018/978-1-7998-8717-1.ch009

Reyes-Torres, A., & Portalés, M. (2020). Multimodal Approach to Foster the Multiliteracies Pedagogy in the Teaching of EFL through Picturebooks: The Snow Lion. *Journal of the Spanish Association of Anglo-American Studies*, *42*(1), 94–119. doi:10.28914/Atlantis-2020-42.1.06

Reyes-Torres, A., Portalés, M., & Torres, C. (2021). The Potential of Sound Picturebooks as Multimodal narratives. *AILA Review*, *34*(2), 300–324. doi:10.1075/aila.21006.rey

Rosenblatt, L. (1938). *Literature as Exploration*. Appleton-Century.

Rosenblatt, L. (1978). *The Reader, the Text, the Poem: The Transactional Theory of the Literary Work*. Southern Illinois University Press.

Salisbury, M. (2005). *Ilustración de libros infantiles* [Illustration of children's books]. Editorial Acanto.

Salisbury, M., & Styles, M. (2012). *Children's picturebooks: The Art of visual storytelling*. Laurence King.

Serafini, F. (2014). *Reading the visual: An introduction to teaching multimodal literacy*. Teachers College Press.

Sís, P. (2000). *Madlenka*. Ediciones Ekaré.

Sobral, C. (2016). *Tão, tão grande* [So, so big]. Orfeu Negro.

Stafford, T. (2011). *Teaching Visual Literacy in the Primary Classroom*. Routledge.

Tabernero Sala, R. (Ed.), *El objeto libro en el universo infantil. La materialidad en la construcción del discurso* [The book object in the children's universe. Materiality in the construction of discourse]. Prensas de la Universidad de Zaragoza.

Tishman, S. (2018). *The Art and Practice of Learning Through Observation*. Routledge.

Torr, J. (2008). Multimodal Texts and Emergent Literacy. In L. Unsworth (Ed.), *New Literacies and the English Curriculum* (pp. 47–66). Continuum.

Tsafarti, E. (2017). *The Neighbours*. Abrams.

Underwood, D. (2020). *Outside In*. Clarion Books - Harper Collins.

Van der Linden, S. (2007). *Lire l'album* [Play the album]. Le Puy-en-Velay: L'Atelier du Poisson Soluble.

Van der Linden, S. (2015). Álbum[es]. [Album[s]]. Barcelona: Ekaré/Banco del Libro/Varipinta Ediciones.

Van Leeuwen, T. (2008). *Discourse and Practice: New Tools for Critical Discourse Analysis*. Oxford University Press. doi:10.1093/acprof:oso/9780195323306.001.0001

Warner, C., & Dupuy, B. (2018). Moving toward Multiliteracies in Foreign Language Teaching: Past and present perspectives ... and beyond. *Foreign Language Annals*, *51*(1), 116–128. doi:10.1111/flan.12316

Westby, C. (2010). Multiliteracies: The changing World of Communication. *Topics in Language Disorders*, *30*(1), 64–71. doi:10.1097/TLD.0b013e3181d0a0ab

ADDITIONAL READING

Arizpe, E., & Ryan, S. (2018). The Wordless Picturebooks: Literacy in Multilingual Contexts and David Wiesner's Worlds. In J. Bland (Ed.), *Using Literature in English Language Education: Challenging Reading for 8-18 Year Olds* (pp. 63–81). Bloomsbury Academic.

Asmundson, J. G., & Taylor, S. (2020, December). Coronaphobia revisted: A state-of-the-art on pandemic-related fear, anxiety, and stress. *Journal of Anxiety Disorders*, *76*, 102326. Advance online publication. doi:10.1016/j.janxdis.2020.102326 PMID:33142124

Sánchez-Villena, A. R., & de La Fuente-Figuerola, V. (2020). COVID-19: Quarantine, isolation, social distancing and lockdown: Are they the same? *Anales de Pediatria (Barcelona, Spain)*, *93*(1), 73–74. doi:10.1016/j.anpedi.2020.05.001 PMID:32507611

KEY TERMS AND DEFINITIONS

COVID-19 and Challenging Picturebooks: Picturebooks read for the sake of reflecting personal and collective experiences during the lockdown can also been considered challenging: because they assume an introspection in what we understand to be our immediate reality (our house, our neighbours, our habits) and, also, different abstract feelings (the fear, the loneliness, the confusion, the bewilderment, etc.).

COVID-19 Pandemic: A global emergency situation caused by virus SARS-CoV-2 which was identified in December 2019 in Wuhan, China and spread very quickly to other countries. The World Health Organization declared the outbreak of a public health emergency of international concern in January 2020 and a pandemic in March 2020.

Isolation During COVID-19 Pandemic: The COVID-19 pandemic is assumed to have caused an increase in the number of socially isolated people. Social Isolation was defined as less frequent contact with people other than co-residing family members. Mental health outcomes of such situation include psychological distress, suicidal ideation, loneliness, and fear of COVID-19.

Lockdown: "Voluntary or mandatory restriction of movement of individuals who have been exposed to the virus or those who are possibly infected. During this time, people must remain in a specific place until the incubation period is over" (Sánchez-Villena & La Fuente-Figuerola, 2020). Lockdowns have significantly disrupted the daily lives of children and adolescents, with increased time at home and limited physical social interaction.

Pedagogy of the Multiliteracies: A more contemporary view of literacy that reflect multiple communication forms and a context of cultural and linguistic diversity within a globalized society. Multiple ways of communicating and making meaning, including such modes as visual, audio, spatial, behavioral, and gestural (Pilgrim & Martínez, 2013, p. 62).

Post-COVID-19 Era: The world after COVID-19 Pandemic.

ENDNOTE

1 The complete video belongs to a Playlist of 6 videos from the Covid-19 stories from people around the world during the pandemic and it can be found at: https://www.bbc.com/reel/playlist/world-in-lockdown

Compilation of References

ʻĀbidīn, N. (2020, May 12). Al-Ḥub fī zaman Corona [Al-Hub is better tan Corona]. *Al-Watan*. https://www.al-watan.com/news-details/id/231225/

Abalakina-Paap, M., Stephan, W., Craig, T., & Gregory, W. (1999). Beliefs in Conspiracies. *Political Psychology*, *20*(3), 637–647. doi:10.1111/0162-895X.00160

Abdelsalam, S. (2021). Understanding balances and its impact on the new events of the Corona pandemic (selected issues). *Mağallat al-Šihāb*, *1*(7), 195-222.

Abed, M. G. (2018). Teachers' Perspectives Surrounding ICT Use amongst SEN Students in the Mainstream Educational Setting. *World Journal of Education*, *8*(1), 6. doi:10.5430/wje.v8n1p6

Abidah, A., Hidaayatullaah, H. N., Simamora, R. M., Fehabutar, D., & Mutakinati, L. (2020). The Impact of Covid-19 on Indonesian Education and Its Relation to the Philosophy of "Merdeka Belajar". *Studies in Philosophy of Science and Education*, *1*(1), 38–49. doi:10.46627ipose.v1i1.9

Acim, R. (2021). Lockdown poetry, healing and the COVID-19 pandemic. *Journal of Poetry Therapy*, *34*(2), 67–76. doi:10.1080/08893675.2021.1899629

Adanti, D. (2017). *Disparen al humorista. Un ensayo gráfico sobre los límites del humor* [Shoot the comedian. A graphic essay on the limits of humor]. Astiberri.

Adnan, M., & Anwar, K. (2020). *Online learning amid the COVID-19 pandemic : Students' perspectives*. Academic Press.

Aggelopoulou, D. (2011). Pedagogical utilization of new technologies and educational software for students with or without special educational needs. In E. Papanis, P. Giavrimis, & A. Vicky (Eds.), *Research and educational practice in special education* (pp. 187–214). Sideris.

Aggelopoulou, D. (2011). Pedagogical utilization of new technologies and educational software for students with/ or without special educational needs. In E. Papanis, P. Giavrimis, & A. Viky (Eds.), *Research and Educational Practice in Special Education* (pp. 187–215). Sideris.

Ahmed, M. (2016). *Openness of Comics: Generating Meaning within Flexible Structures*. University Press of Mississippi. doi:10.14325/mississippi/9781496805935.001.0001

Aichouni, ʻA., & Adjal, A. (2021). The impact of value communication on family bonding in Algerian society during the Covid 19 crisis. *Mağallat al-riwaq li-l-dirāsāt al-iğtimaʻiyya wa-l-insāniyya*, *2*(7), 141-168.

Ainscow, M. (2005). Developing inclusive education systems: What are the levers for change? *Journal of Educational Change*, *6*(2), 109–124. doi:10.100710833-005-1298-4

Ainscow, M. (2005). Understanding the development of an inclusive education system. *Electronic Journal of Research in Educational Psychology*, *3*(3), 5–20. https://www.redalyc.org/pdf/2931/293121928002.pdf

Al-'Ašmāwī, 'A. (2020, April 7). Yā ḫāliqa al-kawni luṭfan anta munqiduna [Oh cosmic affair of Louvain, you are our bound]. *Ǧarīdat al-Umma*. https://al-omah.com/

Al-'Awaḍı, 'A. A. (2020, March 31). Layālī Corona [Corona nights]. *Šabakat Al-Alūka*. https://www.alukah.net/literature_language/0/139424/

Alasona, N. (2021). *ICT and remote methods in border areas: the case of children with learning disabilities* (No. 50070) [Doctoral dissertation, National Kapodistrian University of Athens]. National Archive of Doctoral Dissertations.

Alba, C. (2021). *La primavera de Julio Llamazares* [The spring of Julio Llamazares]. Retrieved from https://www.rtve.es/play/audios/la-estacion-azul/primavera-julio-llamazares-31-01-2021/5775253/

Al-Bašīr, Ḥ. (2020, May 6). Ǧā'iḥat Corona [Corona Cases]. *Alrakoba*. https://www.alrakoba.net/31394213/

Al-Buḫārī. (2002). *Ṣaḥīḥ al-Buḫārī* [Sahih Bukari] (M. Z. Ben Nāṣir, Ed.). Dār Ṭūq al-Naǧāt.

Al-Churà, H. (2020). *Asrār corona: kaifa taḥmī nafsak wa-usratak* [Corona's secrets: How to feed yourself and your family]. Kitāb al-Yawm.

Al-Ǧārim, 'A. (2012). *Dīwān 'Alī al-Ǧārim*. Mu'asasat Hindāwī.

Alghamdi, S. A. (2021, February 10). Acadīmī uṣība bi-Corona. *Akhbar24*. https://akhbaar24.argaam.com/article/detail/531646

Alghamdi, S. A. [@Saad_Alghamdi] (2020, March 5). *Poetic Verses* [Tweet]. Twitter. https://twitter.com/Saad_Alghamdi/status/1505981971595468809?cxt=HHwWkoC58finqeYpAAAA

Al-La'būn, F. [@fawaz_dr]. (2020, March 10). *Ṭāla al-zaman wa-Corona tuṭāriduna* [Time and Corona hit us] [Tweet]. Twiter. https://twitter.com/fawaz_dr/status/1237407639245594628?lang=es

Ally, M., & Prieto-Blázquez, J. (2014). What is the future of mobile learning in education? *RUSC Universities and Knowledge Society Journal*, *11*(1), 142–151. doi:10.7238/rusc.v11i1.2033

Al-Maktaba. (2021). *Plataforma de libros electrónicos* [E-book platform]. https://books-library.net/free-835057225-download

Al-Malā'ika, N. (1986). Dīwān Nāzik al-Malā'ika vol. 2 [Diwan Nazik Angels Vol. 2]. Dar al-'Ūda.

Al-Malā'ika, N. (2019). 'Ašr qasā'id. *Al-Jazeera Documentary*. https://www.youtube.com/watch?v=Ub9CZ_c5fTE&t=268s

Al-Malwānī, A. (2020). *Mā yušbih al-qatl* [What a killer]. Al-Dār al-Miṣriyya al-Lubnāniyya.

Al-Nābulsī, R. (2021). *Imra'a min ṣūf*. Dār al-Warda.

Al-Qarna, M. (2020). *Al-Hurūb min min corona* [The war from Corona]. Dār al-Riwaya al-'Arabiyya.

Al-Qurašī, R. (2020, April 27). Corona fī 'uyūn al-šu'arā' [Corona in the eyes of poets]. *Al-Jazirah*. https://www.al-jazirah.com/2020/20200417/cm4.htm

Alrefai, T. (2020). *Lawn al-ġad: ru'yat al-muṯaqqaf al-'arabī li-mā ba'da Corona* [The color of the return: a vision of Arab attitudes after Corona]. Almutawassit.

Al-Salābī, A. (2020, March 19). Kayfa ta'āmala al-muslimūn ma'a al-awbi'a wa- ātāruhā fī-marāhil tārīḫihim [How do Muslims work with epidemics and Ataroh in the pits of Tarhim]. *Aljazeera*. https://www.aljazeera.net/blogs/2020/3/19/

Al-Samarrā'ī, S. (2016). *Al-'Atabāt al-naṣṣiyya fī riwāyat al-aǧyāl al-'arabiya*. Al Manhal.

Alshawabkeh, A. A., Madhesh, A., Woolsey, M. L., & Kharbat, F. F. (2021). Using online information technology for deaf students during COVID- 19: A closer look from experience. *Heliyon*, *7*(5), e06915. Advance online publication. doi:10.1016/j.heliyon.2021.e06915 PMID:34013080

Altemueller, L, & Lindquist, C. (2017). Flipped classroom instruction for inclusive learning. *British Journal of Special Education, 44*(3), 341-358. doi:10.1111/1467-8578.12177

al-Wardī, I. (1986). *Dīwān Ibn al-Wardī*. Dār al-Qalam.

Anagnostopoulos, B. D., & Delonis, A. (1988). Children's Literature and school. Pataki.

Anastasiadis P. (2020). Η Σχολική Εξ Αποστάσεως Εκπαίδευση στην εποχή του Κορωνοϊού COVID-19: το παράδειγμα της Ελλάδας και η πρόκληση της μετάβασης στο «Ανοιχτό Σχολείο της Διερευνητικής Μάθησης, της Συνεργατικής Δημιουργικότητας και της Κοινωνικής Αλληλεγγύης» [Distance learning in the era of COVID-19, focusing on the Greek Educational System]. *Open Education - The Journal for Open and Distance Education and Educational Technology, 16*(2).

Anastasiadis, P. (2014). Research in e-learning in Greek Primary, Secondary and Higher Education: Review and perspectives. *Open Education - The Journal for Open and Distance Education and Educational Technology, 10*(1), 5-32. https://ejournals.epublishing.ekt.gr/index.php/openjournal/article/view/9809/9933

Anderson, C., Klassen, R., & Georgiou, G. (2007). What teachers say they need and what school psychologists can offer. *School Psychology International, 28*(2), 131–147. doi:10.1177/0143034307078086

Andrade Boué, P. (2000). Quelques aspects de la Merencolie de Charles d'Orléans [Some aspects of Charles d'Orléans' Merencolia]. *Thélème. Revista Complutense de Estudios Franceses, 15*, 167. https://revistas.ucm.es/index.php/THEL/article/view/THEL0000110167A

Androtsopoulou, A. (1997). The choice of modern stories for children as a means of book therapy: Rationale and applications. *Routes*, (49), 12–17.

Angelides, P., Constantinou, C., & Leigh, J. (2009). The role of paraprofessionals in developing inclusive education in Cyprus. *European Journal of Special Needs Education, 24*(1), 75–89. doi:10.1080/08856250802596741

Angell, M. E., Stoner, J. B., & Shelden, D. L. (2008). Trust in Education Professionals: Perspectives of Mothers of Children With Disabilities. *Remedial and Special Education, 30*(3), 160–176. doi:10.1177/0741932508315648

Annahar (Ed.). (2020, November 7). Corona hāǧis al-kuttāb [Corona book pilgrims]. *Al-Ǧarīda*. https://www.annahar.com/arabic/culture/

Antoni, M. H., & Dhabhar, F. S. (2019). The impact of psychosocial stress and stress management on immune responses in patients with cancer. *Cancer, 125*(9), 1417–1431. doi:10.1002/cncr.31943 PMID:30768779

Apple, M. W. (2016). *Εκπαίδευση και εξουσία* [Education and Power]. Epikentro Publishers.

Arab Youth Center. (Ed.). (2021). *Al-Šabāb al-'arabi wa-l-COVID-19: Ḫawāṭir ibdā'iyya arabiyya fī zaman al-wabā* [Al-Habbab Al-Arabi and Covid-19: Arab Creative Paths in the Time of Al-Waba`ah]. Qindeel.

Ardington, C., Wills, G., & Kotze, J. (2021). COVID-19 learning losses: Early grade reading in South Africa. *International Journal of Educational Development, 86*, 102480. doi:10.1016/j.ijedudev.2021.102480

Arizpe, E., Farrar, J., & McAdam, J. (2018). Picturebooks and Literacy Studies. In B. Kümmerling-Meibauer (Ed.), *The Routledge Companion to Picturebooks* (pp. 371–380). Routledge.

Arizpe, E., & Styles, M. (2016). *Children Reading Picturebooks. Interpreting Visual Texts* (2nd ed.). Routledge.

Arkorful, V., & Abaidoo, N. (2014). The Role of e-Learning, the Advantages and Disadvantages of Its Adoption in Higher Education. *International Journal of Education and Research*, *2*(12), 397–410. https://www.ijern.com/journal/2014/December-2014/34.pdf

Asbury, K., Fox, L., Deniz, E., Code, A., & Toseeb, U. (2021). How is COVID-19 Affecting the Mental Health of Children with Special Educational Needs and Disabilities and Their Families? *Journal of Autism and Developmental Disorders*, *51*(5), 1772–1780. doi:10.100710803-020-04577-2 PMID:32737668

Asmundson, J. G., & Taylor, S. (2020, December). Coronaphobia revisted: A state-of-the-art on pandemic-related fear, anxiety, and stress. *Journal of Anxiety Disorders*, *76*, 102326. Advance online publication. doi:10.1016/j.janxdis.2020.102326 PMID:33142124

Ávila, R., & Horvat, S. (Eds.). (2021). *Todo debe cambiar! El mundo después de la Covid-19* [Everything must change! The world after Covid-19]. Rayo Verde.

Avramidis, E., & Norwich, B. (2002). Teachers' attitudes towards integration/inclusion: A review of the literature. *European Journal of Special Needs Education*, *17*(2), 129–147. doi:10.1080/08856250210129056

Awini, S. (2020). *Ḥub fī zaman Corona* [Hub in the time of Corona]. Dar Abaad.

Aziz, R., Susanto, D., Safitri, S. I., Mazida, L. I., & Wijaya, T. (2021). Literacy learning problems: Developing the character of reading fondness in elementary school students during the covid-19. *Premiere Educandum: Jurnal Pendidikan Dasar dan Pembelajaran, 11*(2), 243-253. doi:10.25273/pe.v11i2.10221

Babalis, T., & Xanthakou, G. (2008). School class and socialization of the student. *Education Sciences*, (3), 55–64.

Badi, M. (Director). (1974). *Al-Ḥarīq* [The Hammer] [TV Series]. Télévision Algérienne.

Bajour, C. (2009). *Oír entre líneas* [Hearing between the lines]. Asolectura.

Bakadi, M. (2021). Corona pandemic manifests in the poetry of the poets of the Tamanraset region goumni mobarek in his poems; ya latif, and kalb mounib, as a model. *Mağallat al-Kalim*, *1*(6), 216-234.

Baker, S. (2018). Shifts in the treatment of knowledge in academic reading and writing: Adding complexity to students' transitions between A-levels and university in the UK. *Arts and Humanities in Higher Education*, *17*(4), 388–409. doi:10.1177/1474022217722433

Bakhouche, M. (2021). *Misāḥa li-l-adab* [Maya Literature] [Radio Series]. Al-Iḏā'a al-Ṯaqāfiyya. https://radioalgerie.dz/culture/ar/

Bänziger, T., Grandjean, D., & Scherer, K. R. (2009). Emotion recognition from expressions in face, voice, and body: The Multimodal Emotion Recognition Test (MERT). *Emotion (Washington, D.C.)*, *9*(5), 691–704. doi:10.1037/a0017088 PMID:19803591

Bao, X., Qu, H., Zhang, R., & Hogan, T. P. (2020). *Literacy loss in kindergarten children during COVID-19 school closures*. Academic Press.

Baron, N. S. (2017). Reading in a digital age. *Phi Delta Kappan*, *99*(2), 15–20. doi:10.1177/0031721717734184

Barthes, R. (1973). *Le plaisir du texte* [The pleasure of the text]. Editions du Seuil.

Bartual, R. (2014). *Narraciones gráficas. Del códice medieval al cómic* [Graphic narrations. From medieval codex to comics]. Self Published.

Bassry, A. (2020). *Kağutta fī riwāya būlisiyya* [Kaguta is better than the police]. Al-Dār al-Miṣriyya al-Lubnāniyya.

BBC Playlist. (n.d.). *Lockdown Diaries. Stories from people around the world during pandemic*. Retrieved from: https://www.bbc.com/reel/playlist/world-in-lockdown

Beaton, L. J. (2007). *Stepping stones to success II. Collaboration: Working together for all students.* CTE Resource Center. Commonwealth of Virginia Department of Education.

Beckett, S. L. (2022) Crossing Boundaries of Age, Culture, and Time with Challenging Picturebooks. In Exploring Challenging Picturebooks in Education. International Perspectives on Language and Literature Learning. Routledge.

Beckett, S. L. (2012). *Crossover Picturebooks. A Genre for All Ages*. Routledge.

Beckett, S. L. (2018). Crossover Picturebooks. In B. Kümmerling-Meibauer (Ed.), *The Routledge Companion to Picturebooks* (pp. 209–2019). Routledge.

Beechey T., M. Buchholz M. J., & Keidser G. (2020). *Hearing aid amplification reduces communication effort of people with hearing impairment and their conversation partners*. doi:10.1044/2020_JSLHR-19-00350

Belghelifi, N. (2021). Mass memory and the epidemic's representations in the Machira area: Corona is a model. *Mağallat Wiḥdat al-baḥṯ fī tanmiyat al-mawārid al-bašariyya. CRASC, 3*(16), 98–121.

Benaichouhe, O., & Boussersoub, H. (2020). The role of Facebook in promoting health awareness about Corona Covid 19 A field study of a sample of Facebook users, Corona virus news page, and health education as an example. *Mağallat al-Tamkīn al-Iğtimā'ī, 2*(2), 288-309.

Benedictow, O. J. (2011). La peste negra (1346-1353) [The Black Death (1346-1353)]. In La historia completa, (p. 589). Akal SA.

Benfodil, M. [@Mustapha Benfodil] (2022, February 23). *Mes pièces "End/Igné"* [My "End/Igneous" pieces] [Status update]. Facebook. https://www.facebook.com/benfodilmustapha

Benhadouga, A. (1971). *Rīḥ al-ğanūb* [Alien head]. Sned editions.

Benhadouga, A. (1976). *Le Vent du Sud* [The South Wind] (M. Bois, Trans.). Sned editions. (Original work published 1971)

Benhadouga, A. (1981). *El Viento del sur* [The South Wind] (M. Villegas, Trans.). Instituto Hispano-Árabe de Cultura. (Original work published 1971)

Berger, J. (2015). *Para entender la fotografía* [To understand photography]. Editorial GG.

Bernard, A., Weiss, S., Stein, J. D., Ulin, S. S., D'Souza, C., Salgat, A., Panzer, K., Riddering, A., Edwards, P., Meade, M., McKee, M. M., & Ehrlich, J. R. (2020). Assessing the impact of COVID-19 on persons with disabilities: Development of a novel survey. *International Journal of Public Health, 65*(6), 755–757. doi:10.100700038-020-01433-z PMID:32705300

Bessadi, N. (2020). Al-Muğtama'al-ğazā'irī yašhad izdihāran aṯnā' al-ğā'iḥa. *Ru'ya.* https://www.goethe.de/prj/ruy/ar/covid/21853154.html

Betzalel, N., & Shechtman, Z. (2017). The impact of bibliotherapy superheroes on youth who experience parental absence. *School Psychology International, 38*(5), 473–490. doi:10.1177/0143034317719943

Bianchi, A., Barrios, S., Cabrera, M., Cachia, R., Compañó, R., Malanowski, N., & Centeno, C. (2006). *Revisiting e-Inclusion: From vision to action.* Institute for Prospective Technological Studies, European Commission.

Blais, C., Roy, C., Fiset, D., Arguin, M., & Gosselin, F. (2012). *The eyes are not the window to basic emotions.* doi:10.1016/j.neuropsychologia.2012.08.010

Blanchot, M. (1959). El diario íntimo y el relato [The intimate diary and the story]. *El libro por venir. Madrid. Trotta, 2005*, 219–224.

Boccuti, A. (2020). Pandemia y literatura: variaciones erótico-sentimentales en la imaginación distópica [Pandemic and literature: erotic-sentimental variations in the dystopian imagination]. In *COVID19 – LiTraPan. Literary Training via ICT for Higher Education Improvement, Behavioral Coaching and Discomfort Management during the Coronavirus Pandemic [Branch: UniTo]. II International Symposium "Forbidden Delights: Sex, Eroticism, Beauty, Aesthetics, Pleasure, Law, Sin and Prohibition". 19-20/06/2020.* Retrieved from https://www.youtube.com/watch?v=kQRss0sXAk8, 19

Boccuti, A. (2020). Pandemia y literatura: variaciones erótico-sentimentales en la imaginación distópica [Pandemic and literature: erotic-sentimental variations in the dystopian imagination]. In *COVID19 – LiTraPan. Literary Training via ICT for Higher Education Improvement, Behavioral Coaching and Discomfort Management during the Coronavirus Pandemic [Branch: UniTo]. II International Symposium "Forbidden Delights: Sex, Eroticism, Beauty, Aesthetics, Pleasure, Law, Sin and Prohibition".* Retrieved from https://www.youtube.com/watch?v=kQRss0sXAk8, 19

Boccuti, A. (2022). Contagios narrativos: crónicas y diarios del coronavirus desde América Latina [Narrative infections: chronicles and diaries of the coronavirus from Latin America]. *eHumanista/IVITRA*, 21.

Bonal, X., & González, S. (2021). Educación formal e informal en confinamiento: Una creciente desigualdad de oportunidades de aprendizaje. *Research in Sociology of Education, 14*(1), 44–62. doi:10.7203/RASE.14.1.18177

Bonilla, R. (2021). *Gràcies. Història d'un veïnat* [Thank you. History of a neighborhood]. Animallibres.

Booth, T., Ainscow, M., & Kingston, D. (2006). *Index for inclusion: Developing play, learning, and participation in early years and childcare.* Centre for Studies on Inclusive Education.

Bordería Ortiz, E., Martínez Gallego, F. A., & Gómez Mompart, J. L. (Eds.). (2015). *El humor frente al poder. Prensa humorística, cultura política y poderes fácticos en España (1927-1987).* [Humor versus power. Humorous press, political culture and factual powers in Spain (1927-1987)]. Editorial Biblioteca Nueva.

Borges, J.L. (1984). *Evaristo Carriego.* E.P. Dutton, Inc.

Borges, J.L. (1995). *Premio Cervantes 1979* [Cervantes Prize 1979.] Universidad de Alcalá.

Borges, J. L. (1971). *The Aleph and Other Stories 1933-1969.* Bantam.

Borges, J. L. (1972). *Selected Poems 1923-1967.* Allen Lane The Penguin Press.

Borges, J. L. (1975). *A Universal History of Infamy.* Penguin Modern Classics.

Borges, J. L., & Ferrari, O. (2014). *Conversations* (Vol. 1). Seagull Books.

Bou, E. (1996). El diario: Periferia y literatura [The Journal: Periphery and literature]. Revista de Occidente, (102-103), 121-135.

Boudjedra, R. (2002). *El Repudio* [The Repudiation] (R. Páez, Trans.). Emecé editores. (Original work published in 1981)

Boudjedra, R. (1965). *Pour ne plus rêver* [To stop dreaming]. ÉNA.

Boudjedra, R. (1981). *La Répudiation* [The Repudiation]. Gallimard Folio.

Boudjedra, R. (2001). *Cinq Fragments du désert* [Five Fragments of the Desert]. Barzakh.

Boudjedra, R. (2005). *Para no soñar más, y cinco fragmentos del desierto* [Not to dream anymore, and five fragments of the desert]. (L. Merino, Trans.). Huerga y Fierro Editores. (Original work published 1965)

Bouillet, D. (2013). Some aspects of collaboration in inclusive education - Teachers' experiences. *CEPS Journal*, *3*(2), 93–117. doi:10.26529/cepsj.241

Bourget, L. (2018). *Ma Maison* [My home]. Éditions Les Grands Personnes.

Boutadjin, S. (2020). *Marāyā 'ākisa, al-adab wa-l-awbi'a* [Reflective Mirrors - Literature and Epidemics]. Ministère de la Culture et des Arts. https://www.m-culture.gov.dz/index.php/ar/2-non-categorise/3063-

Bover, A. (2014). *Beabà*, prefaci de Denise Boyer i Eliseu Trenc [*Beaba*, preface by Denise Boyer and Elisha Trenc]. *Tarragona*. Arola Editors.

Bover, A. (2018a). *Tornaveu*. Pròleg de Vicent Pitarch i Almela [*Come back*. Foreword by Vicent Pitarch i Almela]. Tarragona: Arola Editors.

Bover, A. (2018b) Blau marí. Poemes i proses [Navy blue. Poems and prose]. Vilanova i la Geltrú: El Cep i la Nansa Edicions.

Bover, A. (2021). El contagi [Contagion]. Barcelona: Edicions Saldonar.

Bover, A. (2022). Cloc! Pròleg de Màrius Serra [Stop! Prologue by Màrius Serra]. Tarragona: Arola Editors (2nd ed.). Academic Press.

Bowles, S., & Gintis, H. (2013). *A cooperative species: Human reciprocity and its evolution*. Princeton University Press.

Breitenbach, M. M., Armstrong, V. L., & Bryson, S. E. (2013). The implementation of best education practices for a student severely affected by autism. *International Journal of Inclusive Education*, *17*(3), 277–294. doi:10.1080/13603116.2012.676087

Bringel, B., & Pleyers, G. (Eds.). (2020). *Alerta global: políticas, movimientos sociales y futuros en disputa en tiempos de pandemia* [Global alert: policies, social movements and futures in dispute in times of pandemic]. Consejo Latinoamericano de Ciencias Sociales., doi:10.2307/j.ctv1gm027x

Bröckling, U. (2021). *Héroes postheoricos. Un diagnóstico de nuestro tiempo* [Post-Heoric heroes. A diagnosis of our time]. Alianza Editorial.

Broemmel, A. D., Rearden, K. T., & Buckner, C. (2021). Teachers' choices: Are they the right books for science instruction? *The Reading Teacher*, *75*(1), 7–16. doi:10.1002/trtr.1998

Brooks, S. K., Webster, R. K., Smith, L. E., Woodland, L., Wessley, S., Greenberg, N., & Rubin, G. J. (2020). The psychological impact of quarantine and how to reduce it: Rapid review of the evidence. *Lancet*, *395*(10227), 912–920. doi:10.1016/S0140-6736(20)30460-8 PMID:32112714

Brottman, M. (2018). *Contra la lectura: un ensayo dedicado a los lectores que no creen que los libros sean intocables* [Against reading: an essay dedicated to readers who do not believe that books are untouchable]. Blackie Books.

Brownell, M. T., Adams, A., Sindelar, P., Waldron, N., & Vanhover, S. (2006). Learning from collaboration: The role of teacher qualities. *Exceptional Children*, *72*(2), 169–185. doi:10.1177/001440290607200203

Burgin, R. (2013). *Jorge Luis Borges. The Last Interview and other Conversations*. Melville House.

Burnett, J. (1997). *Opening the World to Children: Using Books to Develop Problem-Solving Strategies*. Academic Press.

Cacioppo, J. T., & Cacioppo, S. (2014). Social relationships and health: The toxic effects of perceived social isolation. *Social and Personality Psychology Compass*, *8*(2), 58–72. doi:10.1111pc3.12087 PMID:24839458

Camacho, A. C. L. F., Joaquim, F. L., de Menezes, H. F., & Sant'Anna, R. M. (2020). Tutoring in distance education in times of COVID-19: Relevant guidelines. *Research. Social Development*, *9*(5), 1–12. doi:10.33448/rsd-v9i5.3151

Campagnaro, M. (2019). Do Touch! How Bruno Munari's Picturebooks Work. *Revista di Storia dell'Educazione*, *6*(1), 81-96.

Campagnaro, M., & Dallari, M. (2013). Incanto e racconto nel labirinto delle figure [Enchantment and story in the labyrinth of figures]. In Albii illustrati e relazione educativa. Trento: Erickson.

Campagnaro, M. (2022). Picturebooks and aesthetic Literacy in Early Childhood Education. In *Exploring Challenging Picturebooks in Education. International Perspectives on Language and Literature Learning* (pp. 79–98). Routledge.

Campigotto, R., McEwen, R., & Epp, C. D. (2013). Especially social: Exploring the use of an iOS application in special needs classrooms. *Computers & Education*, *60*(1), 74–86. doi:10.1016/j.compedu.2012.08.002

Camus, A. (2002). *La peste* [Plague]. EDHASA.

Cannon, P. (2018). Rethinking bibliotherapy: A neurorhetoric narratology model for addiction treatment. *Health Information and Libraries Journal*, *35*(4), 331–335. doi:10.1111/hir.12239 PMID:30499173

Carlson, L., Hemmings, B., Wurf, G., & Reupert, A. (2012). The instructional strategies and attitudes of effective inclusive teachers. *Special Education Perspectives*, *21*(1), 7–20.

Carrión, J. (2021). Narrativas de la pandemia [Narratives of the pandemic]. *La Vanguardia, Suplemento Culturals*. Retrieved from https://www.lavanguardia.com/cultura/culturas/20211127/7883333/narrativas-pandemia-libros-covid.html#foto-1

Carrión, J., & Sagar. (2018). *Gótico* [Gothic]. Norma Editorial.

Carrión-Martínez, J. J., Pinel-Martínez, C., Pérez-Esteban, M. D., & Román-Sánchez, I. M. (2021). Family and school relationship during COVID-19 pandemic: A systematic review. *International Journal of Environmental Research and Public Health*, *18*(21), 11710. Advance online publication. doi:10.3390/ijerph182111710 PMID:34770223

Carter, E. W., & Kennedy, C. H. (2006). Promoting Access to the General Curriculum Using Peer Support Strategies. *Research and Practice for Persons with Severe Disabilities*, *31*(4), 284–292. doi:10.1177/154079690603100402

Castillo, A. D. L. (1976). Selección de refranes médicos de la obra de Pedro Valles [Selection of medical sayings from the work of Pedro Valles]. *Medicamenta*, *482*, 455–462.

Catelli, N. (1996). El diario íntimo. Una posición femenina [The intimate diary. A female position]. Revista de Occidente, (102-103), 87-98.

Cavarero, A. (2000). Relating narratives. Storytelling and selfhood (P. A. Kottman, Trans.). Routledge.

Cedefop. (2020a). *Digital gap during Covid-19 for VET learners at risk in Europe. Synthesis report.* https://www.cedefop.europa.eu/bg/toolkits/vet-toolkit-tackling-early-leaving/resources/digitalgap-during-covid-19-vet-learners-risk-europe

Cedefop. (2020b). *How are European countries managing apprenticeships to respond to the Covid-19 crisis? Synthesis report based on information provided by Cedefop community of apprenticeship experts.* https://www.cedefop.europa.eu/files/cedefop_community_apprenticeship_experts_synthesis_ho_ are_european_countries_managing_apprenticeships_to_respond_to_the_coronavirus_crisis.pdf

Christinaki, E., Vidakis, N., & Triantafyllidis, G. (2013). Facial expression recognition teaching to preschoolers with autism: a natural user interface approach. In *BCI '13: Proceedings of the 6th Balkan Conference in Informatics* (pp. 141-148). Association for Computing Machinery. 10.1145/2490257.2490262

Christopher, J. C., Wendt, D. C., Marecek, J., & Goodman, D. M. (2014). Critical Cultural Awareness: Contributions to a Globalizing Psychology. *The American Psychologist*, *69*(7), 645–655. doi:10.1037/a0036851 PMID:24841336

Clark, A. E., Nong, H., Zhu, H., & Zhu, R. (2021). Compensating for academic loss: Online learning and student performance during the COVID-19 pandemic. *China Economic Review*, *68*, 101629. doi:10.1016/j.chieco.2021.101629

Cohn, N. (2013). *The Visual Language of Comics*. Bloomsbury Academic.

Colizzi, M., Sironi, E., Antonini, F., Ciceri, M. L., Bovo, C., & Zoccante, L. (2020). Psychosocial and behavioral impact of COVID-19 in autism spectrum disorder: An online parent survey. *Brain Sciences*, *10*(6), 341. Advance online publication. doi:10.3390/brainsci10060341 PMID:32503172

Collie, R. J., Bostwick, K. C., & Martin, A. J. (2019). Perceived autonomy support, relatedness with students, and workplace outcomes: An investigation of differences by teacher gender. Educational Psychology. *An International Journal of Experimental Educational Psychology*, *40*(3), 253–272.

Collis, B. (1999). *Tele-Learning in a Digital World - The Future of Distance Learning*. International Thompson Computer Press.

Colombo, M., & Santagati, M. (2021). The Inclusion of Students With Disabilities: Challenges for Italian Teachers During the Covid-19 Pandemic. *Social Inclusion (Lisboa)*, *10*(2). Advance online publication. doi:10.17645i.v10i2.5035

Conecta. (2020). *La lectura en tiempos de COVID-19*. https://www.editoresmadrid.org/wp-content/uploads/2020/05/LA-LECTURA-EN-TIEMPOS-DE-COVID-19.pdf

Coneixement en temps de pandèmia, Coneixement en temps de pandèmia. (n.d.). Universitat d'Alacant. Seu Universitària de La Nucia. Retrieved from https://web.ua.es/es/seus/lanucia/documentos/actividades-culturales/2019-2020/cicle-pandemia.pdf

Conejero, P.F.J. (2017). Lletraferides als convents, una escriptura femenina al segle XVI [Letters to convents, a female writing in the sixteenth century]. *Mirabilia/MedTrans. Mirabilia/Mediterranean and Transatlantic Approaches to the Culture of the Crown of Aragon*, (2), 38-70.

Conejero, P.F.J. (2019). Els delits prohibits als cenobis femenins [Forbidden delights in female cenobis]. *Mirabilia/MedTrans: Mirabilia/Mediterranean and Transatlantic Approaches to the Culture of the Crown of Aragon*, (1), 52-76.

Cook, L., & Friend, M. (2004). *Co-Teaching: Principles, practices, and pragmatics*. New Mexico Public Education Department Quarterly Special Education Meeting.

Cope, B., & Kalantzis, M. (2000). *Multiliteracies. Literacy Learning and the Design of Social Futures*. Routledge.

Cope, B., & Kalantzis, M. (2015). *A Pedagogy of Multiliteracies. Learning by design*. Palgrave and Macmillan.

Cortijo Ocaña, A., & Martines, V. (Eds.). (2022). Handbook of Research on Historical Pandemic Analysis and the Social Implications of COVID-19. IGI Global.

Cortijo Ocaña, A., Orazi, V., & Martines, V. (Eds.). (2022). Managing Pandemic Isolation with Literature as Therapy. IGI Global.

Cortijo, A., & Martines, V. (Eds.). (2013). Multilingual Joan Roís de Corella. The Relevance of a Fifteenth-Century Classic of the Crown of Aragon Joan Roís de Corella Multilingüe. La importància d'un clàssic de la Corona d'Aragó del segle XV. Publications of eHumanista-University of California at Santa Barbara.

Costa-Gramunt, T. (2021). Poemes de la pandèmia [Poems from the pandemic]. *Eix Diari*. Retrieved from https://www.eixdiari.cat/opinio/doc/98425/poemes-de-la-pandemia.html

Costa, J. (Ed.). (2018). *Una risa nueva. Posthumor, parodias y otras mutaciones de la comedia* [A new laugh. Post-humor, parodies and other comedy mutations]. Lengua de Trapo.

Courtin, E., & Knapp, M. (2017). Social isolation, loneliness and health in old age: A scoping review. *Health & Social Care in the Community*, *25*(3), 799–812. doi:10.1111/hsc.12311 PMID:26712585

Coyle, C. E., & Dugan, E. (2012). Social isolation, loneliness and health among older adults. *Journal of Aging and Health*, *24*(8), 1346–1363. doi:10.1177/0898264312460275 PMID:23006425

Creswell, J. W. (2009). *Research Design. Qualitative, quantitative and Mixed Methods Approaches*. Sage.

Cuadrada, C. (2012). El llibre de la pesta [The Book of the Plague] (R. Dalmau, Ed.). Academic Press.

Darici, K. (2022a). Marta Sanz, *Parte de mí* (2021) [Marta Sanz, *Part of Me* (2021)]. *eHumanista/IVITRA*, *21*.

Darici, K. (2022b). El tiempo que nos robaron (2021) [The Time They Stole From Us (2021)]. In A. Cortijo Ocaña, V. Orazi, & V. Martines (Eds.), Managing Pandemic Isolation with Literature as Therapy. IGI Global.

Darrow, A.-A. (2009). Barriers to effective inclusion and strategies to overcome them. *General Music Today*, *22*(3), 29–31. doi:10.1177/1048371309333145

Daub, A. C., Villanueva, S., Soares, M. C., & Huber, T. (2021). Educators' Experiences With Teaching During COVID-19 : Journey of a Participatory Action Research Inquiry Team Educators ' Experiences With Teaching During COVID-19 : Journey of a Participatory Action Research Inquiry Team. *Journal of Multicultural Affairs*, *6*(2).

De Naeghel, J., Van Keer, H., Vansteenkiste, M., & Rosseel, Y. (2012). The relation between elementary students' recreational and academic reading motivation, reading frequency, engagement, and comprehension: A self-determination theory perspective. *Journal of Educational Psychology*, *104*(4), 1006–1021. doi:10.1037/a0027800

de Sant Jordi, J. (2011). Poesia [Poetry]. Edició crítica d'Aniello Fratta, versió en català modern de Carles Duarte. Barcelona: Barcino.

de Sant Jordi, J. (2023). Poems (A. Cortijo, A. Cortijo-Rodgers, & V. Martines, Eds.). Academic Press.

De Sousa Santos, B. (2020). *La cruel pedagogía del virus* [The cruel pedagogy of the virus]. Consejo Latinoamericano de Ciencias Sociales. doi:10.2307/j.ctv1gm01nn

Demetrio, D. (2015). *Green Autobiography. La natura è un racconto interiore* [Green Autobiography. Nature is an inner story]. Book Salad.

Denisevich, K. (2020). *Neighbors*. Chronicle Books.

DePauw, K. P., & Doll-Tepper, G. (2000). Toward progressive inclusion and acceptance: Myth or Reality? The inclusion debate and bandwagon discourse. *Adapted Physical Activity Quarterly; APAQ*, *17*(2), 135–143. doi:10.1123/apaq.17.2.135

Dera, J. (2021). Evaluating poetry on COVID-19: Attitudes of poetry readers toward corona poems. *Journal of Poetry Therapy*, *34*(2), 77–94. doi:10.1080/08893675.2021.1899630

Dewey, J. (1938). *Experience and Education*. Kappa Delta Pi.

Dib, M. (1954). *l'Incendie* [The fire]. Le Seuil.

Dib, M. (1979). *El Incendio* [The fire]. Arte y literatura. (Original work published 1954).

Dib, M. (1952). *La Grande Maison* [The Big House]. Le Seuil.

Dib, M. (1959). *Un été africain* [An African summer]. Points.

Dib, M. (1976). *Un verano en África* [A summer in Africa]. (O. C. Alegre, Trans.). Arte y Literatura. (Original work published 1959)

Didier, B. (1996). El diario ¿forma abierta? [The diary, open form?]. Revista de Occidente, (102-103), 39-46.

Didier, B. (1976). *Le journal intime* [The diary]. Presses Universitaires de France.

Didier, B. (1981). *L'écriture-femme* [Women's writing]. Presses Universitaires de France.

Dimitriadis, S. N. (2015). *Learning Theories & Educational Software*. Kallipos.

Djebar, A. (2002). *Les nits a Estrasburg* [Nights in Strasbourg] (A. Casassas, Trans.). Edicions 62. (Original work published in 1997)

Djebar, A. (1980). *Femmes d'Alger dans leur appartement* [Women of Algiers in their apartment]. Éditions des Femmes.

Djebar, A. (1997). *Les Nuits de Strasbourg* [The Nights of Strasbourg]. Actes Sud.

Djebar, A. (2015). *Las noches de Estrasburgo* [The nights of Strasbourg]. (M. S. Crespo, Trans.). Alfaguara. (Original work published 1997)

Djelaoudji, A. (2012). *Al-Masraḥiyya al-ši'riyya fī-l-adab al-maġāribī al-mu'āṣir* [Standard play in warrior literature]. Dār al-Tanwir.

Djelaoudji, A. (2020). *Al-Naṣ al-masraḥī fī-l-adab al-ǧazā'irī* [The Egyptian Naas in Azeri literature]. Dār al-Muntahà.

Djlaodji, A. (2020, June 15). *Ġilaf riwāyatī al-ǧadīda* [Elaf new novels]. Facebook. https://www.facebook.com/265532643874402/posts/908025542958439/

Dost, J. (2020). *Fī qabḍat al-kābūs: ṯalāṯuna yawman mina ḥiṣār Corona*. Dār Ḫuṭūṭ.

Dostoyevski F. (2020). *Mudhillūn muhānūn* [Humiliated and Insulted] (S. Droubi Trans.). Dār al-Tanwīr lil-Ṭibā'ah wa-al-Nashr. (Original work published in 1861)

Drakopoulou, E. (2020). *Inclusive Education and the Impact of COVID-19 on learners with disabilities*. Education Policy - European Disability Forum. https://www.edf-feph.org/content/uploads/2021/06/Inclusive-Education-and-COVID-19_Eleni-Drakopoulou.docx

Drakopoulou, E. (2020). *Inclusive Education and the Impact of COVID-19 on learners with disabilities*. https://www.edf-feph.org/education-policy/

Druker, E., & Kümmerling-Meibauer, B. (Eds.). (2015). *Children's Literature and the Avant-Garde*. John Benjamins. doi:10.1075/clcc.5

Dubuc, M. (2020). *Chez moi, chez toi* [At home, at home]. Casterman.

Eco, U. (1962). *Opera aperta. Forma e indeterminazione nelle poetiche contemporanee* [Open work. Form and indetermination in contemporary poetics]. Bompiani.

eEurope Advisory Group. (2005). *eInclusion. New challenges and policy recommendations*. European Commission.

El Mestari, D. (2020). *Covid-19 en Algérie: enseignements et regards croisés (premiers éléments de réflexion)* [Covid-19 in Algeria: lessons and crossed views (first elements of reflection)]. Centre de Recherche en Anthropologie Sociale et Culturelle CRASC.

Embid, J. (2018). *Con capa y antifaz: la ideología de los superhéroes*. Catarata.

Epstein, J. (1995). School- family- community partnerships: Caring for the children we share. *Phi Delta Kappan, 76*(9), 701–712.

ERI-Lectura. (2020). *Hábitos lectores durante el confinamiento por la covid-19*. https://roderic.uv.es/handle/10550/74797

Escartí, V.J. (1998). Memòria privada [Private memory]. In *Literatura memoralística valenciana dels segles XV al XVIII*. Tres i Quatre.

Escartí, V.J. (2010). Notícia sobre la literatura memorialística al País Valencià, del segle XIV al XIX [News about memorial literature in Valencia, from the fourteenth to the nineteenth century]. *Manuscrits: Revista d'història moderna*, (28), 181-205.

Escartí, V.J. (2021). La memòria de les pestes a l'antic Regne de València: de la nota marginal a la centralitat (s. XV-XVII) [The memory of the plagues in the ancient Kingdom of Valencia: from marginal note to centrality (s. XV-XVII)]. *Mirabilia/MedTrans: Mirabilia/Mediterranean and Transatlantic Approaches to the Culture of the Crown of Aragon, 53*.

Escartí, V. J. (2020). *La pesta a València (1647-1648)* [The plague in Valencia (1647-1648)]. Diputació de València, Institució Alfons el Magànim.

Escartí, V. J., & Ribera, R. J. (2019). *El llibre de memòries de la ciutat de València (1308-1644)* [The book of memoirs of the city of Valencia (1308-1644)]. Edició Ajuntament de València.

Evans, J. (2016). Who am I Why I am here? and Where do I come from? Responding to Philosophical Picturebooks. *Education 3-13, 44*(1), 53-67. doi:10.1080/03004279.2015.1109815

Evans, J. (1998). *What's in the Picture? Responding to Illustrations in Picture Books*. Sage.

Evans, J. (2015b). Picturebooks as Strange, Challenging and Controversial Texts. In J. Evans (Ed.), *Challenging and Controversial Picturebooks: Creative and Critical Responses to Visual Texts* (pp. 3–32). Routledge. doi:10.4324/9781315756912-12

Evans, J. (Ed.). (2015a). *Challenging and Controversial Picturebooks: Creative and Critical Responses to Visual Texts*. Routledge. doi:10.4324/9781315756912

Fang, F. (2020). *Wuhan Diary. Dispatches from a Quarantined City* (M. Berry, Trans.). Ebook.

Farrar, J., Arizpe, E., & McAdam, J. (2022). Challenging Picturebooks and Literacy Studies. In *Exploring Challenging Picturebooks in Education. International Perspectives on Language and Literature Learning* (pp. 43–56). Routledge.

Featherstone, M. (1992). The Heroic Life and Everyday Life. *Theory, Culture & Society, 9*(1), 159–182. doi:10.1177/026327692009001009

Feraoun, M. (1950). *Le fils du pauvre* [The poor man's son]. Cahiers du Nouvel Humanisme.

Feraoun, M. (2001). *El hijo del pobre* [The por man's son] (G. F. Parrilla & M. E. López, Trans.). Ediciones del Oriente y Mediterráneo. (Original work published 1950)

Fernández Prieto, C. (2004). Enunciación y comunicación en la autobiografía [Enunciation and communication in autobiography]. In C. Fernández Prieto & Ma Á. Hermosilla Álvarez (Eds.), Con la colaboración de A. Caballé. Autobiografía en España: un balance. Actas del Congreso Internacional celebrado en La Facultad de Filosofía y Letras de Córdoba del 25 al 27 de octubre de 2001 (pp. 417-432). Madrid: Visor.

Fernández-López, Á., Rodríguez-Fórtiz, M. J., Rodríguez-Almendros, M. L., & Martínez-Segura, M. J. (2013). Mobile learning technology based on iOS devices to support students with special education needs. *Computers & Education, 61*(0), 77–90. https://dx.doi.org/10.1016/j.compedu.2012.09.014

Fidalgo-Blanco, A., Martinez-Nuñez, M., Borrás-Gene, O., & Sanchez-Medina, J. J. (2017). Micro flip teaching – An innovative model to promote the active involvement of students. *Computers in Human Behavior, 72*, 713–723. doi:10.1016/j.chb.2016.07.060

Fioretti, C., Mazzocco, K., Riva, S., Oliveri, S., Masiero, M., & Pravettoni, G. (2016). Research studies on patients' illness experience using the Narrative Medicine approach: A systematic review. *BMJ Open, 6*(7), 112–120. doi:10.1136/bmjopen-2016-011220 PMID:27417197

Flipped Learning Network. (2014). *Definition of flipped learning*. https://flippedlearning.org/definitionof-flipped-learning

Flipped Learning Network. (2014). *Definition of Flipped Learning*. Retrieved from Retrieved March 10, 2022, from https://flippedlearning.org/definition-of-flipped-learning/

Fontdevila, M. (2013). *No os indignéis tanto* [Don't be so unworthy of them]. Astiberri.

Forteza-Forteza, D., Rodríguez-Martín, A., Álvarez-Arregui, E., & Menéndez Álvarez-Hevia, D. (2021). Inclusion, Dyslexia, Emotional State and Learning: Perceptions of Ibero-American Children with Dyslexia and Their Parents during the COVID-19 Lockdown. *Sustainability, 13*(5), 2739. https://dx.doi.org/10.3390/su13052739

Forzani, E., & Leu, D. J. (2012). New Literacies for New Learners: The Need for Digital Technologies in Primary Classrooms. *The Educational Forum, 76*(4), 421–424. https://doi.org/10.1080/00131725.2012.708623

Foucault, M. (1963). Le langage à l'infini [Language to infinity]. *Tel quel, 15*, 44-53. Retrieved from https://www.idixa.net/Pixa/pagixa-1607121915.html

Fox, S., Farrell, P., & Davis, P. (2004). Factors associated with the effective inclusion of primary-aged pupils with Down's syndrome. *British Journal of Special Education, 31*(4), 184–190. doi:10.1111/j.0952-3383.2004.00353.x

Francis, G. L., Blue-banning, M., Turnbull, A. P., & Haines, S. (2016). Culture in Inclusive Schools: Parental Perspectives on Trusting Family-Professional Partnerships. *Education and Training in Autism and Developmental Disabilities, 51*(3), 281–293.

Freeman, C., Mack, T., & Collins, T. (2022, January). Oral Presentation: Intersections: Reading STEM in Tennessee Elementary Schools. *16th Annual Tennessee STEM Education Research Conference*, 36.

Freixas, L. (1996). Auge del diario ¿íntimo? [Rise of the intimate diary?]. Revista de Occidente, (102-103), 6-14.

Freixas, L. (1996). Auge del diario ¿íntimo? en España [Rise of the intimate diary? in Spain]. *Revista de Occidente (Madrid, Spain), 182-183*, 5–14.

Friend, M., & Cook, L. (2016). *Interactions: Collaboration skills for school professionals* (7th ed.). Pearson.

Fundación, S. M. (2021). *Anuario Iberoamericano sobre el Libro Infantil y Juvenil 2021*. Fundación SM. https://www.grupo-sm.com/sites/sm-espana/files/resources/imagenes/COMUNICACION-2021/FUNDACION-SM/AnuarioLIJ_21/Anuario-Iberoamericano-sobre-el-Libro-Infantil-y-Juvenil-2021.pdf

Gaggioli, C. (2018). Digital classroom and students with learning disorders: a study to improve learning processes and teaching practices. *Research on Education and Media, 10*(2) 26-35. doi:10.1515/rem-2018-0012

García Bascuñana, J. F. (2010). *Por otra lectura de Charles d'Orléans: el valor de la imagen* [For another reading of Charles d'Orléans: the value of the image] [Doctoral thesis]. Universitat de Barcelona. https://www.tesisenred.net/handle/10803/1735#page=1

García Márquez, G. (2021). *El amor en los tiempos del cólera* [Love in the time of cholera]. Debolsillo.

García, S. (2010). *La novela gráfica* [The graphic novel]. Astiberri.

Genette, G. (1987). *Seouils* [Seoul.]. Seouil.

Georgiadi, M., Kourkoutas, E., & Kalyva, E. (2007). *Inclusion in Europe.* http://conf2007.edu.uoi.gr/Praktika/1236-1328.pdf

Ghanam, I., & Bensghir, K. (2021). Children's use of electronic screens in light of the Corona epidemic, and its effects on educational values from the points of view of children's parents and teachers. *Mağallat wiḥdat al-Baḥṯ fī Tanmiya al-Mawārid al-Bašariyya, 3*(16), 427-451.

Giannouli, V., Sarris, D., & Papadopoulou, M. (2021). Distance education in the pandemic era: The views of Greek general and special education teachers of secondary education regarding readiness, challenges and the post-covid educational practices. *European Journal of Special Education Research, 7*(4). https://dx.doi.org/10.46827/ejse.v7i4.4050

Gilmour, A. F., Fuchs, D., & Wehby, J. H. (2019). Are Students With Disabilities Accessing the Curriculum? A Meta-Analysis of the Reading Achievement Gap Between Students With and Without Disabilities. *Exceptional Children, 85.* doi:10.1177/0014402918795830

Giordano, P. (2020). *En tiempos de contagio* [In times of contagion]. Penguin Random House Grupo Editorial.

Girard, A. (1996). El diario como género literario [The diary as a literary genre]. Revista de Occidente, (102-103), 31-38.

Glazer, J. (1986). Literature for Young Children. Merrill.

Goethe Institut (Ed.). (2020). Tis'ata 'ašara rābiṭ li-dawarāt tadrībiyya maǧǧāniyyawa-'urūḍ ṯaqāfiyya. *Ru'ya.* https://www.goethe.de/prj/ruy/ar/covid/rethink.html

Goethe Institut (Ed.). (2021). Ibdā': al-fan fī zaman corona. *Ru'ya.* https://www.goethe.de/prj/ruy/ar/covid/rethink.html

Golob, T., Makarovi, M., & Rek, M. (2021). Meta-reflexivity for resilience against disinformation. *Comunicar,* (66), 107-118.

Gomez-Lanier, L. (2018). Building collaboration in the flipped classroom: A case study. *International Journal for the Scholarship of Teaching and Learning, 12*(2), 1–9. doi:10.20429/ijsotl.2018.120207

González Cabeza, I. (2017). *Imágenes de la enfermedad en el cómic actual* [Images of the disease in the current comic]. Servicio de Publicaciones de la Universidad de León - Eolas Ediciones.

Gopegui, B. (2008). *Un pistolazo en medio de un concierto* [A gunshot in the middle of a concert]. Editorial Complutense.

Greco, B. (2020). Amor y cuarentena en la narrativa breve de confinamiento [Love and quarantine in the short narrative of confinement]. In *COVID19 – LiTraPan. Literary Training via ICT for Higher Education Improvement, Behavioral Coaching and Discomfort Management during the Coronavirus Pandemic [Branch: UniTo], II International Symposium Forbidden Delights: Sex, Eroticism, Beauty, Aesthetics, Pleasure, Law, Sin and Prohibition. 19-20/06/2020.* Retrieved from https://www.youtube.com/watch?v=ki5DktWtYoA&feature=youtu.be

Greco, B. (2020). Amor y cuarentena en la narrativa breve de confinamiento [Love and quarantine in the short narrative of confinement]. In *COVID19 – LiTraPan. Literary Training via ICT for Higher Education Improvement, Behavioral Coaching and Discomfort Management during the Coronavirus Pandemic [Branch: UniTo], II International Symposium Forbidden Delights: Sex, Eroticism, Beauty, Aesthetics, Pleasure, Law, Sin and Prohibition*. Retrieved from https://www.youtube.com/watch?v=ki5DktWtYoA&feature=youtu.be

Greco, B. (2022). Pandemic and Literary Creativity. The Spanish Case of Relatos de confinamiento. In A. Cortijo Ocaña & V. Martines (Eds.), Handbook of Research on Historical Pandemic Analysis and the Social Implications of COVID-19 (pp. 80-93). IGI Global. doi:10.4018/978-1-7998-7987-9.ch007

Greco, B. (2022b). Cómic y Covid: *COnVIvienDo 19 días* de David Ramírez [Comics and Covid: *COnVIvienDo 19 days* of David Ramírez]. *eHumanista/IVITRA, 21*.

Greco, B. (2022c). A song to life in pandemic times: *Primavera extremeña* by Julio Llamazares. In A. Cortijo Ocaña, V. Orazi, & V. Martines (Eds.), Managing Pandemic Isolation with Literature as Therapy. *Hershey*. IGI Global.

Greek Ministry of Education. (2020). https://mathainoumestospiti.gov.gr/

Greenberg, G. (1998). Distance education technologies: Best practices for K-12 settings. *IEEE Technology and Society Magazine*, 3. *IEEE Technology and Society Magazine*, *17*(4), 36–40. https://doi.org/10.1109/44.7358626-40

Grieco-Calub, M. T. (2021). COVID-19, Face Masks, and Social Interaction: How a Global Pandemic Is Shining a Light on the Importance of Face-to-Face Communication. *Perspectives of the ASHA Special Interest Groups*, *6*(5), 1097–1105. Advance online publication. doi:10.1044/2021_PERSP-21-00037

Groensteen, T. (1999). *Système de la Bande Dessinée* [Comic Strip System]. Presses Universitaires de France.

Gros, B. (2007). Digital Games in Education: The Design of Games-Based Learning Environments. *Journal of Research on Technology in Education*, *40*(1), 23–38. https://files.eric.ed.gov/fulltext/EJ826060.pdf

Gualano, M. R., Bert, F., Martorana, M., Voglino, G., Andriolo, V., Thomas, R., Gramaglia, C., Zeppegno, P., & Siliquini, R. (2017). The long-term effects of bibliotherapy in depression treatment: Systematic review of randomized clinical trials. *Clinical Psychology Review*, *58*, 49–58. doi:10.1016/j.cpr.2017.09.006 PMID:28993103

Gunawan, J., Juthamanee, S., & Aungsuroch, Y. (2020). Current mental health issues in the era of Covid-19. *Asian Journal of Psychiatry*, *51*, 102103. doi:10.1016/j.ajp.2020.102103 PMID:32361675

Gunnell, D., Appleby, L., Arensman, E., Hawton, K., John, A., Kapur, N., Khan, M., O'Connor, R. C., Pirkis, J., Appleby, L., Arensman, E., Caine, E. D., Chan, L. F., Chang, S.-S., Chen, Y.-Y., Christensen, H., Dandona, R., Eddleston, M., Erlangsen, A., ... Yip, P. S. F.COVID-19 Suicide Prevention Research Collaboration. (2020). Suicide risk and prevention during the COVID-19 pandemic. *The Lancet. Psychiatry*, *7*(6), 468–471. doi:10.1016/S2215-0366(20)30171-1 PMID:32330430

Guo, J. (2021). The Analysis of the Status Quo and Promotion Strategies of Mathematical Reading of Lower Grade Students. *Science Insights Education Frontiers*, *10*(S1), 24. doi:10.15354ief.21.s1.ab054

Gyurko, L. A. (1988). The Metaphysical World of Borges and its Impact on the Novelists of the Boom Generation. *Ibero-amerikanisches Archiv. Neue Folge*, *14*(2), 215–161.

Habgood, M. (2007). *The effective integration of digital games and learning content* (ID: 10385) [Doctoral dissertation, University of Nottingham]. Nottingham ePrints.

Hadi, M. Y. A., Mohamad, B., & Jaafar, M. S. A. (2010). Study of information and communication technology (ICT) usage in the technical and vocational special education programme. *Global Journal of Human Social Science Research, 10*(1), 35-43. https://globaljournals.org/GJHSS_Volume10/ghss_vol10_issue1_ver1_paper11.pdf

Haines, S. J., McCart, A., & Turnbull, A. P. (2013). Family engagement within early childhood response to intervention. In V. Buysse & E. Peisner-Feinberg (Eds.), *Handbook on response to intervention (RTI) in early childhood* (pp. 313–324). Brookes.

Hall, N., Larson, J., & Marsch, J. (Eds.). (2003). *Handbook of Early Childhood Literacy*. Sage. doi:10.4135/9781848608207

Hardiani, H. (2021). Collaboration practices between educators in inclusive education before and during Covid-19. In *Educational Innovation in Society 5.0 Era: Challenges and Opportunities*. doi:10.1201/9781003206019

Hart, J. E., & Whalon, K. J. (2011). Creating Social Opportunities for Students With Autism Spectrum Disorder in Inclusive Settings. *Criminal Justice and Behavior, 46*(5), 1071–1092. doi:10.1177/0093854818771721

Haslam, C., Jetten, J., & Alexander, S. H. (2012). *The social cure: Identity, health and well-being*. Psychology Press.

Hasselbring, T. G., & Glaser, C. H. W. (2000). Use of computer technology to help students with special needs. The Future of Children. *Children and Computer Technology, 10*(2), 102–122. doi:10.2307/1602691

Hatzichristou, C. (2011). Social and Emotional Education at school (vol. 3). Typothito.

Hawton, K., Marzano, L., Fraser, L., Hawley, M., Harris-Skillman, E., & Lainez, Y. X. (2021). Reporting on suicidal behaviour and COVID-19-need for caution. *The Lancet. Psychiatry, 8*(1), 15–17. doi:10.1016/S2215-0366(20)30484-3 PMID:33160581

Heineck, G., & Anger, S. (2010). The returns to cognitive abilities and personality traits in Germany. *Labour Economics, 17*(3), 535–546. doi:10.1016/j.labeco.2009.06.001

Henessy, S., Ruthven, K., & Brindley, S. (2005). Teacher perspectives on integrating ICT into subject teaching: Commitment, constraints, caution, and change. *Journal of Curriculum Studies, 37*(2), 155–192. https://doi.org/10.1080/0022027032000276961

Hernández, D. (2013). La magia del propio andar [The magic of walking itself]. *Entrevista a Julio Llamazares Catharum, 13*, 63–65.

Hodges, C., Moore, S., Lockee, B., Trust, T., & Bond, A. (2020). *The Difference Between Emergency Remote Teaching and Online Learning*. https://er.educause.edu/articles/2020/3/the-difference-between-emergency-remote-teaching-andonline-learning

Hodges, C. B., Moore, S. L., Lockee, B. B., Trust, T., & Bond, M. A. (2020). The Difference Between Emergency Remote Teaching and Online Learning. *Educational Review*.

Holmberg, B. (2003). *Distance education in essence. An overview of theory and practice in the early twenty-first century*. BIS-Verlag, Carl von Ossietzky Universitat Oldenburg.

Holt-Lunstad, J., Smith, T. B., Baker, M., Harris, T., & Stephenson, D. (2015). Loneliness and social isolation as risk factors for mortality: A meta-analytic review. *Perspectives on Psychological Science, 10*(2), 227–237. doi:10.1177/1745691614568352 PMID:25910392

Homans, N. C., & Vroegop, J. L. (2021). Impact of Face Masks in Public Spaces during COVID-19 Pandemic on Daily Life Communication of Cochlear Implant Users. *Laryngoscope Investigative Otolaryngology, 6*(3), 531–539. doi:10.1002/lio2.578 PMID:34195375

Huang, R., Tlili, A., Chang, T.-W., Zhang, X., Nascimbeni, F., & Burgos, D. (2020). Disrupted classes, undisrupted learning during COVID-19 outbreak in China: Application of open educational practices and resources. *Smart Learning Environments*, *7*(1), 19. doi:10.118640561-020-00125-8

Huertas, R. (2019). *Mujeres que leían* [Women who read]. Barcelona: Tres hermanas.

Huertas, R. (2021). *El tiempo que nos robaron* [The time they stole from us]. Barcelona: Tres hermanas.

Huxhold, O., Fiori, K. L., & Windsor, T. D. (2013). The dynamic interplay of social network characteristics, subjective well-being, and health: The costs and benefits of socio-emotional selectivity. *Psychology and Aging*, *28*(1), 3–16. doi:10.1037/a0030170 PMID:23066804

Ibn Anas, M. (1994). *Al-Mudawwana* [Blog]. Dār al-Kutub al-ʻIlmiyya.

Intelligence[2]. (2018). *Intelligence Squared: The Power Of Poetry*. https://intelligencesquared.com/events/the-power-of-poetry/

Išūlā, ʻA. (2020, October 5). Virus Corona. *Šabakat Al-Alūka*. https://www.alukah.net/spotlight/0/142334/

Jakob, M. (2005). *Paesaggio e letteratura* [Landscape and literature]. Olschki.

Jakob, M. (2009). *Il paesaggio* [The landscape]. Il Mulino.

Jenkins, H. (2003). *Transmedia Storytelling. Moving Characters from Books to Films to Video Games can Make them Stronger and more Compelling*. https://www.technologyreview.com/news/401760/transmedia-storytelling

Jewitt, C. (2008). Multimodality and Literacy in School Classrooms. *Review of Research in Education*, *32*(2), 241–267. doi:10.3102/0091732X07310586

Johnston, S. S., McDonnell, A. P., Nelson, C., & Magnavito, A. (2003). Teaching Functional Communication Skills Using Augmentative and Alternative Communication in Inclusive Settings. *Journal of Early Intervention*, *25*(4), 263–280. doi:10.1177/105381510302500403

Judge, S. L. (2000). Computer applications in programs for young children with disabilities: Current status and future directions. *Journal of Special Education Technology*, *16*(1), 29–40. https://doi.org/10.1177/016264340101600103

Jurkowski, S., Ulrich, M., & Müller, B. (2020). Co-teaching as a resource for inclusive classes: teachers' perspectives on conditions for successful collaboration. *International Journal of Inclusive Education*. doi:10.1080/13603116.2020.1821449

Kacimi, M. (2017). Wāqiʻ al-riwāya al-ğazā'irriyya fī-l-kitābāt al-ağnabiyya, al-luġa al-isbāniyya namūdağan [The Protector of the Aghazirian Novel in Foreign Writings, the Spanish Brigade of the Namdani]. In Al-Riwāya wa-l-funūn bayna al-tağrīb wa-l-naqd (pp. 420-428). Mu'assat Tšīcū li-l-Ṭibāʻa wa-l-Našr.

Kalyva, E. (2005). *Autism: Educational and Therapeutic Approaches*. Publications Papazisi.

Karpozilou, M. (1994). The child in the land of books. Kastanioti.

Kaufman, G., & Flanagan, M. (2016). High-low split: Divergent cognitive construal levels triggered by digital and nondigital platforms. In *Proceedings of the 2016 CHI Conference on Human Factors in Computing Systems* (pp. 2773-2777). ACM. 10.1145/2858036.2858550

Kazanopoulos, S., Mouchritsa, M., Tejada, E., & Basogain, O. (2021). Collaboration between In-Service School Teachers and Families in the Context of Inclusive Education : A Review of the Recent Literature. *Journal of Education and Practice*, *12*(6), 47–53. doi:10.7176/JEP/12-6-05

Keck, D., Kammerer, Y., & Starauschek, E. (2015). Reading science texts online: Does source information influence the identification of contradictions within texts? *Computers & Education*, *82*, 442–449. doi:10.1016/j.compedu.2014.12.005

Keegan, D. (2001). *The basic principles of open and distance education*. Metaichmio.

Keegan, D. (Ed.). (1993). *Theoretical Principles of Distance Education* (1st ed.). Routledge.

Kefalaki, M., Rudolph, J., Tan, S., & Diamantidaki, F. (2021). Face masks in education: The cases of Greece and Singapore. *Thesis*, *10*(1), 3-42.

Kern, R. (2000). *Literacy and language teaching*. Oxford University Press.

Kessopoulou, M., & Tsimpidaki, A. (2021). Electronic communication between school and family during the COVID-19 pandemic. *Research in Education*, 137–160.

Khadra, Y. (2006). *Les Sirènes de Bagdad* [The Sirens of Baghdad]. Julliard.

Khadra, Y. (2008). *Ce que le jour doit à la nuit* [What day owes to night]. Julliard.

Khadra, Y. (2009). *Lo que el día debe a la noche* [Whatday owes to night] (W.-C. L. González, Trans.). Ediciones Destino. (Original work published 2008)

Khalil, H., & Ebner, M. (2014). MOOCs completion rates and possible methods to improve retention - a literature review. In J. Viteli & M. Leikomaa (Eds.), *Proceedings of Ed Media 2014—World Conference on Educational Media and Technology* (pp. 1305-1313). Association for the Advancement of Computing in Education (AACE). https://cutt.ly/8omp9lH

Khatibi, S. (2021, August 20). Barāmiğ al-taqāfa fī al-tilivision [Attached software in the phone area]. *Al-Quds Al Arabi*. https://www.alquds.co.uk/

Kheloufi, S. (2021). The impact of the Coronavirus Covid-19 pandemic on global economic indicators during the first quarter of 2020. With reference to the state of the Algerian economy. *OEB Univ. Publish. Co*, *3*(8), 1650–1677.

Khokhar, B. (2007). Widening participation: How can new technologies best be used to enhance, learning and teaching and ensure educational inclusion and engagement for excluded groups? *Proceedings of the 12th forum on Open and Distance Learning*. http://www2.open.ac.uk/r06/conference/

Kirkpatrick, L., Searle, M., Smyth, R. E., & Specht, J. (2020). A coaching partnership: Resource teachers and classroom teachers teaching collaboratively in regular classrooms. *British Journal of Special Education*, *47*(1), 24–47. https://doi.org/10.1111/1467-8578.12296

Klomek, A. B. (2020). Suicide prevention during the COVID-19 outbreak. *The Lancet. Psychiatry*, *7*(5), 390. doi:10.1016/S2215-0366(20)30142-5 PMID:32353271

Koumaki, E., & Haidi, E. (2015). Digital School: Digital learning for children with Special educational needs (EAA) of Special Primary School – Good Practices. *8th Panhellenic Conference of Teachers for ICT: Utilization of Information and Communication Technologies in Teaching Practice*, 1244-1258.

Kourbetis, B., Gelastopoulou, M., & Bombaridou, Ch. (2014). New perspectives in the field of special education: Design and development of accessible educational material for students with disabilities and/or special needs educational needs. In *4th Panhellenic Conference of Educational Sciences* (pp. 9-21). National Documentation Centre - ePublishing.

Kourmousi, N., & Salagianni, M. (2016). Social and Emotional Learning. In Social and Emotional Learning through Children's Literature and the "Steps for Life" Program. Hellenic Committee of the World Preschool Organization.

Krentz, C. (2016). Borges in the Mind's Eye. *Journal of Literary & Cultural Disability Studies*, *10*, 1.

Kress, G. (2003). *Literacy in the New Media Age*. Routledge.

Kress, G. (2009). *Multimodality: A Social Semiotic Approach to Contemporary Communication*. Routledge. doi:10.4324/9780203970034

Kress, G., & Van Leeuwen, T. (2001). *Multimodal discourse: The modes and media of contemporary communication*. Arnold Publishers.

Kucer, S. (2014). *Dimensions of Literacy: A Conceptual Base for Teaching, Reading and Writing in School Settings*. Routledge. doi:10.4324/9780203428405

Kucer, S. (2015). Literacy: Varied, Dynamic and Multidimensional. *Journal of Family Strengths*, *15*(2), 1–35.

Kümmerling-Meibauer, B. (Ed.). (2014). *Picturebooks: Representation and Narration*. Routledge. doi:10.4324/9780203582275

Kümmerling-Meibauer, B. (Ed.). (2018). *The Routledge Companion to Picturebooks*. Routledge.

Kümmerling-Meibauer, B., Meibauer, J., Nachtigäller, K., & Rohlfing, K. J. (Eds.). (2015). *Learning from Picturebooks: Perspectives from Child Development and Literacy Studies*. Routledge. doi:10.4324/9781315866710

Kuper, H., Banks, L. M., Bright, T., Davey, C., & Shakespeare, T. (2020). Disability inclusive COVID-19 response: What it is, why it is important and what we can learn from the United Kingdom's response. *Wellcome Open Research*, *5*, 1–5. https://doi.org/10.12688/wellcomeopenres.15833.1

KuperH.Morgon BanksL.BrightT.DaveyC.ShakespeareT.DickinsonH.WalesS. (2020). *Disability-inclusive COVID-19 response: What it is, why it is important, and what we can learn from the United Kingdom's response*. doi:10.12688/wellcomeopenres.15833.1

Kurata, K., Ishita, E., Miyata, Y., & Minami, Y. (2017). Print or digital? Reading behavior and preferences in Japan. *Journal of the Association for Information Science and Technology*, *68*(4), 884–894. doi:10.1002/asi.23712

Laghresse, S. (2021). Habits and traditions the celebration of the Laylat al-Qadr in Algerian society (Socio anthropological study in the city of Oran). *Mağallat Atropoloğia al-adyān*, *2*(17), 296-312.

Laguna, C. (2020). El libro que recupera la primavera robada de Extremadura en un viaje ilustrado [The book that recovers the stolen spring of Extremadura in an illustrated trip]. *Traveler*. Retrieved from https://www.traveler.es/naturaleza/articulos/julio-llamazares-primavera-extremena-libro-viaje-ilustracion/19682

Lai, C.-L., & Hwang, G.-J. (2016). A self-regulated flipped-classroom approach to improving students' learning performance in a mathematics course. *Computers & Education*, *100*, 126–140. doi:10.1016/j.compedu.2016.05.006

Lakhous, A. (2006). *Scontro di civiltà per un ascensore a Piazza Vittorio* [Clash of civilizations for an elevator in Piazza Vittorio]. Edizioni e/o.

Lakhous, A. (2014). *La zingarata della verginella di Via Ormea* [The Prank of the Good Little Virgin of Via Ormea]. Edizioni e/o.

Lakhous, A. (2008). *Clash of Civilizations Over an Elevator in Piazza Vittorio* (A. Goldstein, Trans.). Europa Editions. (Original work published 2006)

Lakhous, A. (2016). *The Prank of the Good Little Virgin of Via Ormea* (A. Shugaar, Trans.). Europa Editions. (Original work published 2014)

Laredj, W. (2020). *Layliāt Ramada* [Ramada Nights]. Dār al-Ādāb.

Law 3699. (2008). *Special Education and Training for People with Disabilities or Special Educational Needs.* Government Gazette 199.

Law: Special Education and Training of Students with Disabilities or Special Educational Needs, Government Gazette 199 / A. (2008). https://www.e-nomothesia.gr/kat-ekpaideuse/n-3699-2008.html

Lawrence, J. (2011). *An American History of Infamy. Variaciones Borges, 31*, 161–179.

Lee, D. (1998). Yellow Fever and the Slave Trade: Coleridge's "The Rime of the Ancient Mariner." *ELH, 65*(3), 675-700. https://www.jstor.org/stable/300301

Leiter, V. (2007). "Nobody's just normal, you know": The social creation of developmental disability. *Social Science & Medicine, 65*(8), 1630–1641. doi:10.1016/j.socscimed.2007.06.006 PMID:17655995

Leonard, R., Horsfall, D., Noonan, K., & Rosenberg, J. P. (2017). *Identity and the End-of-Life Story: A Role for Psychologists: Identity and EOL.* Academic Press.

León-Nabal, B., Zhang-Yu, C., & Lalueza, J. L. (2021). Uses of Digital Mediation in the School-Families Relationship During the COVID-19 Pandemic. *Frontiers in Psychology, 12*, 12. doi:10.3389/fpsyg.2021.687400 PMID:34248793

Letzel, V., Pozas, M., & Schneider, C. (2020). Energetic Students, Stressed Parents, and Nervous Teachers: A Comprehensive Exploration of Inclusive Homeschooling During the COVID-19 Crisis. *Open Education Studies, 2*(1), 159–170. doi:10.1515/edu-2020-0122

Levinson, M., Cevik, M., & Lipsitch, M. (2020). Reopening Primary Schools during the Pandemic. *New England Journal of Medicine.* https://www.nejm.org/doi/full/10.1056/NEJMms2024920

Lewis, K., Kuhfeld, M., Ruzek, E., & McEachin, A. (2021). *Learning during COVID-19: Reading and math achievement in the 2020-21 school year.* Center for School and Student Progress. https://www.nwea.org/research/publication/learning-duringcovid-19-reading-and-math-achievement-in-the-2020-2021-school-year

Lewis, D. (1990). The Constructedness of Texts: Picture Books and the Metafictive. *Signal, 62*, 31–46.

Lewis, D. (2001). *Reading Contemporary Picturebooks: Picturing Text.* Routledge Falmer.

Liasidou, A., & Symeou, L. (2016). Neoliberal versus social justice reforms in education policy and practice: Discourses, politics and disability rights in education. *Critical Studies in Education, 59*(2), 149–166. doi:10.1080/17508487.2016.1186102

Lichtheim, M. (Ed.). (1978). The Immortality of Writers [M. Lichtheim, Trans.). In Ancient Egyptian Literature, II. The University of California Press.

Liodakis, D. (2000). *Educational programs for the blind.* Atrapos.

Llamazares, J. (2015a). Atlas de la España imaginaria [Atlas of imaginary Spain]. Madrid, Spain: Nórdica Libros.

Llamazares, J. (2020b). Un canto a la vida en medio de la muerte: A song to life in the midst of death. *El País.* Retrieved from https://elpais.com/elpais/2020/11/10/eps/1605008819_369175.html

Llamazares, J. (1997). *Luna de lobos* [Wolf moon]. Seix Barral.

Llamazares, J. (1998). *Trás-os-Montes. Un viaje portugués* [Back-to-back-the-hills. A Portuguese traveler]. Alfaguara.

Llamazares, J. (1999). *Cuaderno del Duero* [Duero Notebook]. Leonesas.

Llamazares, J. (2003). *Memoria de la nieve* [Memory of snow]. Amos.

Llamazares, J. (2006). *El río del olvido* [The river of oblivion]. Alfaguara.

Llamazares, J. (2008). *Las rosas de piedra* [The stone roses]. Alfaguara.

Llamazares, J. (2012). El espejo del agua. Una meditación sobre el paisaje a partir de un cuadro de Juan Manuel Díaz-Caneja [The mirror of water. A meditation on the landscape from a painting by Juan Manuel Díaz-Caneja]. *Cuadernos Hispanoamericanos*, *741*, 15–21.

Llamazares, J. (2013). El viaje como pretexto [Travel as a pretext]. *Catharum*, *13*, 59–61.

Llamazares, J. (2015b). *Distintas formas de mirar el agua* [Different ways of looking at water]. Alfaguara.

Llamazares, J. (2016a). *El viaje de Don Quijote* [The journey of Don Quixote]. Alfaguara.

Llamazares, J. (2016b). *La lluvia amarilla* [The yellow rain]. Cátedra.

Llamazares, J. (2019). *Las rosas del sur* [The roses of the south]. Debolsillo.

Llamazares, J. (2020a). *Primavera extremeña. Apuntes del natural* [Extremaduran spring. Notes of the natural]. Alfaguara.

Locke, V. N., Patarapichayatham, C., & Lewis, S. (2021). *Learning Loss in Reading and Math in US Schools Due to the COVID-19 Pandemic*. Academic Press.

Lozano Sañudo, B. (2011). Borges y la traducción. Análisis de su primera incursión práctica: El príncipe feliz de Oscar Wilde [Borges and translation. Analysis of his first practical foray: Oscar Wilde's The Happy Prince]. *Mutatis Mutandis*, *4*(1), 38–47.

Luque Amo, Á. (2016). *El diario personal en la literatura: teoría del diario literario* [The personal diary in literature: literary diary theory] (Vol. 7). Castilla. Estudios de Literatura., Retrieved from https://revistas.uva.es/index.php/castilla/article/view/315

Luque Amo, Á. (2016). El diario personal en la literatura: teoría del diario literario [The personal diary in literature: literary diary theory]. *Castilla. Estudios de Literatura*, *7*, 273–306.

Luque Amo, Á. (2020). *El diario literario. Poética e historia* [The Literary Journal. Poetics and history]. Peter Lang. doi:10.3726/b17261

Lutz, C. (1978). The Oldest Library Motto: Ψυχῆς Ἰατρεῖον. *The Library Quarterly*, *48*(1). Advance online publication. doi:10.1086/629993

Mackey, M. (2002). *Literacies across Media: Playing the Text*. Routledge Falmer.

Madhesh, A. (2021). Full exclusion during COVID-19: Saudi Deaf education is an example. *Heliyon*, *7*(3), e06536. Advance online publication. doi:10.1016/j.heliyon.2021.e06536 PMID:33842703

Magson, N. R., Freeman, J. Y., Rapee, R. M., Richardson, C. E., Oar, E. L., & Fardouly, J. (2021). Risk and protective factors for prospective changes in adolescent mental health during the COVID-19 pandemic. *Journal of Youth and Adolescence*, *50*(1), 44–57. doi:10.100710964-020-01332-9 PMID:33108542

Mahieddine, H. (2021). Criminal liability for coronavirus (covid-19) transmission in Algerian legislation. *Mağallat al-dirāsāt al-qānūniyya al-muqārana*, *2*(7), 1056-1074.

Majoko, T., & Dudu, A. (2020). Parents' strategies for home educating their children with Autism Spectrum Disorder during the COVID-19 period in Zimbabwe. *International Journal of Developmental Disabilities*, *0*(0), 1–5. doi:10.1080/20473869.2020.1803025 PMID:35937168

Makrodimos, N., Papadakis, S., & Koutsoumba, M. (2017). Distance Education: a case study with the inverted class method for Mathematics of the 5th Primary school. *Open Education: the magazine for Open and Distance Education and Educational Technology, 13*(1), 26-37. doi:10.12681/jode.13975

Maktabat, N. (2021). *Plataforma de libros electrónicos* [E-book platform]. https://www.noor-book.com/

Maldonado, J. E., & De Witte, K. (2022). The effect of school closures on standardised student test outcomes. *British Educational Research Journal, 48*(1), 49–94. doi:10.1002/berj.3754

Mangen, A., Walgermo, B. R., & Brønnick, K. (2013). Reading linear texts on paper versus computer screen: Effects on reading comprehension. *International Journal of Educational Research, 58*, 61–68. doi:10.1016/j.ijer.2012.12.002

Mantzikos, N. C., & Lappa, S. C. (2020). Difficulties and barriers in the education of deaf and hard of hearing individuals in the era of COVID-19: The case of Greece- A viewpoint article. *European Journal of Special Education Research, 6*(3). DOI:57 doi:10.46827/ejse.v6i3.33

Maqableh, M., & Alia, M. (2021). Evaluation online learning of undergraduate students under lockdown amidst COVID-19 Pandemic: The online learning experience and students' satisfaction. Elsevier. *Children and Youth Services Review, 128*, 106160. doi:10.1016/j.childyouth.2021.106160

Marazziti, D., & Stahl, S. M. (2020). The relevance of COVID-19 to Psychiatry. *World Psychiatry, 19*(2), 261. doi:10.1002/wps.20764

Marazziti, D., Avella M. T., Mucci, N., Della Vecchia, A., Ivaldi, T., Palermo, S., & Mucci, F. (2020). Impact of economic crisis on mental health: a ten-year challenge. *CNS Spectrums*, 1-7. doi:10.1017/S1092852920000140

Marazziti, D. (2020). The COVID-19 Outbreak: The Latest Challenge to Psychological and Psychiatric Intervention. *Clinical Neuropsychiatry, 17*(2), 39–40. doi:10.36131/clinicalnpsych20200201 PMID:34908965

Marinoni, G., Land, H., & Jensen, T. (2020). The impact of COVID-19 on higher education around the world. IAU Global Survey Report. International Association of Universities.

Martens, L. (1985). *The Diary Novel*. Cambridge University Press. https://www.merriam-webster.com/dictionary/narrative

Martin, A. (2008). Digital Literacy and the "Digital Society. In C. Lankshear & M. Knobel (Eds.), *Digital Literacies: Concepts, Policies and Practices* (pp. 151–176). Peter Lang Publishing.

Martines, V. (2015). La escritura literaria como terapia y didáctica sentimental [Literary writing as therapy and sentimental didactics]. *Quaderni di didattica della scrittura, 12*(1), 25-37. Doi:10.7369/80660

Martínez-Roig, R., Gavilán-Martín, D., & Merma-Molina, G. (2020). Transmedia storytelling que reporta y supera casos de marginados. Clásicos como muestra de didáctica y psicología social para la superación personal [Transmedia storytelling that reports and overcomes cases of marginalized. Classics as a sample of didactics and social psychology for self-improvement]. In A. Cortijo & J. M. Antolí (Eds.), Approaches to New Trends in Research on Catalan Studies (pp. 235-268). Peter Lang, Romance Literatures & Cultures.

Martínez-Roig, R., Merma-Molina, G., & Urrea-Solano, M. (2020). The power of storytelling. Some aspects of James I's Llibre dels Fets as a transmedia storytelling with educational purposes and social and political psychology. In V.J. Escartí, V. J., & R. Roca (Eds.), En los márgenes de la Historia: marginales y minorías (pp. 261-268). Zaragoza: Pórtico.

Martínez-Roig, R., Urrea-Solano, M., & Hernández-Amorós, M. (2021). Transmedia Storytelling i coneixement en obert. Clàssics i psicología social en favor de les virtuts del bon govern [Transmedia Storytelling and open knowledge. Classics and social psychology in favor of the virtues of good governance]. In A. Cortijo, & E. Sánchez López (Eds.), De la innovació al cànon. Noves tendències de recerca en Filologia Catalana: llengua, literatura, educación i cultura (pp. 395-427). Editorial Afers.

Martin, F., Sun, T., & Westine, C. D. (2020). A systematic review of research on online teaching and learning from 2009 to 2018. *Computers & Education, 159*, 104009. https://doi.org/10.1016/j.compedu.2020.104009

Masalela, R. K. (2008) *Inclusive education and the role of distance education.* http://www.ais.up.ac.za/digi/docs/masalela_paper.pdf

Masra'ī, Ġ. Ğ. [@ryany_2015]. (2020, March 5). *Badā muhīban ğalīlan* [Two loved ones started] [Tweet]. Twiter. https://twitter.com/ryany_2015/status/1235595864036511746?lang=es

Mastrogiannis, A., & Anastopoulos, A. (2012). Dynamics, mathematics environments in Special Education. *6th Panhellenic Conference Hellenic Institute of Applied Pedagogy and Education with international participation and topic "Paideia kalliston Esti Ktima Vrotois: Humanitarian and Positive Sciences: Theory and Practice"*. http://www.elliepek.gr/documents/6o_synedrio_eisigiseis/57_mastrogiannis_anastopoulos.pdf

Matly, M. (2020). *La función del cómic* [The function of the comic]. ACyT Ediciones (Asociación Cultural Tebeosfera).

Matos, D. (2017). *Periodismo cómic. Una historia del género desde los pioneros a Joe Sacco* [Comic journalism. A history of the genre from the pioneers to Joe Sacco]. Comunicación Social Ediciones y Publicaciones.

Mawyer, K. K., & Johnson, H. J. (2019). Eliciting preservice teachers' reading strategies through structured literacy activities. *Journal of Science Teacher Education, 30*(6), 583–600. doi:10.1080/1046560X.2019.1589848

McClain-Nhlapo, C., Singh, R. K., Martin, A., Alasuutari, H., Baboo, N., Cameron, S., … Tucker, M. (2020). Pivoting to Inclusion: Leveraging Lessons from the COVID-19 Crisis for Learners with Disabilities. In Other Education Study. Washington, DC: World Bank Group.

Meek, M. (1988). *How Texts Teach What Readers Learn.* Thimble Press.

Meijer, C., Soriano, V., & Watkins, A. (2003). *Special education in Europe.* European Special Education Agency. https://www.europeanagency.org/sites/default/files/special-needs-education-in europe_sne_europe_el.pdf

Melizi, S. (2020, March 28). Al-Bulaida madīna al-ward [Blida, the city of roses]. *Diwān al- 'Arab.* https://diwanalarab.com/

Mendoza Fillola, A. (2001). *El intertexto lector. El espacio de encuentro de las aportaciones del texto con las del lector* [The reading intertext. The meeting space of the contributions of the text with those of the reader]. Ediciones de la Universidad de Castilla-La Mancha.

Menke, M. R., & Paesani, K. (2019). Analysing Foreign Language Instructional Materials through the Lens of Multiliteracies Framework. *Language, Culture and Curriculum, 32*(1), 34–49. doi:10.1080/07908318.2018.1461898

Mesa Gancedo, D. (2014). Diario y autoficción en la narrativa hispanoamericana contemporánea [Diary and autofiction in contemporary Latin American narrative]. In A. Casas (Ed.), *El yo fabulado* (pp. 191–206). Iberoamericana-Vervuert.

Mildonian, P. (2001). *Alterego. Racconti in forma di diario tra Otto e Novecento* [Alterego. Stories in diary form between the nineteenth and twentieth centuries]. Marsilio.

Miles, S., & Singal, N. (2009). The Education for All and Inclusive Education debate: Conflict, contradiction or opportunity? *International Journal of Inclusive Education, 14*(1), 1–15. https://doi.org/10.1080/13603110802265125

Millard, E., & Marsh, J. (2001). Sending Minnie the Minx Home: Comics and Reading Choices. *Cambridge Journal of Education, 31*(1), 25–38. doi:10.1080/03057640123853

Mississippi Department of Education. (2020). *Updates and Information in Response to COVID-19 (Coronavirus).* https://www.mdek12.org/COVID19

Mitchell, D., & Sutherland, D. (2020). *What really works in special and inclusive education: Using evidence-based teaching strategies*. Routledge.

Mociño-González, I. (2019). Libro-objeto y poesía: construyendo significados a través de los sentidos [Book-object and poetry: constructing meanings through the senses]. In R. Tabernero Sala (Ed.), *El objeto libro en el universo infantil. La materialidad en la construcción del discurso* (pp. 89–108). Prensas de la Universidad de Zaragoza.

Moix, T. (1968). *Los 'comics'. Arte para el consumo y formas pop* [The 'comics'. Art for consumption and pop forms]. Jarama.

Moll, B. I. (2002). Epidemiologia des de l'Edat Mitjana fins a l'actualitat [Epidemiology from the Middle Ages to the present day] *Gimbernat: Revista d'Història de la Medicina i de les Ciències de la Salut, 37*, 21–54.

Monti, S. (Ed.). (2012). *Malattia e scrittura. Saperi medici, malattie e cure nelle letterature iberiche* [Illness and writing. Medical knowledge, diseases and cures in Iberian literature]. Cierre Grafica.

Moore, M. G. (1993). Theory of transactional distance. In D. Keegan (Ed.), *Theoretical principles of distance education* (pp. 22–38). Routledge.

Moore, M. G., & Kearsley, G. (2012). *Distance education: A systems view of online learning*. Wadsworth Cengage Learning.

Morales, M. (2021, February 26). El confinamiento llevó a un máximo histórico el índice de lectura entre los españoles. *El País*. https://elpais.com/cultura/2021-02-26/el-confinamiento-llevo-a-un-maximo-historico-el-indice-de-lectura-entre-los-espanoles.html

Moreillon, J. (2007). *Collaborative Strategies for Teaching Reading Comprehension: Maximizing Your Impact*. ALA Editions.

Mortier, K., Hunt, P., Leroy, M., Van de Putte, I., & Van Hove, G. (2010). Communities of practice in inclusive education. *Educational Studies, 36*(3), 345–355. doi:10.1080/03055690903424816

Mostaghanemi, A. (1993). *Dākirat al-ğasad* [Memory in the flesh]. Dār al-Ādāb.

Mostaghanemi, A. (2000). *Memory in the flesh* (B. A. Sreih, Trans.). American University in Cairo Press. (Original work published 1993)

Mostaghanemi, A. (2002). *Mémoires de la chair* [Memory in the flesh] (M. Mokeddem, Trans.). Albin Michel. (Original work published 1993)

Mosteghanemi, A. [@ahlammostaghaanmy]. (2022, February 28). *Mimma qara'tu* [Status update]. Facebook. https://www.facebook.com/search/posts/?q=ahlem%20mosteghanemi

Mouchritsa, M., Kazanopoulos, S., Romero, A., & Garay, U. (2021). Collaboration between General and Special Education Teachers in Inclusive Classrooms: A Review of the Literature. *Journal of Education and Practice, 12*(6). https://doi.org/10.7176/JEP/12-6-04

Muñoz Molina, A. (2020). Dar testimonio. Prólogo [Bear witness. Prologue]. In F. Fang (Ed.), *Diario de Wuhan. Sesenta días desde una ciudad en cuarentena*. Seix Barral. Trad. de Cheng L. Ning, Aurora Echevarría y Lorenzo Luego.

Mutsvairo, B., & Bebawi, S. (2019). Journalism educators, regulatory realities, and pedagogical predicaments of the "fake news" Era: A comparative perspective on the middle east and Africa. *Journalism & Mass Communication Educator, 74*(2), 143–157. doi:10.1177/1077695819833552

Mylonakou-Keke, H. (2009). *Family and Community School Collaboration, Theoretical Approaches and Practical Applications*. Papazisis.

Nam, C. S., Bahn, S., & Lee, R. (2013). Acceptance of Assistive Technology by Special Education Teachers: A Structural Equation Model Approach. *International Journal of Human-Computer Interaction, 29*(5), 365–377. doi:10.1080/10447318.2012.711990

Nazarian, D., & Smyth, J. M. (2013). An experimental test of instructional manipulations in expressive writing interventions: Examining processes of change. *Journal of Social and Clinical Psychology, 32*(1), 71–96. doi:10.1521/jscp.2013.32.1.71

Neely-Barnes, S. L., Graff, J. C., Roberts, R. J., Hall, H. R., & Hankins, J. S. (2010). "It's our job": Qualitative study of family responses to ableism. *Intellectual and Developmental Disabilities, 48*(4), 245–258. doi:10.1352/1934-9556-48.4.245 PMID:20722475

New London Group. (1996). A Pedagogy of Multiliteracies: Designing social futures. *Educational Review, 66*(1), 60–93.

Nikolajeva, M., & Scott, C. (2000). The Dynamics of Picturebook Communication. *Children's Literature in Education, 31*(4), 225–239. doi:10.1023/A:1026426902123

Nikolajeva, M., & Scott, C. (2003). Verbal and Visual Literacy: The Role of Picturebooks in the Reading Experience of Young Children. In *Handbook of Early Childhood Literacy* (pp. 235–248). Sage. doi:10.4135/9781848608207.n20

Nikolajeva, M., & Scott, C. (2014). *Reading for Learning: Cognitive Approaches to Children's Literature*. John Benjamins. doi:10.1075/clcc.3

Nodelman, P. (1999). Decoding the Images: Illustration and Picture Books. In P. Hunt (Ed.), *Understanding Children's Literature* (pp. 128–139). Routledge.

Norris, S. P., Falk, H., Federico-Agraso, M., Jiménez-Aleixandre, M. P., Phillips, L. M., & Yarden, A. (2009). Reading science texts—epistemology, inquiry, authenticity—a rejoinder to Jonathan Osborne. *Research in Science Education, 39*(3), 405–410. doi:10.100711165-008-9118-5

Norton, D. (2007). Through the eyes of a child. In Introduction to Children's Literature. Epikentro.

Nouri, J. (2016). The Flipped Classroom: For Active, Effective and Increased Learning—Especially for Low Achievers. *International Journal of Educational Technology in Higher Education, 13*(33), 1–10. doi:10.118641239-016-0032-z

Nutbrown, C., Clough, P., Nutbrown, C., & Clough, P. (2007). *Inclusion and exclusion in the early years : conversations with European educators Inclusion and exclusion in the early years : conversations with European educators. 6257*. doi:10.1080/0885625042000262479

OECD. (2020). *TALIS 2018 Results (Volume II): Teachers and School Leaders as Valued Professionals*. TALIS, OECD Publishing. doi:10.1787/19cf08df-en

OECD. (2020a). *Supporting immigrant and refugee students amid the coronavirus pandemic*. https://oecdedutoday.com/immigrant-refugee-studentscoronavirus

OECD. (2020b). *How coronavirus is affecting students with special education needs*. https://oecdedutoday.com/coronavirus-students-special-education-needs/

OECD. (2020c). *Coronavirus school closures: What do they mean for student equity and inclusion?* https://oecdedutoday.com/coronavirus-school-closuresstudent-equity-inclusion/

OECD. (2020d). *OECD Policy Responses to COVID-19. Strengthening online learning when schools are closed: The role of families and teachers in supporting students during the COVID-19 crisis.* https://www.oecd.org/coronavirus/policy-responses/strengthening-online-learning-when-schoolsare-closed-the-role-of-families-and-teachers-in-supporting-students-during-the-covid-19-crisisc4ecba6c/

OECD. (2021). *OECD Skills Outlook 2021: Learning for Life.* OECD Publishing. doi:10.1787/0ae365b4-

Oliver, M. (2009). *Αναπηρία και Πολιτική* [The Politics of Disablement]. Epikentro Publishers.

Oliver, M., & Barnes, C. (2010). Disability studies, disabled people and the struggle for inclusion. *British Journal of Sociology of Education, 31*(5), 547–560. doi:10.1080/01425692.2010.500088

Ommundsen, A. M., Haaland, G., & Kümmerling-Meibauer, B. (Ed.). (2022). Exploring Challenging Picturebooks in Education. International Perspectives on Language and Literature Learning. Routledge.

Ommundsen, A. M. (2022). Cognitively Challenging Picturebooks and the Plesures of Reading. Explorative Learning from Picturebooks in the Classroom. In *Exploring Challenging Picturebooks in Education. International Perspectives on Language and Literature Learning* (pp. 99–121). Routledge.

Orazi, V. (2020a). COVID19 – Literatura, interculturalitat, TIC, entrenament conductal i gestió de l'estrés durant la pandèmia per Coronavirus [COVID19 – Literature, interculturality, ICT, behavioral training and stress management during the Coronavirus pandemic]. In *Coneixement en temps de pandèmia.* Universitat d'Alacant. Seu Universitària de La Nucia. Retrieved from https://www.youtube.com/watch?v=PqVAi9-E2ro&fbclid=IwAR3dbgxgJylCSYOqTbn-BBv80WdVT0XdC-s8KYRHhgy7VRYnbex9PTZc_fQ

Orazi, V. (2020a). COVID19 – Literatura, interculturalitat, TIC, entrenament conductal i gestió de l'estrès durant la pandèmia per Coronavirus [Literature, Interculturality, ICT, behavioral training and stress management during the Covid-19 Pandemic]. In *Coneixement en temps de pandèmia.* Universitat d'Alacant. Seu Universitària de La Nucia. Retrieved from https://www.youtube.com/watch?v=PqVAi9-E2ro&fbclid=IwAR3dbgxgJylCSYOqTbn-BBv80WdVT0XdC-s8KYRHhgy7VRYnbex9PTZc_fQ

Orazi, V. (2020b). Sex and the Pandemic in *#Coronavirusplays.* In *COVID19 – LiTraPan. Literary Training via ICT for Higher Education Improvement, Behavioral Coaching and Discomfort Management during the Coronavirus Pandemic [Branch: UniTo], II International Symposium Forbidden Delights: Sex, Eroticism, Beauty, Aesthetics, Pleasure, Law, Sin and Prohibition.* Retrieved from https://www.youtube.com/watch?v=lp6jOx0EExY&feature=youtu.be

Orazi, V. (2022a). Jordi Casanovas' #Coronavirusplays: Spanish and Catalan microtheatre in the framework of the Project COVID-19 LiTraPan. In A. Cortijo Ocaña & V. Martines (Eds.), Handbook of Research on Historical Pandemic Analysis and the Social Implications of COVID-19 (pp. 175-194). IGI Global.

Orazi, V. (2022b). *Microteatro spagnolo e catalano al tempo della pandemia* [Spanish and Catalan microtheatre at the time of the pandemic]. Torino: Università di Torino. QuadRi – Quaderni di RiCOGNIZIONI XII.

Orazi, V. (2014). El monólogo en el teatro de Max Aub [The monologue in the theater of Max Aub]. *RiCOGNIZIONI, 1*(2), 151–160.

Orazi, V. (2022). Drammatizzare la pandemia. Microteatro spagnolo e catalano attuale [Dramatize the pandemic. Current Spanish and Catalan microtheatre]. *EHUMANISTA, 21*, 22–42.

Orazi, V. (2022). Literature, Language, Art in/and Highher Education in Times of Covid-19 in the Paniberian Context. *eHumanista. Journal of Iberian Studies*, *21*, 1–6.

Orhan, G., & Beyhan, Ö. (2020). Teachers' Perceptions and Teaching Experiences on Distance Education Through Synchronous Video Conferencing During Covid-19 Pandemic. *Social Sciences and Education Research Review, 1*(7), 8–44. https://econpapers.repec.org/RePEc:edt:jsserr:v:7:y:2020:i:1:p:8-44

Østerlie. (2016). Flipped Learning in Physical Education : Why and How? *Physical Education and New Technologies*, 166–176. https://ntnuopen.ntnu.no/ntnu-xmlui/bitstream/handle/11250/2405451/Østerlie-2016-Flipped Learning in Physical Edu %28002%29.pdf?sequence=1

Outka, E. (2019). *Viral Modernism. The Influenza Pandemic and Interwar Literature*. Columbia University Press. doi:10.7312/outk18574

Paesani, K., Allen, H. W., & Dupuy, B. (2016). *Multiliteracies Framework for Collegiate Foreign Language Teaching*. Pearson.

Paleodimou, A. (2017). Complementary distance school education. The case of e-twinning in kindergarten. In Minutes Proceedings of the 9th International Conference on Open and Distance Education (pp. 16–23). https://dx.doi.org/10.12681/icodl.1373

Panhellenic School Network. (2022a). *Electronic School Classroom. E-Class*. https://eclass.sch.gr

Panhellenic School Network. (2022a). *Electronic School Classroom*. E-Class. Retrieved March 10, 2022, from https://eclass.sch.gr

Panhellenic School Network. (2022b). *E-me Digital Education Platform. E-me*. https://e-me.edu.gr

Panhellenic School Network. (2022b). *E-me Digital Education Platform*.E-me. Retrieved March 10, 2022, from https://e-me.edu.gr

Panhellenic School Network. (2022c). *WebEx Teleconference for Teachers*. https://webex.sch.gr/docs.php

Panhellenic School Network. (2022c). *WebEx Teleconference for Teachers*. Retrieved March 10, 2022, from https://webex.sch.gr/docs.php

Panina-Beard, N., & Vadeboncoeur, J. A. (2019). *Narrative therapy*. Salem Press Encyclopedia.

Pantell, M., Rehkopf, D., Jutte, D., Syme, S. L., Balmes, J., & Adler, N. (2013). Social isolation: A predictor of mortality comparable to traditional clinical risk factors. *American Journal of Public Health*, *103*(11), 2056–2062. doi:10.2105/AJPH.2013.301261 PMID:24028260

Papadimitriou S. (2021). Η συμβολή της Εκπαιδευτικής Τηλεόρασης στην εξ Αποστάσεως Σχολική Εκπαίδευση [The contribution of Educational Television to Distance School Education]. *Proceedings of the Conference: Εξ Αποστάσεως Εκπαίδευση και Σχολική Πραγματικότητα*. doi:10.12681/online-edu.3226

Papadopoulou, S. (2004). The Emotional Language. Typothito-George Dardanos.

Papadopoulou, S. (2008). Book Therapy as a Teaching Approach through Linguistic Art and as a Body of Culture. In Education Sciences: Former "School and Life" (pp. 113-118). Academic Press.

Papadopoulou-Mantadaki, S. (2003). The socio-emotional teaching of language through the children's realistic novel. Metaichmio.

Paraskevopoulos, M. (2005). *The contribution of Information Technologies and Communication in the Organization of the Integration Department and in Creation Personalized Programs.* http://www.etpe.eu/new/custom/pdf/etpe211.pdf

Pardeck, J. & Markward, M. (1995). Bibliotherapy: Using books to help children deal with problems. *Early Child Development and Care, 106*(1), 75-90. doi:10.1080/0300443951060108

Pardeck, J. (1995). Bibliotherapy: An Innovative Approach for Helping Children. *Early Child Development and Care, 101*(1), 83-88. doi:10.1080/0300443951100106

Pardede, P. (2019). Print vs Digital Reading Comprehension in EFL. *Journal of English Teaching, 5*(2), 77–90. doi:10.33541/jet.v5i2.1059

Parmigiani, D., Benigno, V., Giusto, M., Silvaggio, C., & Sperandio, S. (2021). E-inclusion : online special education in Italy during the Covid-19 pandemic E-inclusion : online special education in Italy during the Covid-19. *Technology, Pedagogy and Education, 30*(1), 111–124. doi:10.1080/1475939X.2020.1856714

Parmigiani, D., Benigno, V., Giusto, M., Silvaggio, C., & Sperandio, S. (2021). E-inclusion: Online special education in Italy during the Covid-19 pandemic. *Technology, Pedagogy and Education, 30*(1), 111–124. https://doi.org/10.1080/1475939X.2020.1856714

Parrilla, V. F. (2019). La pesta negra del 1348 a la corona d'Aragó. Una revolució social, econòmica i salubrista [The Black Death of 1348 in the Crown of Aragon. A social, economic and health revolution]. *Gimbernat. Revista d'Història de la Medicina i de les Ciències de la Salut.*, (71), 13–22.

Pascual de la Torre, M. (2018). *Malacatú.* Barcelona: A buen paso.

Patera, A. & Tsilimeni, T., (2012). *Literacy and socio-emotional development of the child. Theoretical approaches, activities and games.* Epikentro.

Pedagogical Institute. (2011). *Interdisciplinary Unified Curriculum Framework. The A.P.S. in Informatics.* Pedagogical Institute.

Pellicer Vázquez, A. (2020). En *la* covid-19 [In covid-19]. In P. del Collado Lobatón, G. Nettel & Y. Weiss (Coords.), *Diario de la pandemia.* CulturaUNAM, Revista de la Universidad de México. Retrieved from https://www.revistadelauniversidad.mx/articles/40d935fa-99ad-4d1d-ac3e-2047e0a01421/en-la-covid19

Pengfei, S., Xiaosheng, L., Chao, X., Wenjuan, S., & Bo, P. (2020). Understanding of COVID-19 based on current evidence. *Journal of Medical Virology, 92(6),* 548–551. https://doi:10.1002/jmv.25722

People's Democratic Republic of Algeria. (2020). *Fixant des mesures complémentaires de prévention et de lutte contre la propagation du Coronavirus (COVID-19)* [Laying down additional measures to prevent and combat the spread of Coronavirus (COVID-19)] (Décret exécutif n° 20-70). Journal officiel Algerie. https://www.joradp.dz/FTP/jo-francais/2020/F2020016.pdf

People's Democratic Republic of Algeria. (2020). *Portant mesures supplémentaires au titre du dispositif de prévention et de lutte contre la propagation du Coronavirus (COVID-19)* [Introducing additional measures under the system to prevent and combat the spread of Coronavirus (COVID-19)] (Décret exécutif n° 20-446). Journal officiel Algerie. https://www.joradp.dz/FTP/jo-francais/2021/F2021001.pdf

Perissinotto, C. M., & Covinsky, K. E. (2014). Living alone, socially isolated or lonely—What are we measuring? *Journal of General Internal Medicine, 11*(11), 1429–1431. doi:10.100711606-014-2977-8 PMID:25092012

Pesaro, N. (2021). Fang Fang e le altre: la narrazione femminile del virus in Cina [Fang Fang and the others: the female narrative of the virus in China]. *DEP. Deportate, Esuli, Profughe*, *45*, 227-251. Retrieved from https://www.unive.it/pag/fileadmin/user_upload/dipartimenti/DSLCC/documenti/DEP/numeri/n45/24_Pesaro.pdf

Petscher, Y., Cabell, S. Q., Catts, H. W., Compton, D. L., Foorman, B. R., Hart, S. A., Lonigan, C. J., Phillips, B. M., Schatschneider, C., Steacy, L. M., Terry, N. P., & Wagner, R. K. (2020). How the science of reading informs 21st-century education. *Reading Research Quarterly*, *55*(1), S267–S282. doi:10.1002/rrq.352 PMID:34007089

Petzold, A. M. (2020). Letter to the editor: Resources and recommendations for a quick transition to online instruction in physiology. *Advances in Physiology Education, 44,* 217-219. doi:10.1152/advan.00049.2020

Piccone Stella, S. (2008). *In prima persona. Scrivere un diario* [Firsthand. Write a journal]. Il Mulino.

Pilgrim, J., & Martínez, E. (2013). Defining Literacy in the 21st Century: A guide to Terminology and Skills. *Texas Journal of Literacy Education, 1*(1), 60–69.

Pirkis, J., John, A., Shin, S., DelPozo-Banos, M., Arya, V., Analuisa-Aguilar, P., Appleby, L., Arensman, E., Bantjes, J., Baran, A., Bertolote, J. M., Borges, G., Brečić, P., Caine, E., Castelpietra, G., Chang, S. S., Colchester, D., Crompton, D., Curkovic, M., Deisenhammer, E. A., … Spittal, M. J. (2021). Suicide trends in the early months of the COVID-19 pandemic: an interrupted time-series analysis of preliminary data from 21 countries. *The Lancet. Psychiatry*, S2215-0366(21)00091-2.

Pizzino, C. (2016). *Arresting Development. Comics at the Boundaries of Literature*. University of Texas Press. doi:10.7560/309773

Polychronopoulou, S. (2003). *Children and adolescents with disabilities and abilities. Contemporary trends in education and support*. Route.

Polychronopoulou-Zacharogeorga, S. (2003). *Children and adolescents with special needs and abilities* (Vol. 2). Atrapos.

Porcel, P. (2002). *Clásicos en Jauja. La historia del tebeo valenciano* [The 'comics'. Art for consumption and pop forms]. Edicions de Ponent - Generalitat Valenciana.

Porcel, P., & Pons, A. (2007). *Viñetas a la luna de Valencia. La historia del tebeo valenciano (1965-2006)* [Vignettes to the moon of Valencia. The history of Valencian comics (1965-2006)]. Edicions de Ponent - Generalitat Valenciana.

Porter Abbott, H. (1984). *Diary fiction. Writing as action*. Cornell University Press.

Porto, Â. (2007). Social Representations of Tuberculosis: Stigma and Prejudice. *Revista de Saude Publica*, *41*(Supl.1), 1–7. PMID:18038090

Powell, V., Riglin, L., Hammerton, G., Eyre, O., Martin, J., Anney, R., Thapar, A., & Rice, F. (2020). What explains the link between childhood ADHD and adolescent depression? Investigating the role of peer relationships and academic attainment. *European Child & Adolescent Psychiatry*, *29*(11), 1581–1591. doi:10.100700787-019-01463-w PMID:31932968

Prater, M., Johnstun, M., Dyches, T.T., & Johnstun, M. (2006). Using Children's Books as Bibliotherapy for At-Risk Students: A Guide for Teachers. *Preventing School Failure*, *50*(4), 5-13.

Psifidou, I. (2020a). Challenges and support for VET Teachers and Trainers during Covid-19. In *Croatian Presidency Conference Teachers and Trainers for the Future: Towards the 'New Normal'.* Ministry of Science and Education.

Psifidou, I. (2020b). New roles for VET Teachers and Trainers. *Directors' General for VET (DGVT) online meeting "Paving the way for a better future VET - towards 2030".*

Qandīl, A. (2020). *Corona wa-sinīnu-hā: taḥawwulāt al-'ālam wa-iqtiṣādi-hī wa-ṯawarāti-hī ba'da al-ǧā'iḥa*. Dār al-Taqāfa al-Ǧadīda.

Raḥīm, K. (2020). *Qahwat Ḥabaši* [Abyssinian Coffee]. Dār al-'Ayn.

Raimon. (1993). *Veles e vents* [Sails and winds]. https://www.youtube.com/watch?v=JEpKnkhTj-0

Raimon. (2010a). *Desert d'amics* [Friend Deserts]. https://www.youtube.com/watch?v=lJNRMOXCf50

Raimon. (2010b). *Balada de la garça i l'esmerla* [Ballad of the garza and the emerald]. https://www.youtube.com/results?search_query=raimon+ro%C3%ADs+de+corella

Ramos, A. M. (2017). *Aproximações ao livro objeto: das potencialidades criativas às propostas de leitura* [Approaches to the object book: from creative potential to reading proposals]. Tropelias & Companhia.

Raoul, V. (1989). Women and Diaries: Gender and Genre. *Mosaic: A Journal for the Interdisciplinary Study of Literature*, *22*(3), 57-65. Retrieved from https://www.jstor.org/stable/24780526

Reich, J., Buttimer, C. J., Alison Fang, A., Hillaire, G., Hirsch, K., Larke, L., Littenberg-Tobias, J., Moussapour, R., Napier, A., Thompson, M., & Slama, R. (2020). *Remote Learning Guidance from State Education Agencies during the COVID-19 Pandemic: A First Look*. Massachusetts Institute of Technology - MIT Teaching Systems Lab. doi:10.35542/osf.io/437e2

Reimer, D., Smith, E., Andersen, I. G., & Sortkær, B. (2021). What happens when schools shut down? Investigating inequality in students' reading behavior during Covid-19 in Denmark. *Research in Social Stratification and Mobility*, *71*, 100568. doi:10.1016/j.rssm.2020.100568

Reyes, V. C. R., Paredes, N. C., & Castillo, A. L. G. (2020). Efectos de la COVID-19 en la salud mental de la población [Effects of COVID-19 on the mental health of the population]. *Rev. Haban. Cienc. Méd.*, *1*(19). http://scielo.sld.cu/scielo.php?script=sci_arttext&pid=S1729-519X2020000400008

Reyes-Torres, A., & García-Perera, A. (2022). Influence of Positive Student-Teacher Interaction on the Meaning-Making Process in Virtual Learning: A Study in the Primary English Class. In C. N. Giannikas (Ed.), *Transferring Language Learning and Teaching From Face-to-Face to Online Settings* (pp. 165–188). IGI Global. doi:10.4018/978-1-7998-8717-1.ch009

Reyes-Torres, A., & Portalés, M. (2020). Multimodal Approach to Foster the Multiliteracies Pedagogy in the Teaching of EFL through Picturebooks: The Snow Lion. *Journal of the Spanish Association of Anglo-American Studies*, *42*(1), 94–119. doi:10.28914/Atlantis-2020-42.1.06

Reyes-Torres, A., Portalés, M., & Torres, C. (2021). The Potential of Sound Picturebooks as Multimodal narratives. *AILA Review*, *34*(2), 300–324. doi:10.1075/aila.21006.rey

Riad, M. S. (Director). (1975). *Film Rīḥ al-ǧanūb* [Ronin] [Film]. Television Algerienne.

RIALC-Repertorio Informatizzato della Letteratura Catalana Antica. (n.d.). [RIALC-Computerized Repertoire of Ancient Catalan Literature]. Università degli Studi di Napoli Federico II. http://www.rialc.unina.it/inc-santjordi.html

Rice, M. F., & Dykman, B. (2018). The emerging research base for online learning and students with disabilities. In R. Ferdig & K. Kennedy (Eds.), *Handbook of research on K-12 online and blended learning* (pp. 189–206). ETC Press.

Rilke, R. M. (2009). Del paesaggio [Landscape]. In P. D'Angelo (Ed.), *Estetica e Paesaggio* (pp. 53–64). Il Mulino.

Roldán, L. Á. (2019). Reading, understanding and learning in secondary education: Approaches and perspectives. *Psicologia USP*, *30*. Advance online publication. doi:10.1590/0103-6564e20180126

Román Maestre, B. (2021). Les llibertats i els drets en temps de pandèmia: reflexions des de l'ètica [Freedoms and rights in times of pandemic: reflections from ethics]. *Qüestions de vida cristiana, 270*, 46-56.

Romera Castillo, J. (n.d.). *Literatura y vida en la España actual* [Literature and life in today's Spain]. SELITEN@T. Retrieved from https://www2.uned.es/centro-investigacion-SELITEN@T/pdf/autobio/I2.pdf

Rose, J., Willner, P., Cooper, V., Langdon, P. E., Murphy, G. H., & Stenfert Kroese, B. (2020). The effect on and experience of families with a member who has Intellectual and Developmental Disabilities of the COVID-19 pandemic in the UK: Developing an investigation. *International Journal of Developmental Disabilities, 0*(0), 1–3. doi:10.1080/20473869.2020.1764257 PMID:35309704

Rosenblatt, L. (1938). *Literature as Exploration*. Appleton-Century.

Rosenblatt, L. (1978). *The Reader, the Text, the Poem: The Transactional Theory of the Literary Work*. Southern Illinois University Press.

Rottenberg, B. (2022). Bibliotherapy as an integrative psychotherapeutic channel. *Journal of Poetry Therapy, 35*(1), 27–41. doi:10.1080/08893675.2021.2004371

Rovira-Collado, J. (2017). Canon artístico y criterios de selección de historietas: las propuestas de Unicómic [Artistic canon and comic selection criteria: the proposals of Unicómic]. *Umbral. Literatura para infancia, adolescencia y juventud, 12*(3), 3-19.

Rubio, V.A. (1979). Peste negra, crisis y comportamientos sociales en la España del siglo XIV [Black Death, crisis and social behaviors in fourteenth-century Spain]. In *La ciudad de Valencia (1348 – 1401)* (pp. 22-48). Universidad of Granada.

Ruiz-Bejarano, A. M. (2019). Del placer de la lectura al deseo de leer: el aprendizaje del buen lector. *Revista complutense de educación, 30*(3), 863-878. doi:10.5209/rced.59489

Sabucedo, J.M., Alzate, M., & Hur, D. (2020). COVID-19 y la metáfora de la guerra [COVID-19 and the metaphor of war]. *International Journal of Social Psychology, 35*(3), 618-624. doi:10.1080/02134748.2020.1783840

Saduki, Y. (2018). Maḍāhir wa-natā'iğ al-tanawwu' al-ṯaqāfī fī-l-Ğazā'ir [Maher and the scope of Al-Haqafi diversity on the surface]. *Mağalat dā'irat al-buḥūṯ wa-l-dirāsāt al-qānūniyya wa-siyyāsiyya, 2*(4), 180-193.

Salem, M.O.M. (2020). *Alā'īb ḫālid ma'a Corona*. Al-Mu'asasa al-'Arabiyya li-l-Dirāsāt wa-l-Našr.

Salih, S. S., & Ismail, M. A. (2021). *Corona's Reflections on Contemporary Arabic Poetry (Corona Pandemic Poem by Hashem Al-Bashir As a model)*. Academic Press.

Salisbury, M. (2005). *Ilustración de libros infantiles* [Illustration of children's books]. Editorial Acanto.

Salisbury, M., & Styles, M. (2012). *Children's picturebooks: The Art of visual storytelling*. Laurence King.

Salman, J. (2020). *Corona al-ḥubbu wa-l-ḥarb: malḥama kutibat aṯnā' al-ḥağr*. Al-Dār al-'Arabiyya li-l-'Ulūm.

Samir, A. (Director). (2022, January 5). *Jarka. Ma'a Lila Borsali* [Episodio de serie de televisión]. Televisión Nacional Algerienne 2. https://www.youtube.com/watch?v=YtZ08gDsSYA&t=2181s

Sánchez-Villena, A. R. & V. de La Fuente-Figuerola (2020). COVID-19: Quarantine, isolation, social distancing and lockdown: Are they the same? *Anales de Pediatría, 93*(1), 73-74. doi:10.1016/j.anpedi.2020.05.001

Sanchis Sinisterra, J. (2009). El arte del monólogo [The art of monologue]. *Revista Teatro CELCIT, 35-36*, 162–170.

Santini, Z. I., Koyanagi, A., Tyrovolas, S., Mason, C., & Haro, J. M. (2015). The association between social relationships and depression: A systematic review. *Journal of Affective Disorders, 175*, 53–65. doi:10.1016/j.jad.2014.12.049 PMID:25594512

Santos, S. C. (2019). Art of Questioning (Aq): A Tool in Improving the Reading Comprehension of the BSED-I Majors in English and Science at Holy Child Jesus College. *Ascendens Asia Journal of Multidisciplinary Research Abstracts, 3*(8).

Saunders, B. (2011). Do the Gods Wear Capes? Spirituality, Fantasy, and Superheroes. *Continuum.*

Schimmenti, A., Billieux, J., & Starcevic, V. (2020). The Four Horsemen of Fear: An Integrated Model of Understanding Fear Experiences during the COVID-19 Pandemic. *Clinical Neuropsychiatry, 17*(2), 41-45. doi:10.36131/CN20200202

Schult, J., Mahler, N., Fauth, B., & Lindner, M. A. (2021). Did students learn less during the COVID-19 pandemic? reading and mathematics competencies before and after the first pandemic wave. doi:10.31234/osf.io/pqtgfosf.io/pqtgf

Scolari, C. A. (2013). *Narrativas Transmedia. Cuando todos los medios cuentan* [Transmedia Narratives. When all media counts]. Deusto.

Scully, D., Lehane, P., & Scully, C. (2021). 'It is no longer scary': Digital learning before and during the Covid-19 pandemic in Irish secondary schools. *Technology, Pedagogy and Education, 30*(1), 155–177. https://doi.org/https://doi.org/10.1080/1475939X.2020.1854844

SELITEN@T: A bibliographic guide on (auto)biographical writing. (n.d.). Retrieved from https://www2.uned.es/centro-investigacion-SELITEN@T/escritura_autobio.html

Seppala, E., Rossomando, T., & Doty, J. R. (2013). Social connection and compassion: Important predictors of health and well-being. *Social Research, 80*(2), 411–430. doi:10.1353or.2013.0027

Serafini, F. (2014). *Reading the visual: An introduction to teaching multimodal literacy*. Teachers College Press.

Serrano, M. (2015). Ašr nisā (Ṣ. 'Ilmānī, Trans.). Qatar Foundation Publishing. (Original work published in 2011)

Sfakiotaki, K. K. (2020). Education during a pandemic: International practices. In *1st International Online Training Conference From the 20th to the 21st Century in 15 Days. Attitudes-Perceptions-Scenarios-Perspectives-Proposals* (pp. 451–461). Hellenic Documentation Center.

Sharma, D. (2021). Reading and rewriting poetry on life to survive the COVID-19 pandemic. *Journal of Poetry Therapy, 34*(2), 95–108. doi:10.1080/08893675.2021.1899631

Sharma, U., Loreman, T., & Forlin, C. (2012). Measuring teacher efficacy to implement inclusive practices. *Journal of Research in Special Educational Needs, 12*(1), 12–21. doi:10.1111/j.1471-3802.2011.01200.x

Sharrak, A. (2020). *Corana wa-l-ḫiṭāb: muqaddimāt wa-yawmiyāt*. Mu'assasat Muqārabāt.

Sheridan, S. M., & Kratochwill, T. R. (2008). *Conjoint behavioral consultation*. Springer.

Sibley, M., Comer, J., & Gonzalez, J. (2017). Delivering Parent-Teen Therapy for ADHD through Videoconferencing: A Preliminary Investigation. *Journal of Psychopathology and Behavioral Assessment, 39*(3), 467–485. doi:10.100710862-017-9598-6 PMID:28989230

Simmel, G. (2009). Filosofia del paesaggio [Landscape philosophy]. In P. D'Angelo (Ed.), *Estetica e Paesaggio* (pp. 39–52). Il Mulino.

Singer, J., & Singer, G. H. S. (2008). Writing as Physical and Emotional Healing: Findings from Clinical Research. In *Handbook of Research on Writing: History, Society, School, Individual, Text* (pp. 485–498). Lawrence Erlbaum Assoc.

Singer, L. M., & Alexander, P. A. (2017). Reading across mediums: Effects of reading digital and print texts on comprehension and calibration. *Journal of Experimental Education, 85*(1), 155–172. doi:10.1080/00220973.2016.1143794

Singh, S., Roy, D., Sinha, K., Parveen, S., Sharma, G., & Joshi, G. (2020). Impact of COVID-19 and lockdown on mental health of children and adolescents: A narrative review with recommendations. *Psychiatry Research, 293*, 113429. doi:10.1016/j.psychres.2020.113429 PMID:32882598

Sís, P. (2000). *Madlenka*. Ediciones Ekaré.

Skočić Mihić, S., Maich, K., Belcher, C., Perrow, S., Barišić, A., & Ramić, N. N. (2017). The Role of Bibliotherapy and Therapeutic Storytelling in Creating Inclusive Classroom Communities. In C. M. Curran & A. J. Petersen (Eds.), *Handbook of Research on Classroom Diversity and Inclusive Education Practice*. IGI Global. doi:10.4018/978-1-5225-2520-2.ch016

Sobral, C. (2016). *Tão, tão grande* [So, so big]. Orfeu Negro.

Sofos, A., Costas, A., & Paraschou, B. (2015). Distance Education & Technology. In *Online distance education* (pp. 145–194). Kallipos, Open Academic Publications. https://repository.kallipos.gr/handle/11419/185

Sohrabi, C., Alsafi, Z., O'Neill, N., Khan, M., Kerwan, A., Al-Jabir, A., Iosofidis, C., & Agha, R. (2020). World Health Organization declares global emergency: A review of the 2019 novel coronavirus (COVID-19). *International Journal of Surgery, 76*, 71–76. doi:10.1016/j.ijsu.2020.02.034 PMID:32112977

Solone, C. J., Thornton, B. E., Chiappe, J. C., Perez, C., Rearick, M. K., & Falvey, M. A. (2020). Creating collaborative schools in the united states: A review of best practices. *International Electronic Journal of Elementary Education, 12*(3), 283–292. doi:10.26822/iejee.2020358222

Sontag, S. (1978). *Illness as Metaphor*. Farrar, Straus and Giroux.

Sophos, A., & Kron, F. (2010). *Effective Teaching Using Media. From primary and personal to quaternary and digital Media*. Grigoris.

Sourtzi, M., Ioakeimidou, V., Vlachos, N., Koutsospyrou, Ch., & Chatzimichailidis, V. (2013). A classroom for all. In A. Lionarakis (Ed.), Proceedings of the 7th International Conference on Open & Distance Learning: Learning Methodologies (pp. 161–169). https://doi.org/http://dx.doi.org/10.12681/icodl.649.

Sousanis, N. (2015). *Unflattening*. Harvard University Press.

Spencer-Cavaliere, N., & Watkinson, E. J. (2010). Inclusion understood from the perspectives of children with disability. *Adapted Physical Activity Quarterly; APAQ, 27*(4), 275–293. doi:10.1123/apaq.27.4.275 PMID:20956835

Spink, J. (1990). Children as innovators. Kastanioti.

Srivatsa, S., & Stewart, K. A. (2020). How should clinicians integrate mental health into epidemic responses. *AMA Journal of Ethics, 22*(1), 10–15. doi:10.1001/amajethics.2020.10 PMID:31958385

Stafford, T. (2011). *Teaching Visual Literacy in the Primary Classroom*. Routledge.

Stampoltzi, A., Giannoulas, A., & Kalamatianos, A. (2020). The experience of existence education of students with learning disabilities or disability during COVID-19 period: A pilot study. *Search in Education, 9*(1), 140-157. doi:10.12681/hjre.24497

Staples, K. E., & Diliberto, J. A. (2010). Guidelines for successful parent involvement: Working with parents of students with disabilities. *Teaching Exceptional Children, 42*(6), 58–63. doi:10.1177/004005991004200607

Strogilos, V., Nikolaraizi, M., & Tragoulia, E. (2012). Experiences among beginning special education teachers in general education settings: The influence of school culture. *European Journal of Special Needs Education*, *27*(2), 185–199. https://doi.org/10.1080/08856257.2011.645588

Subramaniam, S., Brunson, L., Cook, J., Larson, N., Poe, S., & St. Peter, C. (2016). Maintenance of Parent-Implemented Discrete-Trial Instruction during Videoconferencing. *Journal of Behavioral Education*, *26*(1), 1–26. doi:10.100710864-016-9258-z

Sullivan, A. & Strang, H. (2002). Bibliotherapy in the classroom: using literature to promote the development of emotional intelligence. *Childhood Education*, *79*(2), 74-80.

Sun, B., Loh, C. E., & Nie, Y. (2021). The COVID-19 school closure effect on students' print and digital leisure reading. *Computers and Education Open*, *2*, 100033. doi:10.1016/j.caeo.2021.100033

Syriopoulou-Delli, C. K., Cassimos, D. C., & Polychronopoulou, S. A. (2016). Collaboration between teachers and parents of children with ASD on issues of education. *Research in Developmental Disabilities*, *55*, 330–345. doi:10.1016/j.ridd.2016.04.011 PMID:27235770

Tabernero Sala, R. (Ed.), *El objeto libro en el universo infantil. La materialidad en la construcción del discurso* [The book object in the children's universe. Materiality in the construction of discourse]. Prensas de la Universidad de Zaragoza.

Tebeosfera. (2020). Tebeos para una pandemia [Comics for a pandemic]. *Asociación Cultural Tebeosfera Blogspot*. https://asociacionculturaltebeosfera.blogspot.com/2020/03/tebeos-para-una-pandemia.html

Telli-Yamamoto, S. G., & Altun, D. (2020). The Coronavirus and the rising of online education. *Journal of University Research*, *3*(1), 25–34. doi:10.32329/uad.711110

The COVID-19 Outbreak. (2020). *Clinical Neuropsychiatry, 17*(2).

The Reading Agency. (2015). *Literature review: The impact of reading for pleasure and empowerment*. BOP Consulting.

Theodoulou, D. (1988). Children's Literature and the Toddler. In *Children's Literature and the Toddler*. Kastaniotis.

Thibodeau M. L., Thibodeau-Nielsen B. R., Quynh Tran C.M. & Tangerino de Souza Jacob R. (2021). *Communicating During COVID-19: The Effect of Transparent Masks for Speech Recognition in Noise*. doi:10.1097/AUD.0000000000001065

Thomas, K. (2009). *"A social worker took the kids away". The power of games to help children learn.* http://archive.futurelab.org.uk/resources/publications-reports-articles/web-articles/Web-Article1507

Tishman, S. (2018). *The Art and Practice of Learning Through Observation*. Routledge.

Tomasello, M., & Vaish, A. (2013). Origins of human cooperation and morality. *Annual Review of Psychology*, *64*(1), 231–255. doi:10.1146/annurev-psych-113011-143812 PMID:22804772

Tomasik, M. J., Helbling, L. A., & Moser, U. (2021). Educational gains of in-person vs. distance learning in primary and secondary schools: A natural experiment during the COVID-19 pandemic school closures in Switzerland. *International Journal of Psychology*, *56*(4), 566–576. doi:10.1002/ijop.12728 PMID:33236341

Torr, J. (2008). Multimodal Texts and Emergent Literacy. In L. Unsworth (Ed.), *New Literacies and the English Curriculum* (pp. 47–66). Continuum.

Trapiello, A. (1998). *El escritor de diarios. Historia de un desplazamiento* [The diary writer. History of a displacement]. Península.

Travagin, G., Margola, D., Dennis, J. L., & Revenson, T. A. (2016). Letting Oneself Go Isn't Enough: Cognitively Oriented Expressive Writing Reduces Preadolescent Peer Problems. *Journal of Research on Adolescence*, *26*(4), 1048–1060. doi:10.1111/jora.12279 PMID:28453210

Trilla, A. (2021). Pròleg [Prologue]. In A. Bover (Ed.), El contagi (pp. 13-15). Barcelona: Saldonar.

Tsafarti, E. (2017). *The Neighbours*. Abrams.

Tsakiridou, H., & Polyzopoulou, K. (2014). Greek teachers' attitudes toward the inclusion of students with special educational needs. *American Journal of Educational Research*, *2*(4), 208–218. doi:10.12691/education-2-4-6

Underwood, D. (2020). *Outside In*. Clarion Books - Harper Collins.

UNESCO. (1994). *The Salamanca Statement and Framework for Action on Special Needs Education. Adopted by the World Conference on Special Needs Education: Access and Quality*. https://unesdoc.unesco.org/ark:/48223/pf0000098427

UNESCO. (2011). *ICTs in education for people with disabilities. Review of innovative practice*. https://unesdoc.unesco.org/ark:/48223/pf0000193655

UNESCO. (2020a). *COVID-19 Educational disruption and response*. https://en.unesco.org/covid19/educationresponse

UNESCO. (2020b). *Global Education Monitoring Report Summary 2020: Inclusion and education. All means all*. https://bit.ly/2020gemreport

UNICEF. (2020). *Protecting the most vulnerable children from the impact of coronavirus: An agenda for action*. Available here: https://www.unicef.org/coronavirus/agenda-for-action

Universal Design and Development of Accessible Digital Educational Materials. (2022). *IEP*. http://www.prosvasimo.iep.edu.gr/el/

Vacalebri Lloret, Ú. (2020). Gestió emocional i ensenyament de Català com a Llengua Estrangera en temps de pandèmia: els tàndems lingüístics en línia UniTo-UA [Emotional management and teaching of Catalan as a Foreign Language in times of pandemic: UniTo-UA online language tandems]. In *COVID19 – LiTraPan. Literary Training via ICT for Higher Education Improvement, Behavioral Coaching and Discomfort Management during the Coronavirus Pandemic [Branch: UniTo], II International Symposium Forbidden Delights: Sex, Eroticism, Beauty, Aesthetics, Pleasure, Law, Sin and Prohibition*. Retrieved from https://www.youtube.com/watch?v=nSH4pT5vpRg&feature=youtu.be

Vacalebri Lloret, Ú. (2022a). Emotional and Psychological Effects of the COVID-19 Pandemic in College Students: A Language Exchange Project as a Tool to Manage Psychological Disorders Related to the COVID-19 Pandemic. In A. Cortijo Ocaña & V. Martines (Eds.), Handbook of Research on Historical Pandemic Analysis and the Social Implications of COVID-19 (pp. 274-287). IGI Global.

Vacalebri Lloret, Ú. (2022b). Les metàfores conceptuals I la pandemia de la COVID-19: una guerra sense bales [Conceptual metaphors and the COVID-19 pandemic: a war without bullets]. *eHumanista/IVITRA, 21*.

Valentine, D. (2002). Distance Learning: Promises, Problems, and Possibilities. *Online Journal of Distance Learning Administration*, *5*(3). https://www.westga.edu/~distance/ojdla/fall53/valentine53.html

Van der Linden, S. (2007). *Lire l'album* [Play the album]. Le Puy-en-Velay: L'Atelier du Poisson Soluble.

Van der Linden, S. (2015). Álbum[es]. [Album[s]]. Barcelona: Ekaré/Banco del Libro/Varipinta Ediciones.

Van Leeuwen, T. (2008). *Discourse and Practice: New Tools for Critical Discourse Analysis*. Oxford University Press. doi:10.1093/acprof:oso/9780195323306.001.0001

Vázquez-Espinosa, E., Laganà, C., & Vazquez, F. (2020). The Spanish Flu and the Fiction Literature. *Revista Espanola de Quimioterapia, 33*(5), 296–312. doi:10.37201/req/049.2020 PMID:32633114

Vinterek, M., Winberg, M., Tegmark, M., Alatalo, T., & Liberg, C. (2022). The Decrease of School Related Reading in Swedish Compulsory School–Trends Between 2007 and 2017. *Scandinavian Journal of Educational Research, 66*(1), 119–133. doi:10.1080/00313831.2020.1833247

Vislie, L. (2003). From integration to inclusion: Focusing global trends and changes in the western European societies. *European Journal of Special Needs Education, 18*(1), 17–35. https://doi.org/10.1080/0885625082000042294

Vogler, E. W., Koranda, P., & Romance, T. J. (2000). Including a Child with Severe Cerebral Palsy in Physical Education: A Case Study. *Adapted Physical Activity Quarterly; APAQ, 17*(2), 161–175. doi:10.1123/apaq.17.2.161

Vuong, Q. H., La, V. P., Nguyen, T. H. T., Nguyen, M. H., Vuong, T. T., Vuong, H. M., & Ho, M. T. (2021). Impacts of parents and reading promotion on creating a reading culture: Evidence from a developing context. *Children and Youth Services Review, 131*, 106311. doi:10.1016/j.childyouth.2021.106311

Vuorikari, R., Velicu, A., Chaudron, S., Cachia, R., & Di Gioia, R. (2020). How Families Handled Emergency Remote Schooling during the COVID-19 Lockdown in Spring 2020: Summary of Key Findings from Families with Children in 11 European Countries. JRC Science for Policy Report. Publications Office of the European Union. doi:10.2760/31977

Vyas, P., & Tandel, B. (2020). The impact of lockdown due to Covid-19 in 2020 on reading habits of academic staff of state open universities: a study. *The Journal of Higher Education, 12*(1), 28–37. doi:10.37867/TE120104

Warner, C., & Dupuy, B. (2018). Moving toward Multiliteracies in Foreign Language Teaching: Past and present perspectives ... and beyond. *Foreign Language Annals, 51*(1), 116–128. doi:10.1111/flan.12316

Wāzan, 'A. (2020). Sab'ata 'ašara kātiban 'arabiyyan yašhadūn alà laḥẓat al-'uzla al-tārīḫiyya fī 'ālam corona. *Independent Arabia.* https://www.independentarabia.com/node/105711/

Westby, C. (2010). Multiliteracies: The changing World of Communication. *Topics in Language Disorders, 30*(1), 64–71. doi:10.1097/TLD.0b013e3181d0a0ab

Whitton, N. (2010). *Learning with digital games: a practical guide to engaging students in higher education.* Routledge.

WHO. Regional Office for Europe. (2020). *Mental Health and Psychological Resilience During the COVID-19 Pandemic.* http://www.euro.who.int/en/health-topics/health-emergencies/coronavirus-covid-19/news/news/2020/3/mental-health-and-psychological-resilience-during-the-covid-19-pandemic

Wiggins, K. C., & Damore, Sh. J. (2006). "Survivors" or "Friends"? A Framework for Assessing Effective Collaboration. *Teaching Exceptional Children, 38*(5), 49–56.

Williams, P. (2005). Using information and communication technology with special educational needs students: The views of frontline professionals. *Aslib Proceedings, 57*(6), 539–553. https://doi.org/10.1108/00012530510634262

Williams, P., Jamali, R. H., & Nicholas, D. (2006). Using ICT with people with special education needs: What the literature tells us. *Aslib Proceedings, 58*(4), 330–345. https://doi.org/10.1108/00012530610687704

Wilson, J. (2006). *Jorge Luis Borges.* Critical Lives. Reaktion Books.

Wilson-Lopez, A., & Gregory, S. (2015). Integrating literacy and engineering instruction for young learners. *The Reading Teacher, 69*(1), 25–33. doi:10.1002/trtr.1351

Woolf, V. (1926). On Being Ill. *The New Criterion, 4*(1), 32–45.

World Health Organization WHO. (2020, March 3). *Joint ICC-WHO statement: An unprecedented call to action for the private sector to tackle COVID-19.* https://www.who.int/es/news/item/16-03-2020-icc-who-joint-statement-an-unprecedented-private-sector-call-to-action-to-tackle-covid-19

Wu, Y., Liu, L., Zheng, W., Zheng, C., Xu, M., Chen, X., Li, W., Xie, L., Zhang, P., Zhu, X., Zhan, C., & Zhou, C. (2021). Effect of prolonged expressive writing on health outcomes in breast cancer patients receiving chemotherapy: A multicenter randomized controlled trial. *Supportive Care in Cancer, 29*(2), 1091–1101. doi:10.100700520-020-05590-y PMID:32601853

Xiang, Y.-T., Yang, Y., Li, W., Zhang, L., Zhang, Q., Cheung, T., & Ng, C. H. (2020). Timely mental health care for the 2019 novel coronavirus outbreak is urgently needed. *Lancet, 7*(3), 228–229. doi:10.1016/S2215-0366(20)30046-8 PMID:32032543

Yıldırım, B. (2021). Preschool Education in Turkey During the Covid-19 Pandemic : A Phenomenological Study. *Early Childhood Education Journal, 49*(5), 947–963. doi:10.100710643-021-01153-w PMID:33519174

Yrigoyen, E. (2020). Con la fuerza de lo real. Pandemia, relato y ficción en época de coronavirus [With the strength of the real. Pandemic, story and fiction in times of coronavirus]. In N. Escutia, B. Fleitas, & T. Oñate y Zubía (Eds.), Pandemia, globalización, ecología. ¿Qué piensa la hermenéutica crítica? 34 filósofas y filósofos responden a estas cuestiones (pp. 149-158). Universidad Nacional de Educación a Distancia (UNED).

Yus Ramos, F. (1997). *La interpretación y la imagen de masas* [The interpretation and the image of masses]. Institut de Cultura «Juan Gil-Albert» - Conselleria de Cultura, Educació i Ciència de la Generalitat Valenciana.

Zachariae, R., & O'Toole, M. S. (2015). The effect of expressive writing intervention on psychological and physical health outcomes in cancer patients: A systematic review and meta-analysis. *Psycho-Oncology, 24*(11), 1349–1359. doi:10.1002/pon.3802 PMID:25871981

Zawād, M. (2020, May 13). *Al-Kātib al-ǧazā'irī Moḥammad Zawād yuhdī al-Bulaida qaṣīda ši'riyya* [Video Archive]. YouTube. https://www.youtube.com/watch?v=ZH3vHuc6KpI

Zhao, N., Zhou, X., Liu, B., & Liu, W. (2020). Guiding Teaching Strategies with the Education Platform during the COVID-19 Epidemic: Taking Guiyang No. 1 Middle School Teaching Practice as an Example. *Science Insights Education Frontiers, 5*(2), 531-539. doi:10.15354/sief.20.rp005

Zhao, Y. (2020). Tofu Is Not Cheese: Rethinking Education Amid the COVID-19 Pandemic. *ECNU Review of Education, 3*(2), 189–203. doi:10.1177/2096531120928082

Zhu, Y. (2021). Reading matters more than mathematics in science learning: An analysis of the relationship between student achievement in reading, mathematics, and science. *International Journal of Science Education, 44*(1), 1–17. doi:10.1080/09500693.2021.2007552

Zidane, M. (2020). Effects of the corona virus pandemic COVID19 on a legal's limits times in algérian law. *Annales de l'Université d'Alger*, (34), 625-642.

Zioga, S. (2021). *Students' perceptions of distance education due to the Covid-19 pandemic* [Unpublished Master's thesis]. University of Ioannina.

Žižek, S. (2020). *Pandemic! COVID-19 Shakes the World.* Polity.

Žižek, S. (2020). *Pandemia. La COVID-19 estremece al mundo* [Pandemic. COVID-19 is shaking the world]. Anagrama.

Zurita, C. (2020). La realidad, la ficción. Apuntes sobre pestes y plagas en la literatura [Reality, fiction. Notes on pests and plagues in literature]. *Trabajo y sociedad: indagaciones sobre el empleo, la cultura y las prácticas políticas en sociedades segmentadas, 35*, 203-208.

About the Contributors

Antonio Cortijo Ocaña is a prof. of medieval and early modern culture at the University of California, Santa Barbara. Author of over 50 monographs and more than 150 articles, Antonio Cortijo Ocaña analyzes in his research the ideological structures and tensions that have forged the Modern Period across the Atlantic and across the languages and cultures of the Iberian Peninsula. He deals with issues such as nation building, power and ideology, religion, and economy in the late medieval through 18th centuries, as well as with the larger topic of the relevance of Humanism in the creation of the modern nations.

Vicent Martines is a Professor at the University of Alicante. He is a member of the Reial Acadèmia de Bones Lletres de Barcelona. He is the Co-director of the Centre Internacional d'Investigació d'Estudis Ibèrics / Internationales Institüt für Iberische Studien (Universitat d'Alacant / Otto-Friedrich Universität Bamberg). He is the chief editor of Series IVITRA Research in Linguistics and Literature, John Benjamin (Amsterdam, The Netherlands / Philadelphia, USA) and co-editor of eHumanista/IVITRA. He also co-directs Mirabilia/MedTrans and Studia Iberica et Americana. Journal of Iberian and Latin American Literary and Cultural Studies. In addition, he directs the "Filología Catalana" & "Clásicos Valencianos" series of the Editorial Atenea-Centro de Lingüística Aplicada and the "European and Mediterranean Classics" series of Peter Lang International Publishing Company. He is the director of the "Textes catalanes modernes" series of the Classiques Garnier (Paris, France) and of the "Textes catalans du Moyen Âge" series of the Textes littéraires du Moyen Âge (Paris, France). He has received the following awards: Rei En Pere el Catòlic d´Investigació (Institut d´Estudis Catalans, 1988), Premi d´Investigació Historicocultural Ibn Al-Abbar (Generalitat Valenciana, Ajuntament d´Onda, 1990), and the Premio de Ensayo de Catalán, Gallego y Vasco de la Fundación Ortega y Gasset (Fundació "La Caixa", 1993). He is the author of over 220 publications.

Veronica Orazi (Florence 1966), PhD in Ibero-Romance Philology, has taught at the Ca' Foscari University of Venice, the University of Bologna and the University of Siena. She is currently Full Professor of Spanish Literature and Catalan Language and Literature at the University of Turin. She is the Director of the Rivista Italiana di Studi Catalani, co-director of the series 'Bibliotheca Iberica' and a corresponding member of the "Institut d'Estudis Catalans" in Barcelona. She was awarded the Premi crítica Serra d'Or de catalanística (2000) and the Premio Città di Monselice per la traduzione letteraria - Sezione Leone Traverso (2002). In 2015 she received the Menció de la Delegació del Govern de la Generalitat de Catalunya a Itàlia for her activity in promoting Catalan culture. Since 2015 she has directed the international research project "Glocal Perspectives in Iberian Studies". Her research interests focus on the study of medieval and contemporary Spanish and Catalan literature and on the Italian translation of Spanish and Catalan literature.

* * *

Juan-Francisco Álvarez-Herrero has a degree in Chemical Sciences from the UV and a doctorate in Educational Technology: e-learning and knowledge management from the URV of Tarragona. He also has a Master's degree in management and management of educational centers as well as the title of University Expert on the Internet and its applications. For more than 25 years, he has been an ESO professor at the Esclavas SCJ-Alcoi school where he also held the position of director between 2014 and 2017. He has been a professor of the University Master's Degree in Technological Innovation in Education at the UCV. At present he is assistant professor-doctor at the Faculty of Education of the University of Alicante, where he works in the areas of Educational Technology and Science Education. He is a trainer of trainers for the INTEF and teacher centers both in the Valencian Community and the rest of Spain. Trainer and speaker at educational centers, universities, congresses and both national and international conferences.

Eduard Baile-López works for the Department of Catalan Language and Literature at Universitat d'Alacant (https://cvnet.cpd.ua.es/curriculum-breve/ca/baile-lopez-eduard/8838). He is part of two research groups: 1. 'Recerca de Literatura Contemporània', VIGROB-109 (https://cvnet.cpd.ua.es/curriculum-breve/grp/ca/recerca-de-la-literatura-contemporania/392); and 2. 'Estudis Transversals: literatura i altres arts en les cultures mediterrànies', VIGROB-232 (https://web.ua.es/va/transversals/). Furthermore, he belongs to a COST Action refered as 'Investigation on Comics and Graphic Novels in the Iberian Cultural Area' (iCOn-MICs, COST Action 19119), for which he works as a co-leader, along with Hugo Almeida (Universidade Nova de Lisboa), of one of its Working Groups, 'Iberian Comics as a Form of Intercultural Dialogue' (https://iconmics.hypotheses.org/). As a teacher, he conducts lessons of Catalan language to future teachers graduating through the Faculty of Educational Sciences. Also, he is in charge, along with José Rovira-Collado, of a module consisting on comics' educational use for secondary school and which is included as a unit in a Master's Degree at Universitat de València named 'Cómic y Educación' (https://postgrado.adeituv.es/es/cursos/area_de_ciencias_de_la_educacion-4/comic-educacion/home.htm). His research interests focus on the educational use of comics and also on cultural studies. For these past few years, he has coordinated two monographs for academic journals and a standalone volume: 1. "Cómic y educación" for Tebeosfera, 10(3) (2019), along with José Rovira-Collado (Universitat d'Alacant) (https://www.tebeosfera.com/numeros/tebeosfera_2016_acyt_-3_epoca-_10.html); 2. "Cambio climático, biodiversidad y ecología en el cómic" for CuCo, Cuadernos de Cómic, 17 (2021), along with José Rovira-Collado and Laura Caraballo (Université Clermont Auvergne) (https://erevistas.publicaciones.uah.es/ojs/index.php/cuadernosdecomic/issue/view/101; and 3. Renovación del cómic en español. Lecturas de España a Hispanoamérica (Le Grimh, 2022), along with Viviane Alary (Université Clermont Auvergne) and José Rovira-Collado (https://iconmics.hypotheses.org/1399). He is one of Unicòmic's academic coordinators (https://web.ua.es/es/unicomic2021/congreso-unicomic-2021.html), a research association on comics and didactics at Universitat d'Alacant (since 2011) and, moreover, he is the director of the 'Aula de Cómic' (https://web.ua.es/es/aulacomic/aula-de-comic-universidad-de-alicante.html) for the same institution (since 2017).

Xabier Basogain is a professor at the University of the Basque Country - Euskal Herriko Unibertsitatea. Telecommunications Engineer from the Polytechnic University of Madrid, and Doctor of Telecommunications Engineering from the University of the Basque Country - Euskal Herriko Unibertsitatea. Member of the Department of Systems Engineering and Automation of the School of Engineering of Vitoria-Gasteiz. He has taught courses in digital systems, microprocessors, digital control, systems engineering, discrete event modeling and simulation, machine learning, and synchronous collaboration tools in education. His research activities include the areas of soft computing and cognitive sciences for STEM/STEAM, learning and teaching technologies applied to online education, virtual and augmented reality with mobile technologies.

Margarida Castellano Sanz is a Valencian teacher and essayist . She is a secondary school teacher of Valencian and English in public education in the Valencian Country and, currently, a teacher in the Department of Language and Literature Teaching at the University of Valencia. In 2013, she obtained a doctorate in Philology at the University of Valencia with a thesis with international mention on post-colonial literature and migrant identities: The construction of the female autobiographical subject in Catalan immigration literature, with which he obtained an excellent cum laude. In 2017 she won the Joan Fuster Prize for Essay with the essay Les otres catalanes: Memory, identity and autobiographical self in immigration literature which takes as reference the work of Catalan women writers of immigrant origin (Agnès Agboton, Asha Miró, Laila Karrouch, and Najat El Hachmi) that expand the meaning of Catalan identity in the 21st century. She has been director of the specific CEFIRE for Multilingualism (2017-2019) and General Director of Educational Innovation and Organization of the Generalitat Valenciana (2019-2021). (Katiuscia Darici - Contributing Author) Katiuscia Darici is Lecturer in Spanish Literature and Catalan Language and Literature at the University of Turin. She holds a Ph.D. in Foreign Literatures and Literary Studies from the University of Verona and in Humanities from the Pompeu Fabra University of Barcelona. Her academic interests focus on Iberian Studies as well as Contemporary Literature in Spanish and Catalan. She authored the books «"La piel fría" de Albert Sánchez Piñol: una novela "in limine"» (2020) and «Traslaciones. Identidades híbridas en las literaturas ibéricas» (2021). She has published articles or book chapters on Iberian Studies in Italy, Eduardo Mendoza, Albert Sánchez Piñol, Najat El Hachmi, Andrés Neuman, among others. She has co-edited the volume «Historieta o Cómic. Biografía de la narración gráfica en España» (2017).

Urtza Garay Ruiz is Dean of the Faculty of Education of Bilbao (UPV/EHU). Principal researcher of the educational technology research group WebLearner at the University of the Basque Country. Two six-year research periods recognised and lecturer in the Department of Didactics and School Organisation.

Evangelia Gkigkelou is a Greek middle and high school teacher, Special Education Teacher, PhD Candidate at University of the Basque Country in Spain.

Mourad Kacimi is a professor in the Area of Arab and Islamic Studies, both with a broad profile in teaching and research. He has a specialized training in Arab and Islamic Studies. His training enables him to investigate in different research camps in the Area of Arab and Islamic Studies. In particular, on issues related to Islamic thought, science and Arab-Islamic cultural traditions, medieval Arab-Islamic history, historiography, medieval and contemporary Arab literature, Islamic law and institutions, and the Islamic economic system. His work experience consists of exercising the activity of intercultural mediator, and professor of literature and Arabic language.

Spyridon Kazanopoulos works as a science teacher at Greek High School. His postgraduate specialization is in educational leadership, and he is a Ph.D. candidate at the University of the Basque Country. His scientific interests concern inclusive education in Greek secondary schools, intercultural education, and effective educational leadership.

Christos Lalos was born in Athens, Greece. Graduated in Computer Science in Management and Economics, holds 2 Master's Degrees in Digital Systems and Business Administration, graduate of the School of Pedagogy and Technological Education and years Adult educator. He is a PhD candidate in the field of Informatics and education. From 2005 until today, he has worked in various companies and public organizations.

Belén Lozano Sañudo obtained her degree in Translation and Interpreting at the University of Alicante in June 1999. Between September 2004 and January 2020 she was an associate professor, first in the German area of the Department of Integrated Philologies and later in the area of German from the Department of Translation and Interpretation of the University of Alicante. In July 2019, she obtained a Doctorate degree from the aforementioned university with the thesis entitled: "The translation of the LIJ: creative challenges, socio-cultural conditions and influence on the national LIJ and the authorial idiolect". Since February 2021 she is an Assistant Professor in the Department of English and German Philology at the University of Valencia. Likewise, from September 2014 to January 2017. She is a member of ISIC-IVITRA and the Institute of Modern Applied Languages (IULMA) of Valencia. It is part of the DITAPE project, Teaching and Research in Automatic Translation and Post-Editing (2021/GV/080), an R&D project financed by the Conselleria d'Innovació, Universitats, Ciència i Societat Digital, of the Generalitat Valenciana. Her lines of research are the translation of English and German children's and youth literature into Spanish and Catalan studied from the perspective of polysystems, legal translation, translation teaching and machine translation.

Maria Mouchritsa is a Greek language teacher at a Greek Secondary school. Her master's degree specialization is in Special Education and in the last few years, she has been working as an integration class teacher and as a parallel support teacher in the context of inclusive education in Greece. She is currently a PhD candidate at the University of the Basque and her scientific interests are Inclusive Education and Intercultural Education.

Francisco José Pascual is a graduate in Spanish Philology (Valencian philology section) (1995) by the University of Valencia and Investigative Sufficiency Recognition (2001) by the Catalan Philology Department of the University of Valencia. He is also a graduate in Spanish Philology (2006) by UNED (National University distance education). Master in Applied Research in Feminist Gender and Citizenship Studies by the Jaume I University of Castellón (2014).

Ainara Romero Andonegui is a lecturer and researcher at the Department of Didactics and Educational Organisation of the Faculty of Education of Bilbao, University of the Basque Country (UPV/EHU), PhD in Education. She teaches undergraduate and postgraduate studies in educational technology and didactics. Her research interests are related to emerging educational technologies, teaching-learning methodologies and learning difficulties. She is a member of the consolidated research group of the Basque Research System "WebLearner".

Eneko Tejada is a doctor at the UPV/EHU and member of the Department of Didactics and School Organization at the Faculty of Education of Bilbao. His work as a teacher at the university has focused on Didactics and educational technology. He is also Professor of the master's degree in Technology, Learning and Education (UPV / EHU). He has carried out uninterrupted research activity in the area of education, mainly focused on the application of new technologies to education.

Index

"El Contagi" 63

A

Academic Reading 200, 206, 209
Ailment 104
Algeria 126-130, 134, 136-137, 141-142
Anger 86, 88-89, 91-92, 94, 121, 162, 180, 185
Asynchronous 145, 149, 154, 159-160, 163, 173-174, 176
August Bover 63-65, 70, 81

B

Bibliotherapy 1, 9-12, 85, 125
Black Death 14-15, 25-26, 104, 113
Book Therapy 85, 118-119, 121, 123-125
Bruguera School 92, 102-103

C

Catalan Contemporary Poetry 63
Challenging Picturebooks 213-215, 217, 229-231, 233, 235
Charles d'Orléans 1, 4-8, 10-11
Children's Literature 118-119, 123-125, 217, 227, 231-233
Cognitive Development 118-120
Colonialism 104-105, 108-109
Comics 68, 83, 86-92, 94, 96-103, 198-199, 201-204, 206-207, 209, 232
Communication 1, 26, 35, 58, 61, 69, 73, 76, 85, 114, 136-138, 144-145, 147-152, 154, 157-163, 166-167, 169-174, 176, 178-182, 185-186, 193-194, 215-216, 232, 234-235
Confined or Pandemic Narrative 61
Confinement 22, 24, 28-30, 32, 38, 43-44, 48-50, 52-58, 74-79, 82, 86-88, 90, 97-98, 105, 198-203, 205-208, 214, 220, 223
Cooperation 60-61, 125, 147, 149, 154-155, 171-172, 174, 177, 181, 192-193
Coronaphobia 57, 61, 234
Coronavirus Pandemic 57-59, 63, 67, 70, 74, 81-84, 102, 133, 144-145, 148, 151, 155, 168, 215, 233
COVID-19 14-15, 18-21, 23-27, 41, 43-46, 48, 57-61, 67-71, 77, 81-86, 97, 101-102, 122, 126, 129-136, 139, 141-148, 151-155, 159, 161-172, 180-190, 193-196, 198-199, 201, 206, 208-213, 219, 223, 227, 230-231, 233-235
COVID-19 and Challenging Picturebooks 235
COVID-19 Pandemic 14, 24-27, 41, 43-46, 59-61, 67, 69, 71, 77, 84-86, 97, 101-102, 126, 129-130, 141, 144, 146, 148, 152, 154-155, 159, 161-163, 165, 168-172, 180-184, 186-190, 199, 201, 206, 209-213, 219, 223, 227, 230, 235
Crisis 16, 24, 26, 39, 45, 67-68, 74, 80-81, 83, 86, 98, 102-103, 130-132, 134-136, 138, 145-147, 149, 151, 154-155, 159, 162, 167-168, 172, 182, 186, 190-191, 193-196
Culture 3, 25, 37, 44, 65-66, 92-93, 98-100, 114, 121, 125-126, 130, 132, 139-140, 169, 185, 208, 212, 230, 232

D

Daily Life 52, 130, 152
Deaf 144-152
Diary 28-29, 31-34, 37-50, 52-61, 64, 89, 91-92
Diary Fiction 46, 54, 59, 61
Digital Divide 155, 158
Digital Reading 200-201, 204, 206-208, 211
Distance Education 144-147, 149, 151, 155, 159-161, 164-168, 170-174, 180-181, 185-186, 188-189, 192-193, 195
Distance Learning 145, 147-148, 151, 154-155, 159-163, 167, 169-173, 179-180, 182, 184, 189, 195, 212
Divide 155, 158

Dreams 46, 50, 53, 55, 104-105, 112, 115-116

E

E-Books 126
Educators 26, 146-148, 154-155, 162-163, 166, 172, 175, 179, 181, 184, 187, 192, 195-196
El Tiempo Que Nos Robaron 43-44, 58, 82
Emotional Development 118, 120, 147, 155, 181
Epic Destiny 104, 106

F

Face Masks 145, 147, 150-152
Fear 3, 15, 18, 22, 24, 30, 49-50, 52, 57, 61, 67-69, 71-72, 75, 77-78, 80, 84-89, 92, 94, 121, 131-133, 150, 215, 234-235

G

Graphic Medicine 88, 103
Graphic Novel 67, 87, 89, 91-92, 97-98, 100, 103, 122

H

Healing 1, 10, 12, 45, 71, 81, 85-86, 88-89, 94, 201, 207-209
Hearing Impairments 144-145, 149, 151, 161
Hearing Loss 144, 150
Hero's Journey 86, 88-89, 94
Humor 86, 99

I

Iconic Solidarity 96, 103
ICT 57-59, 68, 81-85, 155, 157-159, 166-167, 170, 172-173, 179, 182-183, 194, 226, 233
ICT in Education 85, 157
Influenza 14, 104-107, 111, 117
Integration 7, 146, 154, 156-160, 163, 166, 169-172, 178, 181, 184, 189, 192
Isolation 20-21, 56, 60, 63, 67-71, 75-83, 85, 88, 122, 124, 130-131, 133, 137, 144-149, 151, 163, 182, 214, 217, 234-235
Isolation During COVID-19 Pandemic 85, 235

J

Joan Roís de Corella 1, 3, 9-11
Jordi de Sant Jordi 1, 5-10
Julio Llamazares 28, 39-41, 83

L

Landscape 28-30, 32-42, 65, 76, 78, 88, 97-98, 173
Learning Benefits 158, 198
Lifelong Training 189
Literature 1-3, 9-12, 14, 16-17, 25, 28-30, 36-37, 39-40, 42-49, 56-61, 63-64, 66-67, 81-83, 87, 98, 101-102, 104-108, 111-128, 130-132, 136, 138-140, 145, 147, 152, 156-157, 168, 170, 173, 182, 184-185, 200, 207, 213-214, 217, 225, 227, 230-234
Literature as Therapy 2, 10, 82-83, 213, 217
Lockdown 1, 28-30, 39, 42-45, 49, 52, 54, 60-61, 63, 67, 70, 126, 129-130, 132, 134-136, 145, 148, 152, 160, 165, 173, 182, 188, 198, 209, 211-215, 217, 219-220, 223-224, 227, 230, 234-235
Loneliness 45, 50, 52, 60, 67, 78, 85, 97, 122, 124, 131, 135, 137, 144-147, 151, 215, 235

M

Media 3, 16, 22, 87-88, 96, 98, 101, 103, 126-127, 130-131, 136-137, 149, 152, 155, 159, 165, 169, 176, 180, 232
Middle Age 14
Multiliteracies 213-219, 222-223, 227, 230-235
Multimodality 215, 217, 231-232

N

Narrative Therapy 118, 121-122, 124
National Applause for Coronavirus Health Workers (Aplauso por los trabajadores de la salud) 61
Necessary Other 49-50
New Valencian School 89, 92, 103

O

On-Line 171
Opera Aperta 87, 100, 103

P

Pandemic 1, 9, 14-16, 19, 21, 23-31, 36-37, 39, 41, 43-46, 48, 52, 54, 57-64, 67-71, 74-75, 77-78, 80-86, 88-89, 93, 96-99, 101-102, 104-108, 112, 116-118, 122-123, 126-127, 129-139, 141, 143-146, 148-149, 151-152, 154-155, 159-163, 165, 168-173, 179-184, 186-190, 192, 195, 199-201, 206-215, 217, 219, 223-224, 227, 230-231, 233, 235
Pandemic Literature 28
Parents 7, 51, 113-114, 118, 123, 141, 146-148, 160,

162, 165, 167, 171-172, 178-183, 186, 188, 193, 208, 212
Pedagogy of the Multiliteracies 213-214, 216-217, 219, 223, 230, 235
Personal Protective Equipment (PPE) 85
Plague 15, 18-22, 24-25, 72-73, 77, 104-105, 107, 109, 133, 140
Post-COVID-19 Era 44, 61, 235
Primavera Extremeña 28-29, 33, 36-37, 39-40, 42, 83
Psychological Consequences 63, 86, 88

R

Reader Intertext 103
Reader Involvement 85
Reading 1, 3, 9-11, 39-40, 54, 60, 64-65, 71, 76, 79, 84-85, 87, 96, 99-103, 105, 109, 112-114, 116, 118-121, 123, 125, 130, 144, 146-148, 166, 168, 174, 198-212, 214-215, 217, 219-223, 225-227, 230, 232-234
Rituals 15, 21, 30, 43, 52, 56-57
Romance Literature 1, 9
Rosa Huertas 43, 46, 48-49

S

Science Students 198
Secondary Education 145, 165, 174, 193, 198, 200-201, 205, 211, 223
Slice of Life 89, 103
Social Development 118, 120, 164, 178
Socio-Educational Therapy 126
Soliloquy 75, 77, 85
Spanish Literature 28-29, 48
Special Needs 147, 154, 156, 158, 161, 164, 166-167, 169-170, 181, 183-184
Students 53, 55, 84-85, 121-122, 125, 144-149, 151-152, 154-183, 185-186, 188, 190-193, 195-196, 198-211, 214-218, 220, 222-230
Synchronous 146, 151, 159, 168, 173, 175-176, 179

T

Teachers and Trainers 190, 192-196
Technology 15, 20, 46, 127, 131, 136-137, 148-149, 151-152, 154, 158-159, 161, 164-167, 169-173, 179, 181-182, 186-188, 192-193, 199-200, 208, 210
Therapeutic Effects 198
Trainees at Risk Early Retirement 191
Travel Literature 29-30, 37, 42
Travelogue 28-29, 36, 38
Tuberculosis 14, 104-108, 116-117

V

Valencian Annals 14, 17-18, 22
Valencian Historiography 14, 17-18
Valencian School 89, 92, 103
Virus 14-16, 18, 21, 24, 29-30, 34, 52, 59, 68, 70-71, 74-78, 80-81, 86, 97, 100, 108, 131-135, 139, 141, 143-144, 235
Visual Literacy 213-214, 218, 232, 234

W

Women's Diaries 47, 53
Word is Mighty 1
Writing Therapy 1

Y

Yellow Fever 104-105, 108-110, 116-117

www.ingramcontent.com/pod-product-compliance
Lightning Source LLC
LaVergne TN
LVHW080526300926
849162LV00007B/1547